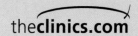

RADIOLOGIC CLINICS

OF NORTH AMERICA

Imaging of the Upper Extremity

July 2006 • Volume 44 • Number 4

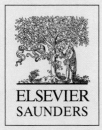

ELSEVIER
SAUNDERS

An imprint of Elsevier, Inc
PHILADELPHIA LONDON TORONTO MONTREAL SYDNEY TOKYO

W.B. SAUNDERS COMPANY
A Division of Elsevier Inc.

1600 John F. Kennedy Boulevard • Suite 1800 • Philadelphia, Pennsylvania 19103-2899

http://www.theclinics.com

RADIOLOGIC CLINICS OF NORTH AMERICA Volume 44, Number 4
July 2006 ISSN 0033-8389, ISBN 1-4160-3901-5

Editor: Barton Dudlick

Radiologic Clinics of North America (ISSN 0033-8389) is published in January, March, May, July, September, and November by W.B. Saunders, 360 Park Avenue South, New York, NY 10010-1710. Business and editorial offices: 1600 John F. Kenedy Boulevard, Suite 1800, Philadelphia, Pennsylvania 19103-2899. Accounting and circulation offices: 6277 Sea Harbor Drive, Orlando, FL 32887-4800. Periodicals postage paid at New York, NY, and additional mailing offices. Subscription prices are USD 235 per year for US individuals, USD 350 per year for US institutions, USD 115 per year for US students and residents, USD 275 per year for Canadian individuals, USD 430 per year of Canadian institutions, USD 320 per year for international individuals, USD 430 per year for international institutions and USD 155 per year for Canadian and foreign students/residents. To receive student and resident rate, orders must be accompanied by name of affiliated institution, date of term, and the signature of program/residency coordinatior on institution letterhead. Orders will be billed at individual rate until proof of status is received. Foreign air speed delivery is included in all Clinics subscriptionprices. All prices are subject to change without notice. **POSTMASTER:** Send address changes to *Radiologic Clinics of North America*, Elsevier Periodicals Customer Service, 6277 Sea Harbor Drive, Orlando, FL 32887-4800. **Customer Service: 1-800-654-2452 (US). From outside of the US, call (+1) 407-345-4000.**

Radiologic Clinics of North America also published in Greek Paschalidis Medical Publications, Athens, Greece.

Radiologic Clinics of North America is covered in *Index Medicus, EMBASE/Excerpta Medica, Current Contents/Life Sciences, Current Contents/Clinical Medicine, RSNA Index to Imaging Literature, BIOSIS, Science Citation Index,* and *ISI/BIOMED*.

Printed in the United States of America.

GOAL STATEMENT

The goal of the *Radiologic Clinics of North America* is to keep practicing radiologists and radiology residents up to date with current clinical practice in radiology by providing timely articles reviewing the state of the art in patient care.

ACCREDITATION

The *Radiologic Clinics of North America* is planned and implemented in accordance with the Essential Areas and Policies of the Accreditation Council for Continuing Medical Education (ACCME) through the joint sponsorship of the University of Virginia School of Medicine and Elsevier. The University of Virginia School of Medicine is accredited by the ACCME to provide continuing medical education for physicians.

The University of Virginia School of Medicine designates this educational activity for a maximum of 15 AMA PRA Category 1 Credits™. Physicians should only claim credit commensurate with the extent of their participation in the activity.

The American Medical Association has determined that physicians not licensed in the US who participate in this CME activity are eligible for 15 AMA PRA Category 1 Credits™.

Category 1 credit can be earned by reading the text material, taking the CME examination online at http://www.theclinics.com/home/cme, and completing the evaluation. After taking the test, you will be required to review any and all incorrect answers. Following completion of the test and evaluation, your credit will be awarded and you may print your certificate.

FACULTY DISCLOSURE/CONFLICT OF INTEREST

The University of Virginia School of Medicine, as an ACCME accredited provider, endorses and strives to comply with the Accreditation Council for Continuing Medical Education (ACCME) Standards of Commercial Support, Commonwealth of Virginia statutes, University of Virginia policies and procedures, and associated federal and private regulations and guidelines on the need for disclosure and monitoring of proprietary and financial interests that may affect the scientific integrity and balance of content delivered in continuing medical education activities under our auspices.

The University of Virginia School of Medicine requires that all CME activities accredited through this institution be developed independently and be scientifically rigorous, balanced and objective in the presentation/discussion of its content, theories and practices.

All authors/editors participating in an accredited CME activity are expected to disclose to the readers relevant financial relationships with commercial entities occurring within the past 12 months (such as grants or research support, employee, consultant, stock holder, member of speakers bureau, etc.). The University of Virginia School of Medicine will employ appropriate mechanisms to resolve potential conflicts of interest to maintain the standards of fair and balanced education to the reader. Questions about specific strategies can be directed to the Office of Continuing Medical Education, University of Virginia School of Medicine, Charlottesville, Virginia.

The authors/editors listed below have identified no financial or professional relationships for themselves or their spouse/partner:
Javier Beltran, MD; Jenny T. Bencardino, MD; Brian J. Bigoni, MD; Christine B. Chung, MD; Barton Dudlick, Acquisitions Editor; Keir A. B. Fowler, MD; Paula A. Habib, BA; Juerg Hodler, MD, MBA; Marlena Jbara, MD; Ara Kassarjian, MD, FRCPC; Faaiza Kazmi, MD; Michel De Maeseneer, MD, PhD; William E. Palmer, MD; Madhavi Patnana, MD; Hollis G. Potter, MD; Joel Rosner, MD; Maryam Shahabpour, MD; Peter Van Roy, PhD; Joseph S. Yu, MD; and Marco Zanetti, MD.

The authors/editors listed below have identified financial or professional relationships for themselves or their spouse/partner:
Liat J. Kaplan, MD, is an independent contractor for Nighthawk Radiology.
Michael B. Zlatkin, MD, is on the Advisory Committee/Board and has speaker's bureau/teaching engagements for GE Healthcare.

Disclosure of discussion of non-FDA approved uses for pharmaceutical and/or medical devices.
The University of Virginia School of Medicine, as an ACCME provider, requires that all authors identify and disclose any "off label" uses for pharmaceutical and medical device products. The University of Virginia School of Medicine recommends that each physician fully review all the available data on new products or procedures prior to clinical use.

TO ENROLL

To enroll in the Radiologic Clinics of North America Continuing Medical Education program, call customer service at 1-800-654-2452 or sign up online at http://www.theclinics.com/home/cme. The CME program is available to subscribers for an additional annual fee USD 205.

IMAGING OF THE UPPER EXTREMITY

CONTRIBUTORS

JAVIER BELTRAN, MD, Chairman, Department of Radiology, Maimonides Medical Center, Brooklyn, New York

JENNY T. BENCARDINO, MD, Head, Musculoskeletal Radiology, Medical Arts Radiology Group, P.C.; and Department of Radiology, Huntington Hospital, North Shore Long Island Jewish Health System, Huntington, New York

BRIAN J. BIGONI, MD, Assistant Clinical Professor on the Volunteer Faculty, Department of Radiologic Sciences, University of California Los Angeles; and Staff Radiologist, Naval Hospital, Camp Pendleton, California

CHRISTINE B. CHUNG, MD, Assistant Professor, Department of Radiology, Veterans Affairs Medical Center, University of California, San Diego, California

KEIR A. B. FOWLER, MD, Musculoskeletal Fellow, Department of Radiology, Veterans Affairs Medical Center, University of California, San Diego, California

PAULA A. HABIB, BA, Department of Radiology, The Ohio State University Medical Center, Columbus, Ohio

JUERG HODLER, MD, MBA, Professor of Radiology and Chief, Department of Radiology, University Hospital Balgrist, Zü rich, Switzerland

MARLENA JBARA, MD, Clinical Adjunct Professor, Department of Radiology, Maimonides Medical Center, Brooklyn, New York

LIAT J. KAPLAN, MD, Department of Radiology and Imaging, Division of Magnetic Resonance Imaging, Hospital for Special Surgery, New York, New York

ARA KASSARJIAN, MD, FRCPC, Director, Musculoskeletal MRI, Massachusetts General Hospital; and Instructor in Radiology, Harvard Medical School, Boston, Massachusetts

FAAIZA KAZMI, MD, Resident, Department of Radiology, Maimonides Medical Center, Brooklyn, New York

MICHEL DE MAESENEER, MD, PhD, Professor of Radiology and Anatomy, Faculty of Medicine, and Director, Section of Musculoskeletal Radiology, Department of Radiology, Vrije Universiteit Brussel, Jette, Belgium

WILLIAM E. PALMER, MD, Director, Musculoskeletal Radiology, Massachusetts General Hospital; and Associate, Professor of Radiology, Harvard Medical School, Boston, Massachusetts

MADHAVI PATNANA, MD, Resident, Department of Radiology, Maimonides Medical Center, Brooklyn, New York

HOLLIS G. POTTER, MD, Department of Radiology and Imaging, Division of Magnetic Resonance Imaging, Hospital for Special Surgery, New York, New York

JOEL ROSNER, MD, Musculoskeletal Radiologist, National Musculoskeletal Imaging, Sunrise, Florida

MARYAM SHAHABPOUR, MD, Director, Musculoskeletal MRI, Department of Radiology, Vrije Universiteit Brussel, Jette, Belgium

PETER VAN ROY, PhD, Professor of Anatomy and Applied Biomechanics, Faculty of Medicine and Physical Therapy, Department of Experimental Anatomy, Vrije Universiteit Brussel, Jette, Belgium

JOSEPH S. YU, MD, Professor of Radiology; Director of Musculoskeletal Radiology; and Director of Residency Program, Department of Radiology, The Ohio State University Medical Center, Columbus, Ohio

MARCO ZANETTI, MD, Privatdozent and Deputy Chief, Department of Radiology, University Hospital Balgrist, Zü rich, Switzerland

MICHAEL B. ZLATKIN, MD, President, National Musculoskeletal Imaging, Sunrise, Florida; and Voluntary Professor of Radiology, University of Miami School of Medicine, Miami, Florida

IMAGING OF THE UPPER EXTREMITY

Volume 44 · Number 4 · July 2006

Contents

> The shoulder is commonly imaged using MR imaging, with or without intraarticular contrast medium. Some anatomic structures, such as the rotator cuff tendons and bony components, can be assessed without arthrographic technique, whereas the glenohumeral ligaments and labrum require arthrographic technique for more accurate assessment. In either case, an understanding of the normal anatomy of the shoulder with regard to bony and soft tissue structures is essential for MR imaging interpretation. In this article we discuss normal anatomy and variations of the glenohumeral joint (bone and soft tissues), rotator cuff tendons, and coracoacromial arch.

> The glenohumeral ligaments, particularly the inferior one, are the major passive stabilizers of the joint, and the labrum functions as a site of ligamentous attachment. The strong union between the collagen fibers of the glenohumeral ligaments and the glenoid labrum is more resistant to injury than the union between the glenoid rim and the labrum. Labral tears associated with glenohumeral instability are therefore usually secondary to avulsion rather than impaction. This article reviews the normal MR imaging anatomy, variants and pitfalls of the glenohumeral ligaments, and the basic biomechanics of the glenohumeral ligaments. Examples of injuries involving these structures are provided.

> MR imaging is the optimal method for evaluating suspected rotator cuff pathology. Current techniques of fast spin-echo imaging without and with fat suppression allow accurate identification and characterization of tendinous and myotendinous abnormalities of the rotator cuff. Impingement disorders, tendon degeneration, instability, and trauma comprise the multifactorial nature of rotator cuff disease. This article addresses the role of MR imaging in evaluating the rotator cuff and the importance of MR imaging in identifying other lesions that may mimic rotator cuff pathology.

A rationale for protocol design, including MR arthrography and the use of specialized positioning, such as abduction and external rotation (ABER), are discussed.

MR Imaging of the Rotator Cuff Interval   525

Brian J. Bigoni and Christine B. Chung

The rotator cuff interval is defined as the space between the anterior aspect of the supraspinatus tendon and the superior aspect of the subscapularis tendon. Knowledge of the anatomy, an understanding of the commonly encountered pathology, and an approach for the systematic inspection of the rotator cuff interval is crucial for the accurate characterization and diagnosis of pathology of this region. This article reviews the basic normal anatomy of the rotator cuff interval, imaging considerations unique to this area, and commonly encountered pathology.

MR Imaging of the Shoulder After Surgery   537

Marco Zanetti and Juerg Hodler

This review article describes postoperative MR findings relating to surgery in shoulder impingement syndrome, including rotator cuff lesions, shoulder instability, and arthroplasty. Potentially misleading postoperative findings are emphasized. Because standard MR imaging may not always be the method of choice for postoperative imaging, alternative imaging techniques have been included (MR arthrography, CT arthrography, and sonography).

Normal MR Imaging Anatomy of the Elbow   553

Keir A. B. Fowler and Christine B. Chung

The functional complexity achieved at the elbow is a reflection of the sophisticated architecture that embodies this articulation. In addition to challenging anatomic relationships to conceptualize, there are many anatomic variations that exist in the osseous, capsular, and muscular structures. This article offers a detailed description of the structural and imaging anatomy of the elbow, information that establishes the foundation of imaging interpretation of internal derangements.

Normal MR Imaging Anatomy of the Wrist and Hand   569

Joseph S. Yu and Paula A. Habib

MR imaging is widely used in the evaluation of internal derangement of joints. In the past, the use of hand and wrist MR imaging lagged behind imaging of larger joints, largely because of technical limitations of spatial resolution and signal-to-noise ratio when imaging the small anatomic structures. However, with recent technical advances in extremity coil design, MR imaging has provided us with new insights into the difficult anatomy of the wrist by allowing improved visualization of the relationship of the muscles, ligaments, tendons, and bone. Although the limits of spatial resolution afforded by specialized surface coils and signal processing methods may not have yet been completely realized at 1.5 Tesla, the potential for significant improvements in hand and wrist imaging is likely to rest with the advent of higher strength magnets.

ELSEVIER
SAUNDERS

RADIOLOGIC
CLINICS
OF NORTH AMERICA

Radiol Clin N Am 44 (2006) 479–487

Normal MR Imaging Anatomy of the Rotator Cuff Tendons, Glenoid Fossa, Labrum, and Ligaments of the Shoulder

Michel De Maeseneer, MD, PhD[a],*, Peter Van Roy, PhD[b],
Maryam Shahabpour, MD[a]

- Bony structures of the glenohumeral joint
- Soft tissues of the glenohumeral joint
- Coracoacromial arch
- Rotator cuff and bursae

- Neurovascular structures
- Acknowledgements
- References

The shoulder is commonly imaged using MR imaging, with or without intraarticular contrast medium. Some anatomic structures, such as the rotator cuff tendons and bony components, can be assessed without arthrographic technique, whereas the glenohumeral ligaments and labrum require arthrographic technique for more accurate assessment. In either case, an understanding of the normal anatomy of the shoulder with regard to bony and soft tissue structures is essential for MR imaging interpretation. In this article we discuss normal anatomy and variations of the glenohumeral joint (bone and soft tissues), rotator cuff tendons, and coracoacromial arch.

Bony structures of the glenohumeral joint

The shape of the glenoid fossa may vary considerably. Some glenoid fossae are pear shaped with a narrower superior portion compared with the inferior portion. A small bony indentation may be present along the anterior border of the glenoid fossa. As a result, the anterosuperior portion of the labrum may remain unattached to the glenoid fossa, creating a sublabral hole [1].

The concavity of the bony glenoid fossa also may vary. Some may be shallow, others more concave. Some 18% to 25% of individuals may present with a blunted posterior margin, also designated as posterior glenoid rim deficiency, predisposing to posterior subluxation. The shape of the cartilage and labrum, however, may compensate for the bony deficiency. Usually the glenoid cavity reveals a 5- to 7-degree retroversion relative to the mediolateral axis of the scapula. When retroversion becomes more important, this may also predispose to posterior luxation, although scientific evidence remains controversial [2].

Dysplasia of the scapular neck is a rare condition usually showing a shallow glenoid fossa with an

---

This article was previously published in *Magnetic Resonance Imaging Clinics of North America* 2004;12:1–10.
[a] Division of Radiologic Sciences, Wake Forest University Hospital, Medical Center Boulevard, Winston-Salem, NC 27157, USA
[b] Department of Experimental Anatomy, Vrije Universiteit Brussel, Laarbeeklaan 101, 1090 Jette, Belgium
* Corresponding author.
E-mail address: mdemaes2@wfubmc.edu (M. De Maeseneer).

doi:10.1016/j.rcl.2006.04.002

anterior bony notch. Usually the cartilage is markedly hypertrophied in such patients [2].

The biceps groove offers a stable sulcus for the biceps tendon. The groove may be continuous with a supratubercular extension, the ridge of Meyers. The presence of the ridge of Meyers predisposes to the formation of traction spurs at the edges of the biceps groove, as shown by specimen studies [3].

Soft tissues of the glenohumeral joint

The biceps tendon attaches to the supraglenoid tubercle, but fibers also insert on the superior labrum and the base of the coracoid process (Figs. 1 and 2) [4]. In its intraarticular position the biceps tendon may be surrounded by a synovial layer of cells. It may attach to the capsule by means of a mesentery-like fold (Fig. 3) [5]. Rarely, the intraarticular part of the tendon may be missing and the origin may be in the intertubercular sulcus. Up to three accessory heads of the biceps muscle may originate from the lesser tuberosity or from the anterior aspect of the capsule [6]. The short head of the biceps muscle originates from the coracoid process. It may be broadened by a lateral extension that runs over the coracoacromial ligament.

The glenoid labrum is made of fibrous tissue and enlarges the glenoid cavity (Fig. 4). The labrum contains only sparse chondrocytes. Normally the labrum is larger at its superior aspect than at its inferior aspect, and is also larger at its posterior aspect than at its anterior aspect. Variations between individuals in the width and thickness of the labrum vary from 2 to 14 mm. Significant variations in

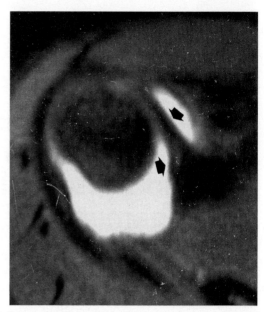

Fig. 2. Attachment of biceps to superior labrum is shown on transverse fat-saturated MR arthrogram (*short arrows*).

the morphology of the labrum are also present [4,7,8]. On transverse sections the labrum may be triangular, rounded, crescent shaped, or blunted (Fig. 5). Between the cartilage and the labrum a sublabral recess may be evident. This is especially so at the level of the superior labrum (Fig. 6). In contradistinction to what many radiologists tend to think, such a recess may also be found along other portions of the labrum. Some authors have attempted to identify characteristic distributions that would allow differentiation of these recesses from traumatic dehiscence. Unfortunately, differentiation from traumatic dehiscence may be difficult on all imaging modalities, even arthroscopy [4,8].

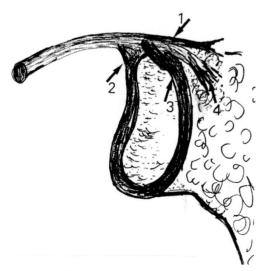

Fig. 1. Line drawing shows attachment of biceps tendon to supraglenoid tubercle (*1, arrow*), to superior labrum (*2,3, arrows*), and fibers coursing toward coracoid (*4, arrow*).

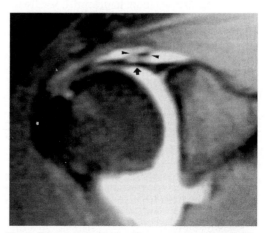

Fig. 3. Fat-saturated MR arthrogram. Arrow points to biceps tendon. Note mesentery-like fold attaching to the biceps tendon (*arrowheads*).

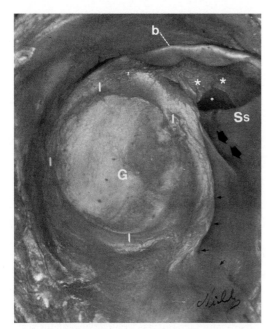

Fig. 4. Anatomic dissection after removal of head of humerus. Photograph of glenoid fossa. Note labrum (l), glenoid cavity (G), and biceps tendon (b). Superior glenohumeral ligament is shown (*asterisk*), middle glenohumeral ligament (*black short arrows*). Also note inferior glenohumeral ligament (*small arrows*). Opening (°) is seen between superior glenohumeral ligament and subscapularis muscle. Ss, subscapularis tendon.

At the level of the superior labrum three types of attachments are recognized (Fig. 7). In a type 1 attachment there is no cleft between the labrum and cartilage. In contradistinction in a type 2 attachment, a small recess may be present between labrum and cartilage. In a type 3 attachment a large

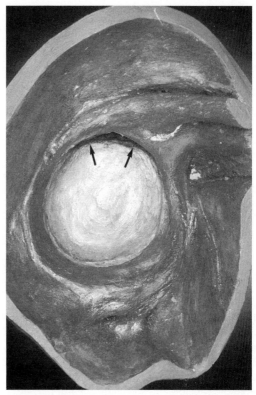

Fig. 6. Photograph of model showing typical superior sublabral recess (*arrows*).

recess is evident (Fig. 8). As mentioned previously such large superior sublabral recesses may be difficult to differentiate from traumatic lesions, designated superior labrum anterior to posterior (SLAP) lesions [4].

The sublabral hole or foramen is different from the sublabral recess. It is present in 11% of

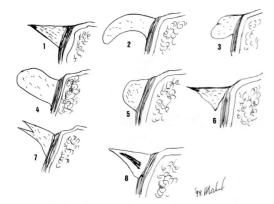

Fig. 5. Line drawing of different shapes of glenoid labrum on transverse section. Note triangular shape (*1*), blunted shape (*2–5*), recess under labrum (*6*), pseudosplitting of labrum caused by adjacent ligament (*7*), and heterogenous signal or calcification in labrum (*8*).

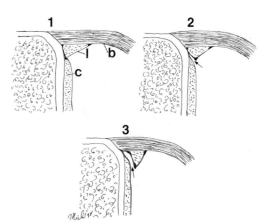

Fig. 7. Line drawing shows labrum (l), biceps (b), and cartilage (c). Note type 1 superior labrum (no recess present), type 2 (small recess), type 3 (large sublabral recess).

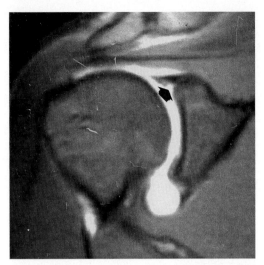

Fig. 8. Type 2 recess is seen on coronal MR arthrogram (*small arrow*).

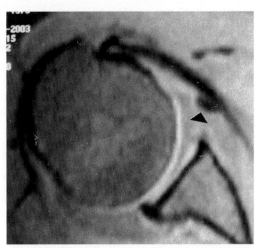

Fig. 9. Transverse gradient echo MR image. Note thick cordlike middle glenohumeral ligament (*arrowhead*).

individuals but may coexist with a superior sublabral recess [5]. A sublabral hole is typically found at the 2 o'clock position and is often seen when the glenoid cavity is pear shaped, becoming smaller above the equator. Measuring the width of the glenoid cavity below and above the equator may be an additional clue to the diagnosis of a sublabral hole. In about 2% of individuals the anterosuperior labrum is entirely absent. In some of these individuals the middle glenohumeral ligament may show a cordlike thickening. This situation is often designated the Buford complex, and is seen in 1.5% of persons [4].

On the anterior aspect of the scapula the attachment of the capsule was differentiated in three types by Zlatkin et al [9]. In type 1 the capsule attaches adjacent to the glenoid labrum. In type 2 the capsule attaches at the level of the neck of the scapula, and in type 3 the insertion is situated at the transition area between neck and body of the scapula. The precise level of attachment may occasionally be misinterpreted related to a large overhanging subcoracoid or digitiform joint recess [9]. In the axillary region the capsule may be partially fused with the tendon of the triceps muscle that inserts on the infraglenoid tubercle. At the level of the humerus the capsule inserts on the anatomical neck. On the posterior side a small bare area is present between the cartilage and the insertion of the capsule on the humerus. The capsule of the glenohumeral joint has three enlargements: the subcoracoid, axillary, and intertubercular recesses [7]. Openings are present in the capsule through which the joint cavity is in direct continuity with these expansions. A constant recess surrounds the long tendon of the biceps muscle in the intertubercular groove (Fig. 9).

The subscapularis bursa is located between the scapula and subscapularis muscle. It communicates with the joint through openings between the glenohumeral ligaments and also through the sublabral foramen. A capsular reinforcement, designated as the rotator cable, may be found on the posterosuperior aspect of the capsule, presenting as a vertically oriented fold [10].

The glenohumeral ligaments reinforce the anterior and inferior portions of the capsule (Figs. 10 and 11). Their appearance may vary from well-developed ligaments to bundles of collagen fibers in the capsule with an orientation different from other

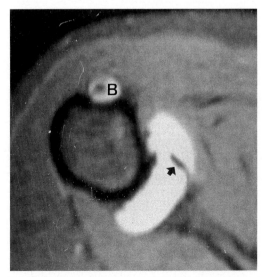

Fig. 10. Note inferior glenohumeral ligament (*arrow*) on transverse MR arthrogram. Biceps tendon surrounded by peribicipital recess also is seen (B).

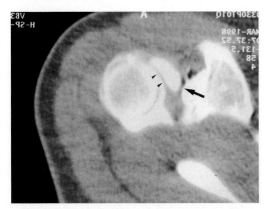

Fig. 11. Transverse CT arthrogram shows common origin of biceps (*arrowheads*) and superior glenohumeral ligament (*arrow*).

capsular fibers. In this situation the capsular folds are only evident with certain arm positions. The superior glenohumeral ligament originates from the superior part of the glenoid cavity, anteriorly to the origin of the biceps tendon. Its origin may be shared with the biceps tendon or middle glenohumeral ligament. On transverse images the ligament courses parallel to the lateral aspect of the coracoid process. The superior glenohumeral ligament is a fairly constant structure, present in most persons [4].

The middle glenohumeral ligament attaches on the anterosuperior labrum or the neck of the scapula. It then courses in an inferolateral direction, inserting on the humerus medial to the lesser tuberosity. It is the most variable ligament in size and presence. It may be absent in 8% to 30% of shoulders. It may have a cordlike appearance or may correspond to a capsular fold. Openings above and below the middle glenohumeral ligaments have been reported in 36% to 46% of shoulders. One single opening superior to the middle glenohumeral ligament is reported in 6% to 18% of individuals. When the middle glenohumeral ligament is absent a large communication may be found between the joint and subscapular bursa [11–13].

The inferior glenohumeral ligament has an anterior and a posterior band and an intermediate portion, the axillary recess. All structures together are sometimes referred to as the "inferior glenohumeral ligament complex." The anterior band originates on the anterior labrum at the 2 to 4 o'clock position. The anterior band is thicker than the posterior band in 75% of individuals. The posterior band originates on the posterior labrum at the 7 to 9 o'clock position. The anterior band attaches inferiorly to the humeral head. It plays an important role in the stability of the shoulder [14].

The coracohumeral ligament originates from the lateral aspect of the base of the corocoid process. It inserts on the tuberosities of the humerus on both sides of the intertubercular groove. In 20% of individuals fibers from the pectoralis minor tendon may insert on to the coracohumeral ligament. The coracohumeral ligament is therefore a rudimentary insertion of the pectoralis minor muscle [15].

Coracoacromial arch

The supraspinatus outlet corresponds to an osteoligamentous ring formed by the spina scapula, the acromion, the coracoacromial ligament, and the corocoid process.

The dimensions and orientation of the acromioclavicular joint surfaces varies significantly among individuals. A fibrous plica or cartilaginous meniscus may be present in the joint space, also altering joint configuration. The shape of the acromion may show considerable interindividual variation. The undersurface of the acromion, as seen on oblique sagittal MR images, has been classified into different types. It may show a flattened, concave, convex, or hooked appearance (Fig. 12). Although it has been suggested that the convex and hooked types may predispose to rotator cuff tears, there also appears to be high interobserver variation in the classification of acromial types. In the oblique sagittal plane, anterior downsloping of the acromion may be assessed, and has also been listed as a cause of impingement. At the anterior aspect of the acromion spur formation may occur in the coracoacromial ligament as a result of humeroacromial conflict [2,16].

In the oblique-coronal plane, lateral downsloping of the acromion may be evaluated. The slope and the length of the acromial process in this plane may result in limited subacromial space, although

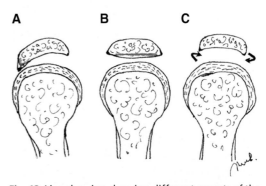

Fig. 12. Line drawing showing different aspects of the undersurface of the acromion in the oblique sagittal plane. Hooked acromion with marked downsloping limiting subacromial space (*A*), convex undersurface (*B*), concave undersurface with wide subacromial space (*C*).

again the relationship with impingement remains unclear. The scapular spine root angle, the slope of the acromion in the sagittal plane, and the acromial offset all are factors determining the superoposterior bony coverage of the humeral head.

Most of these variations have been studied with conflicting results, and precise values that allow differentiation of the normal from the abnormal are still lacking [2]. Dynamic MR studies may be performed with the arm in different positions, preferably those that provoke the pain caused by impingement. The clinical relevance of the results of such studies remains to be proven [17].

The os acromiale is an accessory ossicle between the distal aspects of clavicle and acromial process (Fig. 13). It is reported to be present in 1% to 15% of persons. It often results in clinical symptoms of impingement, although in some cases it may be asymptomatic. The presence of secondary MR findings, such as rotator cuff tendinopathy and bone marrow edema, suggest the clinical relevance of the os acromiale [18,19].

The coracoclavicular ligament is comprised of the laterally situated trapezoid ligament and the medial and posterior conoid ligament. The coracohumeral interval lies between the humeral head and coracoid process. In normal individuals this space averages 6.7 to 8.7 mm. Several morphologic variations may predispose to anterior impingement [20]. These coracoid changes include coracoid slope in the sagittal and transverse planes, length of the coracoid process, and coracoid offset. These factors determine the available space between the anterior aspect of the humeral head and the coracoid process.

Rotator cuff and bursae

The rotator cuff is comprised of the subscapularis, biceps, supraspinatus, infraspinatus, and teres minor muscles (Fig. 14). The subscapularis muscle may be divided into nine bellies (Fig. 15). The most inferior belly may insert separately on the humerus distally form the main insertion on the minor trochanter [6]. Occasionally a belly may insert on the coracoid process. The supraspinatus tendon contains a single large tendon and inserts on the greater tubercle and superolateral aspect of the humerus (Figs. 16 and 17). The most cranial portion of the tendon appears more rounded and is also twice as long as the remainder of the tendon. It constitutes the posterior margin of the rotator cuff interval [6]. A fusion between the infraspinatus and teres minor tendons is so common that the latter is sometimes considered the inferior belly of the infraspinatus. Hence, the presence of a separate teres minor tendon should be considered a variation (Fig. 18) [6].

Bursae about the shoulder joint are divided into communicating and noncommunicating types. The communicating bursae include the subcoracoid bursa, the subscapular bursa and the peribicipital recess. Noncommunicating bursae include a bursa superior to the acromioclavicular joint, a bursa near the inferior tip of the scapula, and

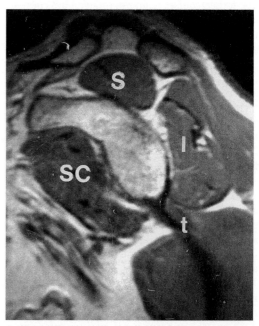

Fig. 14. Oblique sagittal T1 weighted MR image at level of coracoid process. Supraspinatus (S), infraspinatus (I), and subscapular muscle (SC) are seen, as well as attachment of triceps tendon (t) to inferior glenoid.

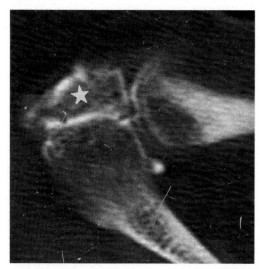

Fig. 13. Transverse CT image shows os acromiale (*star*).

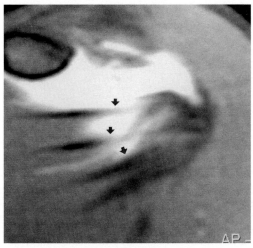

Fig. 15. Oblique coronal MR arthrogram. The different tendons arising from the subscapularis muscle belly are seen (*arrows*).

another between scapula and ribs. Still others are located at the insertion sites of the latissimus dorsi, teres major, and pectoralis major muscles [21].

The subacromial and subdeltoid bursae are usually fused to form to subacromiodeltoid bursa (Fig. 19). This primary bursa has a typical synovial layer.

Neurovascular structures

Neurovascular structures about the shoulder include the brachial plexus and axillary artery and

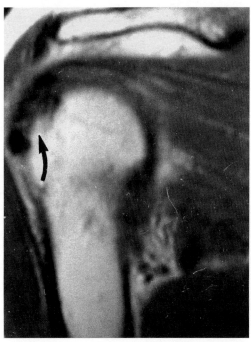

Fig. 17. Coronal T1-weighted MR image. Note insertion of infraspinatus tendon and teres minor tendon on posterior aspect of humerus (*curved arrow*).

vein. Twenty-nine variations of the brachial plexus and its emerging nerves have been described. Many of these variations predispose to thoracic outlet syndrome [22]. Accessory scalenus muscles are frequent (28% of the population) and may lead to

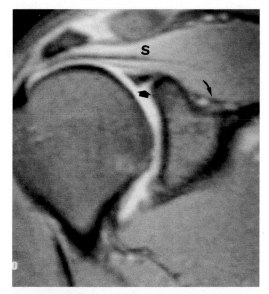

Fig. 16. Note single supraspinatus tendon (S). Superior sublabral recess is also seen (*short arrow*) as well as suprascapular notch (*curved arrow*). Note that suprascapular notch is covered by ligament.

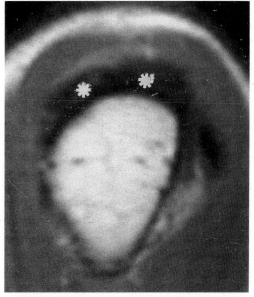

Fig. 18. Sagittal oblique T1-weighted MR image. Note insertion of supraspinatus tendon (*asterisks*).

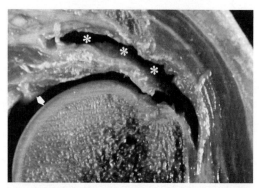

Fig. 19. Coronal anatomic slice. Joint space is seen (*short white arrow*). Also note subacromiosubdeltoid bursa (*asterisks*). Communication between joint space and bursa is present as a result of ruptured supraspinatus tendon (Courtesy of D. Resnick, MD, San Diego, CA.)

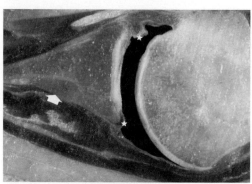

Fig. 20. Transverse anatomic slice. Note anterior and posterior labrum (*stars*). Spinoglenoid fossa containing nerves for infraspinatus muscle is shown (*white short arrow*). (Courtesy of D. Resnick, MD, San Diego, CA.)

neurovascular compression when hypertrophied, such as in respiratory disease and certain sports. Because of the tremendous anatomic variability, most surgeons are reluctant to operate in this region out of concern for inadvertently injuring neurovascular structures, with catastrophic consequences.

Langer's muscular arch of the axilla consists of a tendinous or muscular connection between the latissimus dorsi and pectoralis major muscles. The arch may exert compression on neurovascular structures in the axilla [23].

The suprascapular nerve passes through the scapular notch and contains motor branches for the supraspinatus and infraspinatus muscles (Fig. 20). The scapular notch is covered by the transverse scapular ligament. In some individuals the notch may be covered by a fibrous or bony bridge, resulting in nerve compression [24]. Also, an accessory ligament (50%) may be present anteroinferiorly to the transverse scapular ligament, with the suprascapular nerve passing inferior to it. Hence significant friction is exerted on the nerve in case of sudden shoulder movements [25]. Of the suprascapular nerve, two motor branches are directed to the supraspinatus fossa innervating the supraspinatus muscle, and two other motor branches are directed to the infraspinatus fossa innervating the infraspinatus muscle. Depending on the location of compression, a particular type of compressive neuropathy may result (Fig. 21). Labral cysts are one such cause of nerve branch compression, and may be easily diagnosed with MR imaging [26].

The quadrilateral space is located between the humerus, triceps, teres minor, and teres major tendons (see Fig. 18) [27]. The axillary nerve and posterior humeral circumflex artery pass through this space and compression may occur here, especially in athletes. Instead, the axillary nerve may pierce the subscapularis muscle, leading to entrapment. Other accessory muscles may be present in the axilla and exert compression on diverse neurovascular structures.

Acknowledgements

The authors thank Eric Barbaix, MD, Lecturer, Department of Anatomy, Rijks Universiteit Gent, Belgium, for his knowledge of classic anatomic textbooks and anatomic variations. This work was

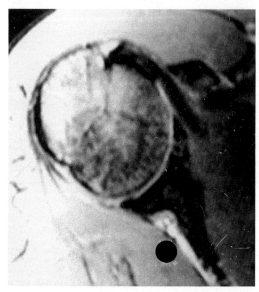

Fig. 21. Spinoglenoid notch often contains marked vascular structures (*black circle*) not to be confused with labral cysts.

financially supported by Prijs Professor Dr. A. Baert, Katholieke Universiteit Leuven.

References

[1] Presher A, Klümpen T. The glenoid notch and its relation to the shape of the glenoid cavity of the scapula. J Anat 1997;190:457–60.

[2] Mellado JM, Calmet J, Domènech S, Sauri A. Clinically significant variations of the shoulder and the wrist: role of MR imaging. Eur Radiol 2003;13:1735–43.

[3] Hitchcock HH, Bechtol CO. Painful shoulder, observations on the role of the long head of the biceps brachii on its causation. J Bone Joint Surg 1948;2A:263–73.

[4] De Maeseneer M, Van Roy F, Lenchik L. CT and MR arthrography of the normal and pathologic anterosuperior labrum and labral-bicipital complex. Radiographics 2000;20:S67–81.

[5] Wall MS, O'Brien SJ. Arthroscopic evaluation of the unstable shoulder. Clin Sports Med 1995; 14:817–40.

[6] Testut L. Les anomalies musculaires chez l'homme. Paris: Masson; 1884.

[7] Hata Y, Nakatsuchi Y, Saitoh S, Hosaka M, Uchiyama S. Anatomic study of the glenoid labrum. J Shoulder Elbow Surg 1992;74A: 491–500.

[8] Detrisac DA, Johnson LL. Arthroscopic shoulder anatomy: pathologic and surgical implications. Thorofare (NJ): Sack; 1986.

[9] Zlatkin MB, Ianotti JP, Schnall MD. MRI of the shoulder. New York: Raven Press; 1991.

[10] Burkhart SS. Shoulder arthroscopy: new concepts. Clin Sports Med 1996;15:635–54.

[11] Palmer WE, Caslowitz PL, Chew FS. MR arthrography of the shoulder: normal intraarticular structures and common abnormalities. AJR Am J Roentgenol 1995;164:141–6.

[12] Stoller DW. MR arthrography of the glenohumeral joint. Radiol Clin North Am 1997;1:97–115.

[13] Beltran J, Rosenberg ZS, Chandnani VP, Cuomo F, Beltran S, Rokito A. Glenohumeral instability: evaluation with MR arthrograpy. Radiographics 1997;17:657–73.

[14] O'Brien SJ, Neves MC, Arnoczky SP, et al. The anatomy and histology of the inferior glenohumeral ligament complex of the shoulder. Am J Sports Med 1990;18:449–56.

[15] Cooper DE, O'Brien SJ, Arnoczky SP, Warren RF. The structure and function of the coracohumeral ligament: an anatomic and microscopic study. J Shoulder Elbow Surg 1993;2:70–7.

[16] Farley TE, Neumann CH, Steinbach LS, Petersen S. The coracoacromial arch: MR evaluation and correlation with rotator cuff pathology. Skel Radiol 1994;23:641–5.

[17] Roberts CS, Davila JN, Hushek SG, et al. Magnetic resonance imaging of the subacromial space in the impingement sign positions. J Shoulder Elbow Surg 2002;11:595–9.

[18] Uri DS, Kneeland BJ, Herzog R. Os acromiale:evaluation of markers for identification on sagittal and coronal oblique MR images. Skel Radiol 1997;26:31–4.

[19] Farley TE, Neumann CH, Steinbach LS, Petersen S. The coracoacromial arch: MR evaluation and correlation with rotator cuff pathology. Skel Radiol 1994;23:641–5.

[20] Dines DM, Warren RF, Inglis AE, Pavlov H. The coracoid impingement syndrome. J Bone Joint Surg 1990;72B:314–6.

[21] Testut L, Latarjet A. Traite d'anatomie humaine. Tome I Osteologie, Arthrologie, Myologie. 9th edition. Paris: Doin et Cie; 1948.

[22] Kerr AT. The brachial plexus of nerves in man, the variations in its formation and branches. Am J Anat 1919;23:285–95.

[23] Clarijs JP, Barbaix E, Van Rompaey H, Caboor D, Van Roy P. The muscular arch of the axilla revisited: its possible role in thoracic outlet and shoulder instability syndromes. Man Ther 1996;1:133–9.

[24] Fisher H. Quelques considerations sur la morphologie de l'omoplate. Echancrure coracoidienne transformée en un canal par un pont osseux. Comptes Rendus des Anatomistes 1927;5:96–8.

[25] Avery BW, Pilon FM, Barclay JK. Anterior coracoscapular ligament and suprascapular nerve entrapment. Clin Anat 2002;15:383–6.

[26] Tung GA, Entzian D, Stern JB, Green A. MR imaging and MR arthrography of paraglenoid labral cysts. AJR Am J Roentgenol 2000;174:1707–15.

[27] Linker CS, Helms CA, Fritz RC. Quadrilateral space syndrome: findings at MR imaging. Radiology 1993;188:675–6.

RADIOLOGIC
CLINICS
OF NORTH AMERICA

Radiol Clin N Am 44 (2006) 489–502

MR Imaging of the Glenohumeral Ligaments

Jenny T. Bencardino, MD[a],*, Javier Beltran, MD[b,c]

The shoulder is the most commonly dislocated major joint in the body. The discrepancy between the small size of the glenoid fossa and the large size of the humeral head provides the glenohumeral joint with the largest mobility among the human articulations [1]. This also makes this joint particularly vulnerable for dislocation. The stability of the shoulder joint is maintained by passive and active mechanisms, depending on whether muscle energy is required. The glenohumeral ligaments, glenoid labrum, capsule, and bony restraints (acromion, coracoid process) are among the passive stabilizing mechanisms. The rotator cuff muscles and the long head of biceps tendon provide dynamic stabilization to the shoulder.

The glenohumeral ligaments (GHL) are infoldings of the glenohumeral capsule, extending from the anterior and inferior glenoid margin of the joint to the region of the anatomical neck of the humerus. Three ligaments have been described: the superior GHL, the middle GHL, and the inferior GHL complex, formed by the anterior band, the

posterior band, and the axillary recess of the joint [2–4]. The GHL, particularly the inferior one, are the major passive stabilizers of the joint and the labrum functions as a site of ligamentous attachment [1,5]. The strong union between the collagen fibers of the GHL and the glenoid labrum is more resistant to injury than the union between the glenoid rim and the labrum itself. Labral tears associated with glenohumeral instability are therefore usually secondary to avulsion rather than impaction. This article reviews the normal MR imaging anatomy, variants, and pitfalls of the GHL to discuss the basic biomechanics of the GHL and to illustrate examples of injuries involving these structures.

Normal anatomy and variants

Understanding of the complex anatomy and normal anatomic variations of the GHL is essential for accurate interpretation of standard and arthrographic MR images [6–8].

This article was previously published in *Magnetic Resonance Imaging Clinics of North America* 2004;12:11–24.
[a] Musculoskeletal Radiology, Medical Arts Radiology Group, PC, Huntington Hospital, North Shore-Long Island Jewish Health System, 270 Park Avenue, Huntington, NY 11743, USA
[b] Department of Radiology, Maimonides Medical Center, 4802 Tenth Avenue, Brooklyn, NY 11219, USA
[c] Department of Radiology, SUNY Downstate Medical Center, 450 Clarkson Avenue, Brooklyn, NY 11203, USA
* Corresponding author.
E-mail address: jennybencardino@yahoo.com (J.T. Bencardino).

Superior GHL

Anatomy

The superior GHL extends from the superior glenoid margin and base of the coracoid process, just anterior to origin of the long head of the biceps tendon, to the fovea capitis line, just superior to the lesser tuberosity, where it blends with the coracohumeral ligament [1]. On arthroscopic examination, this ligament is found in 97% of patients [1]. Palmer et al [9] identified the superior GHL in 98% of 48 patients undergoing MR arthrography of the shoulder. The superior GHL is consistently visualized in the axial plane as a thick bandlike structure arising from the superior glenoid tubercle, parallel to the coracoid process (Fig. 1A) [10]. Oblique sagittal MR arthrographic images show the superior GHL located underneath the coracohumeral ligament and coracoid process (Fig. 1B). A normal foramen or opening exists between the superior GHL and the middle GHL, allowing communication with the subscapularis bursa (Fig. 2) [11].

An important anatomic area is the rotator interval, a space located between the anterior margin of the supraspinatus tendon and the superior margin of the subscapularis tendon [12,13]. The joint capsule that covers this space is reinforced by fibers emanating from the coracohumeral ligament and the superior GHL. The superior GHL forms a fold having the macroscopic appearance of a U-shaped anterior stabilizing sling for the long head of the biceps tendon [14]. Thus, the rotator interval roofs and, more importantly, lends support to the long head of biceps tendon [15]. A lesion of the superior GHL might lead to anterior instability of the biceps tendon. This anatomic space is closely related to the superior labrum and the middle GHL as well [16].

Variants

The superior GHL may originate with the long head of the biceps tendon, alone, or with the middle GHL (Fig. 3) [17,18]. A rare variant of a superior GHL overriding the biceps origin, extending to the superior labrum posteriorly without attachments to the middle GHL or anterior labrum, has been reported recently [19]. The superior GHL is normally thin, but it can become thick, in which case the middle GHL may be absent or underdeveloped [7].

Middle GHL

Anatomy

The middle GHL shows the greatest variation of all the GHL [1]. It was absent in up to 30% of the cases in cadaver dissections, and it was not identified in 12% to 21% of patients surveyed with MR arthrography [7,9,20]. Arthroscopically, the middle GHL has been described as being attached to the

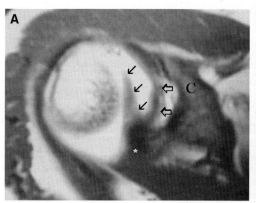
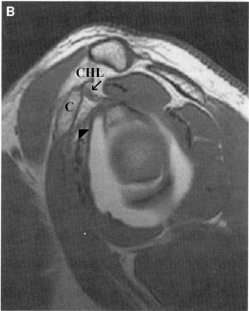

Fig. 1. (A) Axial MR arthrogram shows the superior GHL (*open arrows*) originating from the superior glenoid tubercle (*asterisk*), parallel to the coracoid process (C). A joint origin with the long head of the biceps tendon (*arrows*) is noted. (B) Oblique sagittal MR arthrogram demonstrates the superior GHL (*arrowhead*) underneath the coracoid process and the coracohumeral ligament (CHL) (*arrow*).

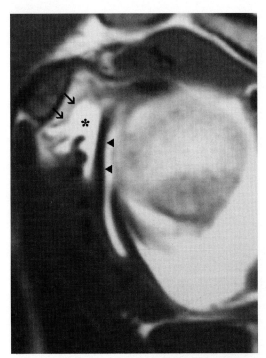

Fig. 2. Oblique sagittal MR arthrogram shows normal foramen (*asterisk*) between the superior GHL (*arrows*) and the middle GHL (*arrowheads*), allowing communication with the subscapularis recess.

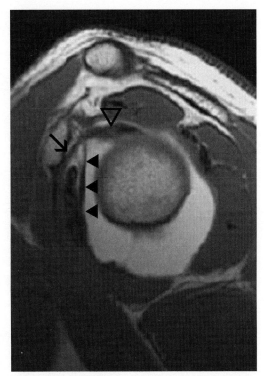

Fig. 3. Oblique sagittal MR arthrograms depict the superior GHL (*arrow*) in continuity with the biceps tendon (*open arrowhead*). The middle GHL (*solid arrowheads*) also originates form the biceps tendon.

anterior surface of the scapula, medial to the articular margin. It then lies obliquely, posterior to the superior margin of the subscapularis muscle and blends with the anterior capsule (Fig. 4A). Distally it is attached to the anterior aspect of the proximal humerus, below the insertion of the superior GHL. Using MR arthrography, the scapular insertion of the middle GHL is seen more often at the level of the anterior superior labrum rather than at the level of the scapula as was suggested arthroscopically [21,22]. The middle GHL can be seen on axial MR images as a hypointense structure separated from the anterior superior labrum by a small cleft. Axial images obtained more inferiorly will demonstrate the middle GHL as a flat or round structure attached or completely separated from the joint capsule (Fig. 4B) [7]. Oblique sagittal images obtained with full capsular distension demonstrate the middle GHL as a hypointense band crossing the anterior capsular space from its labral attachment proximally to its capsular merge distally (Fig. 4C). Oblique coronal images following intraarticular injection of contrast material rarely show the middle GHL, unless it is redundant and thick.

The middle GHL may originate with the superior GHL, alone, or with the inferior GHL [7]. It inserts at the humerus at the base of the lesser tuberosity, although it can also blend with the subscapularis

tendon before reaching the tuberosity. As it passes anterior to the glenoid labrum, a labral tear or displaced fragment may be simulated on axial images if contiguous slices are not examined [7,23]. The position of the middle GHL is closely related to the degree of rotation of the arm during scanning [7]. With the arm in external rotation, the middle GHL becomes stretched and blends with the capsule [24]. With the arm in internal rotation, the middle GHL becomes redundant and migrates medially, anterior to the scapular neck, mimicking a loose body or stripped anterior capsule (Fig. 5).

Variants

The middle GHL presents the largest multiplicity of normal variants. In one anatomical study, the ligament was absent in 30% of the specimens [25]. In a series of 108 MR arthrograms obtained in 95 asymptomatic volunteers, Park et al [20] found that the superior GHL and the inferior GHL were present in 99% of the cases, but the middle GHL was present in only 79% of the cases. In Chandnani et al's series [21], the middle GHL was identified with MR arthrography in 85% of their cases. Absence of the middle GHL is often associated with a prominent subscapularis recess (Fig. 6).

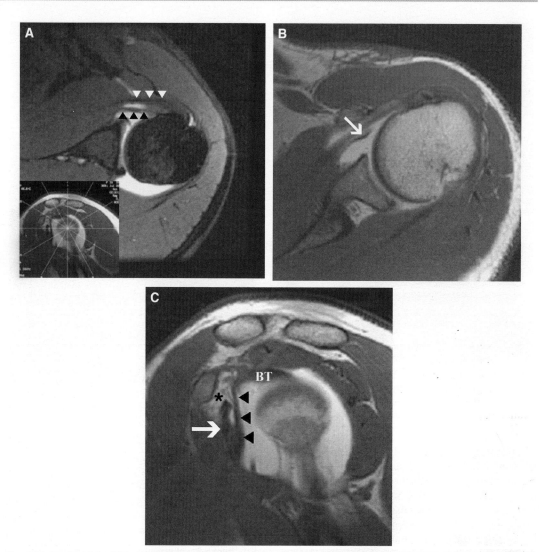

Fig. 4. Normal middle GHL. (*A*) Oblique axial MR arthrogram demonstrates the middle GHL (*black arrowheads*) in its entire extent, posterior to the subscapularis tendon (*white arrowheads*). (*B*) Axial MR arthrogram shows normal flattened appearance of the middle GHL (*arrow*). Note is made of attenuated anterior labrum and Hill-Sachs lesion. (*C*) Oblique sagittal MR arthrogram demonstrates the middle GHL (*arrowheads*) as a hypointense band crossing the anterior capsular space posterior to the subscapularis tendon (*white arrow*). Incidentally noted is absent superior GHL. BT, biceps tendon.

The origin of the middle GHL is a frequent location of normal variants, the most common being a joint origin of the middle GHL with the superior GHL, less frequently a joint origin with the superior GHL and long biceps tendon, or joint origin with the long biceps tendon, absent the superior GHL (see Fig. 4B).

A well-recognized variant is the so-called "Buford complex," which represents a cordlike thickening of the middle GHL, with absence of the anterior superior portion of the labrum [4,17,26]. This variant is seen in up to 6.5% of patients [27]. On axial MR images obtained at the level of the superior half of the glenoid cavity, a thickened middle GHL close to the glenoid margin with an absent labrum may simulate a labral tear (Fig. 7A). Differentiation with labral tear is achieved by following the thickened middle GHL on consecutive axial MR images from its origin in the anterior superior labrum to its blending with the anterior joint capsule and subscapularis tendon. Also, identification of a thick middle GHL on oblique sagittal images helps one avoid this pitfall (Fig. 7B). A high association of Buford complex, sublabral foramen, superior

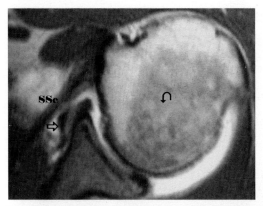

Fig. 5. Axial MR arthrogram in internal rotation of the humeral head (*curved arrow*) depicts the middle GHL (*open arrow*) as a redundant structure migrated medially, anterior to the scapular neck and posterior to the subscapularis tendon (*arrow*).

GHL injuries, and superior labrum anterior to posterior (SLAP) lesions has recently been described [27,28].

A few cases of longitudinal split or duplicate middle GHL have been reported [4,29]. In these cases, oblique sagittal images demonstrate a double-parallel line, and axial images show a U-shaped structure that may simulate a labral cleft or tear. This may represent a true normal variant or a healed longitudinal tear of the middle GHL.

Inferior GHL

Anatomy

The inferior GHL complex is composed of an anterior band, a posterior band, and an axillary recess [1]. The anterior band of the inferior GHL inserts in the anterior glenoid rim about the midglenoid notch, whereas the posterior band attaches to the posterior inferior glenoid quadrant. The humeral insertion of the inferior GHL complex has two distinct patterns: (1) the collar-like attachment in which the entire inferior GHL inserts slightly inferior to the articular edge of the humeral head (Fig. 8), and (2) the V-shaped attachment in which the anterior and posterior bands of the inferior GHL attach adjacent to the articular edge of the humeral head, and the axillary pouch attaches at the apex of the V distal to the articular edge [30]. With the arm held in adduction and external rotation (ABER position), the anterior band of the inferior GHL becomes taut and can be visualized in its entire extent (Fig. 9) [25].

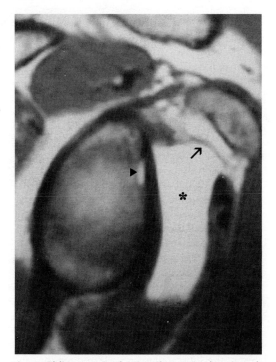

Fig. 6. Oblique sagittal MR arthrogram showing absent middle GHL, with a prominent anterior capsular recess (*asterisk*). Incidentally noted are the superior GHL (*arrow*) and sublabral foramen (*arrowhead*).

Variants

The anterior band of the inferior GHL is usually thicker than the posterior band, although the opposite situation may exist. The insertion of the axillary recess, along with the anterior and posterior bands at the neck of the humerus, creates a jagged appearance on axial MR images that should not be misconstrued as fraying or tearing of this structure (see Fig. 8) [7]. Also, synovial folds emanating from the capsule of the axillary recess may be prominent, simulating loose bodies or intraarticular debris on axial and oblique coronal MR images [7].

A new anterior GHL was described by Kolts et al [31] in their anatomic study of 12 cadaver shoulder joints. This ligament was coined the "spiral ligament" as the course of its fibers is spiral with the shoulder in external rotation and abduction. The "spiral ligament" is located in the anterior shoulder joint capsule. It extends from the axillary component of the inferior GHL and the infraglenoid tubercle coursing upward laterally and fusing with the middle GHL (Fig. 10). Superiorly, the ligament melted into the superior portion of the subscapularis, inserting together with its tendon into the lesser tuberosity. To the authors' knowledge, this ligament has not yet been described in the radiological literature.

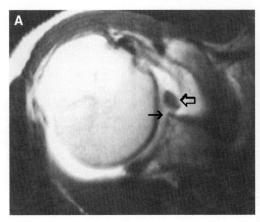
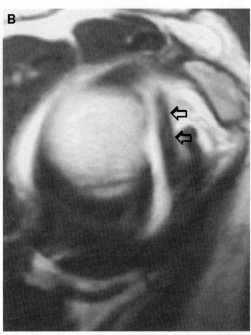

Fig. 7. Buford complex. (*A*) Axial MR arthrogram shows absence of the anterosuperior labrum (*arrow*); the posterior labrum is normal. The middle GHL (*open arrow*) is unusually thick. (*B*) Oblique sagittal MR arthrogram shows a thick middle GHL (*arrows*).

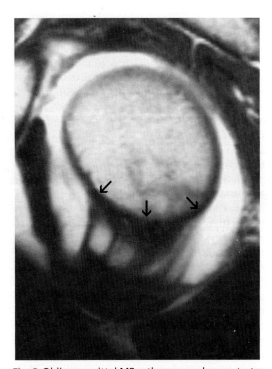

Fig. 8. Oblique sagittal MR arthrograms demonstrates collar-like attachment of the entire inferior GHL (*arrows*), inserting slightly inferior to the articular edge of the humeral head.

Basic biomechanics

The glenohumeral joint is the articulation of the human body with the greatest range of motion (over 180 degrees in several planes). The large articular surface of the humeral head compared with the small articular surface of the glenoid cavity explains the extended mobility of the joint. Because of its wide range of motion, the glenohumeral joint is also more susceptible to dislocations, subluxations, and lesions related to chronic stress in the surrounding soft tissues.

The stability of the glenohumeral joint is provided by a series of active (rotator cuff and long biceps tendon) and passive mechanisms, including shape and tilt of the glenoid fossa, adhesion and cohesion of the articular surfaces, negative intracapsular pressure, and integrity of the capsule, labrum, and the GHL [32,33].

The capsular mechanism provides the most important contribution to the stability of the glenohumeral joint. The anterior capsular mechanism [3] includes the fibrous capsule, the GHL, the synovial membrane and its recesses, the fibrous glenoid labrum, the subscapularis muscle and tendon, and the scapular periosteum. The anterior capsular insertion can be divided into three types depending on the proximity of the capsular insertion to the

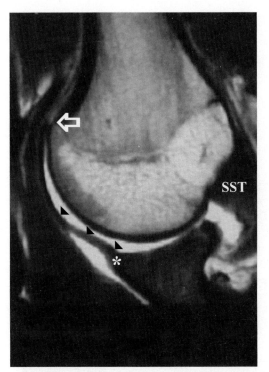

Fig. 9. ABER position. Oblique sagittal MR arthrogram along the longitudinal axis of the humerus shows a normal glenohumeral joint in the ABER position. Note the stretched anterior band of the inferior GHL (*arrowheads*) attached to the anteroinferior labrum (*asterisk*) and humeral neck (*open arrow*). Note also the supraspinatus tendon (SST) inserting into the greater tuberosity.

glenoid margin [2]. In type I, the capsule inserts at the glenoid margin, in type II it inserts at the glenoid neck, and in type III the insertion is more medial, at the scapula [6]. When performing MR arthrography, the capsule is overdistended, and this produces a false appearance of type III insertion. In general, the further the anterior capsular insertion from the glenoid margin, the more unstable will be the glenohumeral joint (type III).

The posterior capsular mechanism [34] is formed by the posterior capsule, the synovial membrane, the glenoid labrum and periosteum, and the posterior superior tendinous cuff and associated muscles (supraspinatus, infraspinatus and teres minor). The long head of biceps tendon inserting in the superior aspect of the labrum, and the triceps tendon inserting in the infraglenoid tubercle inferiorly, constitute additional supportive structures of the glenohumeral joint.

The GHL contribute to a different degree to the stability of the glenohumeral joint, depending on the position of the arm. The relative contribution of each individual GHL to joint stability has been

the subject of debate. Matsen et al [32] and Caspari et al [22] indicated that the superior GHL and middle GHL are absent in a high percentage of individuals, and therefore they must not be important structures in maintaining stability. Turkel et al [33] studied the contribution of each of the GHL by means of selectively cutting these structures in cadavers and then assessing the stability of the joint at different degrees of abduction and external rotation. They concluded that the inferior GHL is the most important structure in the prevention of dislocation with the arm at 90 degrees of abduction and external rotation. Other researchers, arguing that selectively cutting the GHL alters the synergy of the individual structures in the intact shoulder, questioned this conclusion [35].

In a classic experiment, O'Connell et al [35] measured the tension of the GHL in cadavers after application of a controlled external torque. They concluded that at 90 degrees of arm abduction, the inferior GHL and the middle GHL developed the most strain, whereas with the arm at 45 degrees of abduction, the most strain was also developed by the inferior GHL and middle GHL, though some strain occurred at the superior GHL. The superior GHL may provide some degree of stability to the shoulder in 0 degrees of arm abduction and aid in the prevention of inferior subluxation [33,35,36].

Pathology

The anterior band of the inferior GHL is the most frequently injured capsule-ligamentous structure [9,37,38]. In a series of 121 patients studied by Palmer et al [18], 31 of 37 unstable shoulders had discrete inferior labral-ligamentous lesions at surgery. Labral tears are frequently associated with partial or complete tears of the GHL in patients with glenohumeral instability, as demonstrated arthroscopically following a single episode of dislocation or recurrent episodes of instability [39–41] and by MR imaging [9]. The accuracy of MR arthrography for the evaluation of the GHL specifically was reported by Chandnani et al [21] in a series of 46 patients with arthroscopic correlation. Lesions of the superior, middle, and inferior GHL were depicted with sensitivity and specificity of 100%/94%, 89%/88%, and 88%/100% respectively.

Superior GHL

Based on the peculiar anatomy of the rotator cuff interval, lesions of the superior GHL are closely related to those affecting this space. The rotator interval exists as a consequence of the interposition of the coracoid process between the supraspinatus and the subscapularis tendons. The rotator interval,

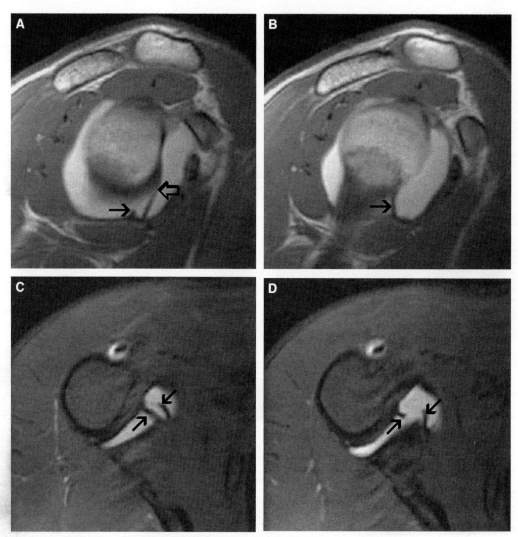

Fig. 10. (A, B) Oblique sagittal MR arthrograms demonstrate the anterior band of the inferior GHL (*arrows*) and a separate hypointense band (*open arrow*) extending anteriorly and upward toward the origin of the middle GHL. (*C, D*) Axial MR arthrograms show two distinct hypointense bands inserting into the inferior glenoid rim, likely corresponding to the anterior band of the inferior GHL and the spiral ligament (*arrows*).

therefore, does not have tendinous fibers. The space is a ligamentous region covered superiorly by the coracohumeral ligament and the superior GHL [12]. These two ligaments come together at the superior margin of the bicipital groove to form a restraining pulley mechanism for the tendon of the long head of the biceps. The long head of biceps tendon is situated deep in the rotator interval as it traverses from its intraarticular portion into the bicipital groove. Rotator interval tears have been associated with glenohumeral instability [13]. Chronic multidirectional instability and shoulder dislocations may result in enlargement of the interval in response to chronic trauma [42]. In these cases, the rotator interval may be depicted as an area of contrast collection protruding between the subscapularis and supraspinatus tendons on sagittal MR arthrographic images (Fig. 11). When a true isolated rotator interval is present, fluid signal or arthrographic contrast solution extends through the rent into the subacromial subdeltoid bursa. These tears are typically thin and longitudinal, and are not associated with tendon retraction [13,43]. Some individuals with rotator interval abnormalities do not have glenohumeral instability [43]. Anterior extension of supraspinatus tearing through the rotator cuff interval involving the cranial fibers of the subscapularis may be caused by anterosuperior internal impingement during flexion and internal rotation of the shoulder [44]. A recent report suggested an association between subcoracoid bursal effusions and tears of the

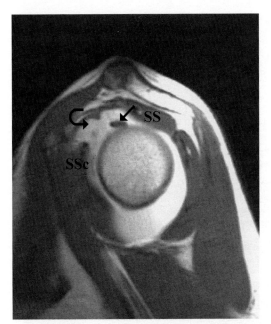

Fig. 11. Capacious rotator interval. Oblique sagittal T1-weighted MR-arthrographic image demonstrates a prominent rotator interval (*curved arrow*) in this patient with chronic glenohumeral instability. Note the intraarticular portion of the long head of biceps tendon (*arrow*). SS, supraspinatus; SSc, subscapularis.

anterior rotator cuff and the rotator interval [15]. Tears of the superior GHL in the rotator interval have also been described in association with tears of the middle GHL [16].

Middle GHL

Tears of the middle GHL are unusual lesions in patients with glenohumeral instability, but their frequency may be higher than previously recognized. In their series, Chandnani et al [21] reported that the middle GHL was abnormal in 52% of 33 patients with history of glenohumeral instability undergoing MR arthrography and arthroscopy in which the middle GHL could be identified. In this publication, a case of middle GHL tear was illustrated with an axial image that demonstrated a thickened and irregular middle GHL. In another series of 83 patients with glenohumeral instability treated arthroscopically, Terry et al [45] found that GHL injuries where present in 58% of the shoulders, with the superior GHL and the middle GHL the most commonly involved. These two reports are in contradiction to the widely held notion that the inferior GHL is the most commonly injured ligament.

Two different patterns of middle GHL have been identified [16]. The first is detachment of the ligament from its scapular insertion. In this case, the ligament is interrupted, foreshortened, thickened, and wavy, and it appears to be floating within the anterior capsular space. The second pattern of rupture of the middle GHL is a split longitudinal tear, extending from the scapular origin into the distal portion of the ligament but without complete interruption of the fibers (Fig. 12). The ruptured ligament is better demonstrated in the oblique sagittal and axial planes.

The most commonly associated lesion is a tear of the superior labrum, extending anteriorly into the fibers of the middle GHL, the superior labrum anterior to posterior lesion (SLAP VII lesion) (see Fig. 12). The labral tear may be extensive with a flap of labral tissue, which appears to be floating within the joint. The middle GHL tear also may be associated with a tear of the coracohumeral ligament, a rotator cuff interval tear and a SLAP lesion extending anteriorly and inferiorly, beyond the labral origin of the middle GHL (SLAP V and SLAP VII) [46].

The mechanism of injury of the middle GHL is difficult to ascertain. Some patients have associated SLAP lesions. SLAP lesions may result from compression forces to the shoulder, usually after a fall onto an outstretched arm or from traction on the arm, either secondary to violent contraction of the biceps muscle leading to excessive traction of the superior labrum or repeated overhead motion [47–49]. In atraumatic cases, tears of the superior labrum are probable related to degeneration [50]. It is conceivable that the mechanisms of injury in patients presenting with a combination of rotator interval tear, SLAP lesion, and coracohumeral ligament tear along with a tear of the middle GHL may involve a vectorial force directing the humeral head anteriorly and superiorly. Only two reports, by Maffet et al [51] and Shankman et al [46], have described an association between superior labral tear and middle GHL tear (SLAP VII lesion). The infrequency of reports involving the MGHL may be related to the relative rarity of the lesion, the lack of familiarity of the interpreting radiologist with these injuries, and the diversity of normal variants, making assessment of integrity of the middle GHL more difficult.

Inferior GHL

Injuries to the inferior GHL can occur without an associated labral tear. Humeral avulsion of the GHL (HAGL) is less often seen than classic Bankart lesions, but may also cause anterior shoulder instability [46]. HAGL can present as a pure soft tissue injury or as a "bony" HAGL. The latter comprises an avulsion fracture from the medial cortex of the humeral neck. Bui-Mansfield's literature search

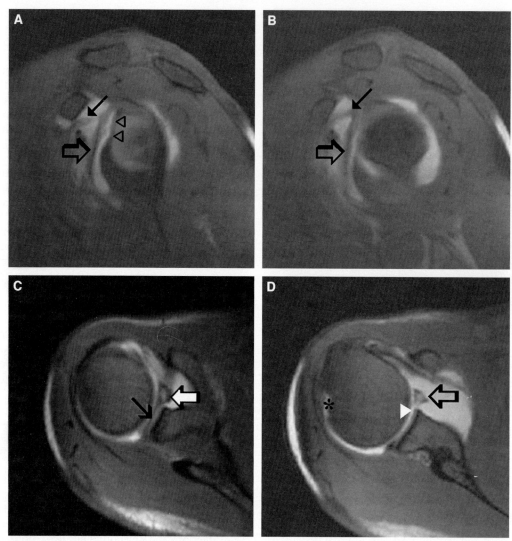

Fig. 12. Middle GHL tear. (*A, B*) Oblique sagittal MR arthrograms demonstrate split longitudinal tearing of the middle GHL (*open arrow*) superimposed on Buford complex. Absent anterosuperior labrum (*arrowheads*) and associated superior GHL tear (*arrow*) are noted. (*C– F*) Axial and oblique coronal MR arthrograms in the same patient show tear of the superior labrum anterior to posterior (SLAP lesion) (*arrow*). Split longitudinal tear of a thickened middle glenohumeral ligament (*open arrow*) is noted. Note is made of absent anterosuperior labrum (*arrowhead*) and Hill-Sachs lesion (*asterisk*).

found 59 reported cases of HAGL injury [30]. In this recently published series [30], 67% of patients with HAGL lesions presented with history of prior shoulder dislocation. The HAGL lesion demonstrated strong male predominance (97%). The lesion was commonly seen among athletes, rugby players being the most frequently affected. Also noted was an unclear association of HAGL lesions with a clinical history of prior surgery.

Isolated lesions to the anterior capsule in patients who had suffered shoulder dislocation were first described by Nicola et al [52]. This lesion was considered to occur as a result of hyperabduction and external rotation to distinguish it from the classical Bankart lesion, which often occurs as the result of hyperabduction of the shoulder associated with impaction. Although mechanical failure of the labral-ligamentous complex was proven to take place most commonly at the junction of the labrum and the glenoid rim based on study of cadaver specimens, failure at the humeral insertion site of the GHL was not uncommonly observed (up to 25% of cases) [53]. The reported incidence of HAGL lesion in the literature ranges from 2% to as high as 9.4% [30,54,55]. The discrepancy between clinical and biomechanical studies may be explained by

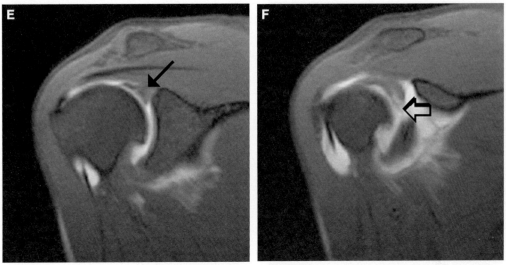

Fig. 12 (continued)

differences in testing conditions or failure to recognize these lesions based on arthroscopy or open surgery [30]. HAGL lesions can be overlooked if the appropriate area is not searched specifically for this condition [56]. Detection of an HAGL lesion requires careful blunt dissection to separate the subscapularis muscle from the capsule. Otherwise, exposure of the HAGL lesion may be misconstrued as an iatrogenic breach of the capsule rather than an injury [30]. HAGL lesion is located below the level of the subscapularis muscle in the inferior pouch of the shoulder, and appears as a thickened,

roughed edge in the capsular defect. Diagnostic criteria for HAGL injury based on arthroscopy includes visualization of the fibers of the subscapularis muscle through the avulsed inferior joint capsule, exposed subscapularis muscle, and loss of the "wave" that is formed by the reflection of the anterior capsule onto the humeral neck [54,55].

Half of the patients reported in Bui-Mansield's series showed pathologic findings on radiologic examinations, either at radiography or MR imaging [30]. The HAGL lesion is detected on conventional

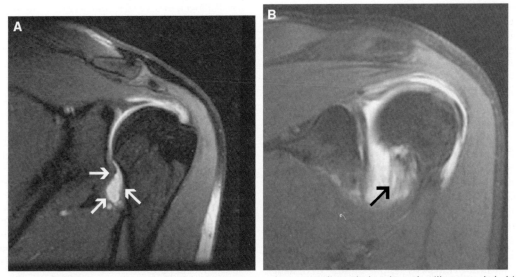

Fig. 13. (A) Oblique coronal MR arthrogram shows normal contrast-distended U-shaped axillary pouch (white arrows). (B) Oblique coronal MR arthrogram through the anterior band of the inferior GHL demonstrates irregularity and fraying at its humeral insertion (arrow). The axillary pouch appears as an inverted J-shaped structure.

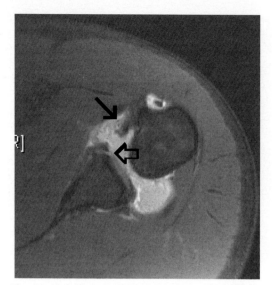

Fig. 14. Floating anterior inferior GHL. Axial MR arthrogram in same patient as Fig. 13B shows thickening and fraying of the anterior band of the inferior GHL at its humeral insertion (*arrow*) associated with Bankart lesion (*open arrow*).

radiographs only when there is associated bony avulsion from the humeral neck, known as bony HAGL [57]. Other radiographic features included bony Bankart, comminuted fracture of the clavicle, greater tuberosity fracture, and osteochondral fracture of the humeral head. MR identification of HAGL lesions requires joint distension either by effusion or MR arthrography. Otherwise, humeral detachment of the inferior GHL may not be detected on routine MR examinations of the shoulder. Main MR diagnostic criteria on oblique coronal fat-suppressed T2-weighted MR images or MR arthrographic images included conversion of a fluid-distended U-shaped axillary pouch into a J-shaped structure and extravasation of joint effusion or arthrographic solution across the torn humeral attachment (Fig. 13). On oblique sagittal fat-suppressed MR images, fluid extravasation, edema, or both are seen anterior to the humeral neck. Subacute and chronic injuries in which scar tissue may affix the ligament to the humeral neck can be overlooked on MR imaging. A large number of patients with HAGL lesions present with associated abnormalities. These include rotator cuff tears (94% of which involve the subscapularis), Bankart lesion (the association of HAGL lesion and Bankart injury has been denoted the "floating anterior inferior GHL") (Fig. 14), osteochondral injury of the humeral head, Hill-Sachs lesion, middle GHL avulsion, partial tear of the long head of the biceps tendon, and clavicular fracture.

HAGL lesions are typically treated surgically. An isolated HAGL lesion may occasionally be treated conservatively using a sling immobilizer followed by a shoulder-strengthening program. In general, HAGL lesions in young patients with first-time traumatic anterior shoulder dislocation or recurring dislocations are treated with arthroscopy or open repair. The goal is to secure good healing of the capsule to the bone, particularly inferiorly [57].

References

[1] Rockwood CA, Matsen FAI. The shoulder. Philadelphia: Saunders; 1990. p. 17–27.
[2] Zlatkin MB, Bjorkengren AG, Gylys-Morin V, et al. Cross-sectional imaging of the capsular mechanism of the glenohumeral joint. AJR Am J Roentgenol 1988;150:151–8.
[3] Rafii M, Firooznia H, Golimbu C, et al. CT arthrography of capsular structures of the shoulder. AJR Am J Roentgenol 1986;146:361–7.
[4] Yeh LR, Kwak S, Kim YS, et al. Anterior labroligamentous structures of the glenohumeral joint: correlation on MR arthrography and anatomic dissection in cadavers. AJR Am J Roentgenol 1998;171:1229–36.
[5] O'Connell PW, Nuber GW, Mileski RA, Lautenschlager E. The contribution of the glenohumeral ligaments to anterior stability of the shoulder joint. Am J Sports Med 1990;18:579–84.
[6] Massengill AD, Seeger LL, Yao L, et al. Labrocapsular ligamentous complex of the shoulder: normal anatomy, anatomic variation, and pitfalls of MR imaging and MR arthrography. Radiographics 1994;14:1211–23.
[7] Beltran J, Bencardino J, Mellado J, et al. MR arthrography of the shoulder: variants and pitfalls. Radiographics 1997;17:1403–12.
[8] Kwak SM, Brown RR, Resnick D, et al. Anatomy, anatomic variations, and pathology of the 11- to 3-o'clock position of the glenoid labrum: findings on MR arthrography and anatomic sections. AJR Am J Roentgenol 1998;171:235–8.
[9] Palmer WE, Brown JH, Rosenthal DJ. Labral ligamentous complex of the shoulder: evaluation with MR arthrography. Radiology 1994;190:645–51.
[10] Sanders TG, Morrison WB, Miller MD. Imaging techniques in the evaluation of glenohumeral instability. Am J Sports Med 2000;28:414–34.
[11] Stoller DW. MR arthrography of the shoulder joint. Radiol Clin N Am 1997;35:97–116.
[12] Petersilge CA, Witte DH, Sewell BO, et al. Normal regional anatomy of the shoulder. Magn Reson Imaging Clin N Am 1993;1:1–18.
[13] Seeger LL, Lubowitz J, Thomas BJ. Case report 815: tear of the rotator interval. Skeletal Radiol 1993;22:615–7.
[14] Werner A, Mueller T, Boehm D, Gohlke F. The stabilizing sling for the long head of the biceps

tendon in the rotator cuff interval. A histoanatomic study. Am J Sports Med 2000;28:28–31.

[15] Grainger AJ, Tirman PF, Elliott JM, et al. MR anatomy of the subcoracoid bursa and the association of subcoracoid effusion with tears of the anterior rotator cuff and the rotator interval. AJR Am J Roentgenol 2000;174: 1377–80.

[16] Beltran J, Bencardino J, Padron M, et al. The middle GHL: normal anatomy, variants and pathology. Skeletal Radiol 2002;31:253–62.

[17] Snyder SJ. Diagnostic arthroscopy: normal anatomy and variations. In: Snyder SJ, editor. Shoulder arthroscopy. New York: McGraw-Hill; 1994. p. 179–214.

[18] Palmer WE, Caslowitz PL, Chew FS. MR arthrography of the shoulder: normal intraarticular structures and common abnormalities. AJR Am J Roentgenol 1995;164:141–6.

[19] Pradhan RL, Itoi E, Watanabe W, et al. A rare anatomic variant of the superior GHL. Arthroscopy 2001;17:E3.

[20] Park YH, Lee JY, Moon SH, et al. MR arthrography of the labral capsular ligamentous complex in the shoulder: imaging variations and pitfalls. AJR Am J Roentgenol 2000;175: 667–72.

[21] Chandnani VP, Gagliardi JA, Murnane TG, et al. Glenohumeral ligaments and shoulder capsular mechanism: evaluation with MR arthrography. Radiology 1995;196:27–32.

[22] Caspari RB, Geissler WB. Arthroscopic manifestations of shoulder subluxation and dislocation. Clin Orthop 1993;291:54–66.

[23] Neumann CH, Petersen SA, Jahnke AH. MR imaging of the labral-capsular complex: normal variations. AJR Am J Roentgenol 1991;157: 1015–21.

[24] Kwak SM, Brown RR, Trudell D, Resnick D. Glenohumeral joint: comparison of shoulder positions at MR arthrography. Radiology 1998;208: 375–80.

[25] Moseley HF, Overgaard B. The anterior capsular mechanism in recurrent anterior dislocation of the shoulder. J Bone Joint Surg Br 1962;44: 913–27.

[26] Tirman PF, Feller JF, Palmer WE, et al. The Buford complex—a variation of normal shoulder anatomy: MR arthrographic imaging features. AJR Am J Roentgenol 1996;166:869–73.

[27] Ilahi OA, Labber MR, Cosculluela P. Variants of the anterosuperior glenoid labrum and associated pathology. Arthroscopy 2002;18:882–6.

[28] Rao AG, Kim TK, Chronopoulos E, McFarland EG. Anatomical variants in the anterosuperior aspect of the glenoid labrum: a statistical analysis of seventy-three cases. J Bone Joint Surg Am 2003; 85:653–9.

[29] Matsen FA III, Thomas SC, Rockwood CA Jr. Anterior glenohumeral instability. In: Rockwood CA, Matsen FA III, editors. The shoulder. Philadelphia: Saunders; 1990. p. 526–622.

[30] Bui-Mansfield LT, Taylor DC, Uhorchak JM, Tenuta JJ. Humeral avulsions of the GHL: imaging features and a review of the literature. AJR Am J Roentgenol 2002;179:649–55.

[31] Kolts I, Busch LC, Tomusk H, et al. Anatomical composition of the anterior shoulder joint capsule. A cadaver study on 12 glenohumeral joints. Ann Anat 2001;183:53–9.

[32] Matsen FA, Harryman DT, Sidles JA. Mechanics of glenohumeral instability. Clin Sports Med 1991;10:783–8.

[33] Turkel SJ, Panio MW, Marshall JL, Girgis FG. Stabilizing mechanisms preventing anterior dislocations of the glenohumeral joint. J Bone Joint Surg Am 1981;63:1208–17.

[34] Garneau RA, Renfrew DL, Moore TE, et al. Glenoid labrum: evaluation with MR imaging. Radiology 1991;179:519–22.

[35] O'Connell PW, Nuber GW, Mileski RA, Lautenschlager E. The contributions of the glenohumeral ligaments to anterior stability of the shoulder joint. Am J Sports Med 1990;18: 579–84.

[36] Debski RE, Wong EK, Woo SL, et al. An analytical approach to determine the in situ forces in the glenohumeral ligaments. J Biomech Eng 1999; 121:311–5.

[37] Schweitzer ME. MR arthrography of the labral-ligamentous complex of the shoulder. Radiology 1994;190:641–3.

[38] Gagey O, Gagey N, Boiserenault P, et al. Experimental study of dislocations of the scapulohumeral joint. Rev Chir Orthop Reparatrice Appar Mot 1993;79:13–21.

[39] Hintermann B, Gachter A. Arthroscopic findings after shoulder dislocation. Am J Sports Med 1995; 23:545–51.

[40] Hintermann B, Gachter A. Theo van Rens Priza: arthroscopic assessment of the unstable shoulder. Knee Surg Sports Traumatol Arthrosc 1994; 2:64–9.

[41] Taylor DC, Arciero RA. Pathologic changes associated with shoulder dislocations: arthroscopic and physical examination findings in the first-time, traumatic anterior dislocations. Am J Sports Med 1997;25:306–11.

[42] Nohubara K, Hitoshi I. Rotator interval lesion. Clin Orthop 1987;223:44.

[43] Steinbach LS. Rotator cuff disease. In: Steinbach LS, Tirman PFJ, Peterfy CG, Feller JF, editors. Shoulder magnetic resonance imaging. Philadelphia: Lippincott Williams & Wilkins; 1998. p. 99–133.

[44] Paulson MM, Watnik NF, Dines DM. Coracoid impingement syndrome, rotator interval reconstruction, and biceps tenodesis in the overhead athlete. Orthop Clin North Am 2001;32:485–93.

[45] Terry GC, Hammon D, France P, Norwood LA. The stabilizing function of passive shoulder restraints. Am J Sports Med 1991;19:26–34.

[46] Shankman S, Bencardino J, Beltran J. Glenohumeral instability: evaluation using MR

arthrography of the shoulder. Skeletal Radiol 1999;28:365–82.

[47] Snyder S, Karzel R, Del Pisso W, et al. SLAP lesions of the shoulder. Arthroscopy 1990; 14:274–9.

[48] Snyder SJ, Banas MP, Karzel RP. An analysis of 140 injuries to the superior glenoid labrum. J Shoulder Elbow Surg 1995;4:243–8.

[49] Tung GA, Entzian D, Green A, Brody JM. High-field and low-field MR imaging of superior glenoid labral tears and associated tendon injuries. AJR Am J Roentgenol 2000; 174:1107–14.

[50] DePalma A, Gallery G, Bennett G. Variational anatomy and degenerative lesions of the shoulder joint. In: American Academy of Orthopedic Surgeons, editors. Instructional course lectures 6. St. Louis: Mosby; 1949. p. 225–81.

[51] Maffet MW, Gartsman GM, Moseley B. Superior labrum-biceps tendon complex lesions of the shoulder. Am J Sports Med 1995;23:93–8.

[52] Nicola T. Anterior dislocation of the shoulder: the role of the anterior capsule. J Bone Joint Surg Am 1942;25:614–6.

[53] Bigliani LU, Pollock RG, Soslowsky LJ, et al. Tensile properties of the inferior GHL. J Orthop Res 1992;10:187–97.

[54] Wolf EM, Cheng JC, Dickson K. Humeral avulsion of glenohumeral ligaments as a cause of anterior shoulder instability. Arthroscopy 1995;11:600–7.

[55] Bokor DJ, Conboy VB, Olson C. Anterior instability of the glenohumeral joint with humeral avulsion of the GHL: a review of 41 cases. J Bone Joint Surg Br 1999;81:93–6.

[56] Field LD, Bokor DJ, Savoie FH III. Humeral and glenoid detachment of the anterior inferior GHL: a cause of anterior shoulder instability. J Shoulder Elbow Surg 1997;6:6–10.

[57] Bach BR, Warren RF, Fronek J. Disruption of the lateral capsule of the shoulder: cause of recurrent dislocation. J Bone Joint Surg Br 1988; 70:274–6.

ELSEVIER
SAUNDERS

RADIOLOGIC
CLINICS
OF NORTH AMERICA

Radiol Clin N Am 44 (2006) 503–523

MR Imaging of the Rotator Cuff

Ara Kassarjian, MD, FRCPC[a],*, Jenny T. Bencardino, MD[b],
William E. Palmer, MD[a]

Repetitive overhead motions, such as those commonly employed in tennis, baseball, swimming, and football, can lead to primary rotator cuff impingement [1]. Primary impingement is often seen in middle-aged athletes who present with chronic pain and weakness associated with overhead sporting activities. Conversely, secondary impingement is typically a manifestation of glenohumeral instability and is more common in young athletes who employ overhead or throwing motions. Although less common, secondary impingement may also be seen in the setting of posterior superior impingement and scapulothoracic instability. Prompt and accurate diagnosis of impingement syndromes helps ensure timely and appropriate treatment of recreational and professional athletes.

MR imaging is an accurate method of evaluating the rotator cuff, coracoacromial arch, and the subacromial-subdeltoid bursa [2,3]. In addition, MR imaging can often identify lesions responsible for instability and secondary impingement. This article addresses the role of MR imaging in evaluating the rotator cuff and the importance of MR imaging in identifying other lesions that may mimic rotator cuff pathology. A rationale for protocol design, including MR arthrography and the use of specialized positioning, such as abduction and external rotation (ABER), are discussed.

MR imaging protocol

Although there are innumerable ways of performing MR imaging of the shoulder, a few fundamental principles should be applied. Use of a local surface coil, such as a dedicated phased array coil, is mandatory to ensure adequate spatial resolution and signal to noise and thereby achieve high-quality imaging. The patient is typically in the supine position with the arm slightly externally rotated at their side. To ensure mild external rotation, we place a rolled towel under the elbow, which typically results in a comfortable slightly externally rotated position, thereby reducing motion artifact resulting from patient discomfort.

This article was previously published in *Magnetic Resonance Imaging Clinics of North America* 2004;12:39–60.
[a] Musculoskeletal MRI, Massachusetts General Hospital, 15 Parkman Street, Suite 515, Boston, MA 02114, USA
[b] Musculoskeletal Radiology, Medical Arts Radiology Group, PC, Huntington Hospital, North Shore-Long Island Jewish Hospital Health System, 270 Park Avenue, Huntington, NY 11743, USA
* Corresponding author.
E-mail address: akassarjian@partners.org (A. Kassarjian).

doi:10.1016/j.rcl.2006.04.005

Our current protocol includes coronal oblique, sagittal oblique, and axial imaging planes. Axial proton density (2500/20) or gradient echo (550/15, flip angle 20) images should extend from the top of the acromioclavicular joint though the inferior glenoid margin. Coronal oblique proton density (2500/20), fast spin-echo T2-weighted (3800/100, ETL 8), and fast spin-echo intermediate TE (2700/50, ETL 6) fat-suppressed images are prescribed perpendicular to the glenoid cavity. Alternatively, these can be prescribed parallel to the supraspinatus tendon. The oblique coronal images extend form the subscapularis anteriorly to the infraspinatus and teres minor posteriorly. Oblique sagittal images are oriented perpendicular to the oblique coronal images (ie, parallel to the glenoid cavity). T1-weighted and fast-inversion recovery or fat-suppressed T2-weighted images in the oblique sagittal plane extend from the body of the scapula through the greater tuberosity. It is critical to ensure that the most lateral image covers the distal fibers of the supraspinatus and infraspinatus as they insert on the greater tuberosity. Although this protocol produces excellent imaging of the rotator cuff, partial-thickness undersurface tears and small full-thickness tears may not be visible in the absence of an effusion because of insufficient signal differences between the rotator cuff and the adjacent humeral head.

MR arthrography exploits the advantages gained from the presence of a joint effusion. Dilution of commercially available gadolinium formulations to a concentration of approximately 2 mmol ensures optimization of paramagnetic effects on T1-weighted imaging. To obtain this concentration, 0.4 mL of gadopentate dimeglumine (Magnevist, Berlex Laboratories, Wayne, New Jersey) are added to 50 cc of normal saline. Ten milliliters of this solution are mixed with 5 mL of nonionic iodinated contrast and 5 mL of preservative free lidocaine 1%, resulting in a final gadolinium dilution of 1:250. A 22-gauge 3.5-in spinal needle is advanced into the glenohumeral joint under fluoroscopic guidance, and 12 to 15 mL of this solution is injected to achieve adequate capsular distention. The addition of iodinated contrasted into the solution allows for fluoroscopic confirmation of intra-articular injection. Also, standard pre- and postexercise fluoroscopic images can be obtained. MR imaging is initiated within 30 minutes of injection to avoid loss of capsular distention as the fluid is absorbed out of the joint. Some institutions add a small quantity of epinephrine to the solution to achieve vasoconstriction and thus delay resorption of the contrast from the glenohumeral joint. This technique may be beneficial if there is a potential for delay between injection and initiation of MR scanning.

The MR arthrographic protocol takes advantage of the T1 shortening effects of gadolinium. We employ routine three-plane spin-echo frequency selective fat-suppressed T1-weighted sequences, a coronal oblique fast spin-echo T2-weighted sequence, and a sagittal oblique spin-echo T1-weighted sequence. For younger patients and patients suspected of having posterior superior impingement and partial-thickness undersurface tears, the arm is placed in the abduction and external rotation (ABER) position with the patient's palm under the head. Oblique axial fat-suppressed T1-weighted images of the glenohumeral joint are then obtained. The ABER position is valuable in demonstrating lesions of posterior superior impingement and undersurface tears of the rotator cuff as well as nondisplaced tears of the anterior inferior labrum in patients with glenohumeral instability [4].

Anatomic considerations

The tendons of the supraspinatus, infraspinatus, subscapularis, and teres minor comprise the rotator cuff. The subscapularis inserts on the lesser tuberosity, with superficial fibers extending to the greater tuberosity and thus contributing to the transverse humeral ligament, which forms the roof of the intertubercular (bicipital) groove. The supraspinatus, infraspinatus, and teres minor insert onto the superior, middle, and inferior facets of the greater tuberosity, respectively. The rotator interval is a triangular-shaped space between the anterior fibers of the supraspinatus and the superior fibers of the subscapularis. The coracoid process forms the base of this space, and the transverse humeral ligament forms the apex. The coracohumeral ligament, the superior glenohumeral ligament, and the tendon of the long head biceps brachii are intimately related to the rotator interval (Fig. 1). All four muscles of the rotator cuff act as stabilizers of the glenohumeral joint. The supraspinatus is primarily a shoulder abductor. The infraspinatus and teres minor externally rotate the shoulder, with the former also being an abductor and the latter being a weak adductor. The subscapularis is a strong adductor and internal rotator [5,6].

The supraspinatus muscle originates along the dorsal surface of the scapula within the supraspinous fossa. The muscle fibers course along a lateral orientation and converge to form a dominant single tendon along the anterior aspect of the muscle. The myotendinous junction is typically at the 12 o'clock position above the humeral head, although there is some slight variation in this position (Fig. 2) (see later discussion) [7]. The supraspinatus tendon is bordered superiorly by the subacromial-subdeltoid

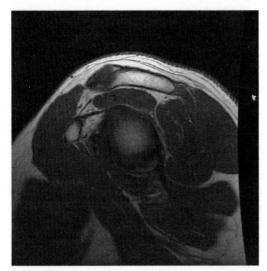

Fig. 1. Rotator interval. Sagittal oblique T1-weighted image shows normal rotator interval between the supraspinatus and the subscapularis.

bursa and inferiorly by the joint capsule. Anteriorly, the more distal supraspinatus tendon converges with the coracohumeral ligament, and posteriorly it merges with the anterior fibers of the infraspinatus tendon. The supraspinatus tendon is best evaluated in the coronal oblique plane and the sagittal oblique plane, with the latter being helpful in evaluating the most anterior fibers of the supraspinatus. The region just medial to the convergence of the posterior fibers of the supraspinatus and the anterior fibers of the infraspinatus has been referred to as the posterior rotator interval. The supraspinatus is innervated by the suprascapular nerve (C5 and

C6), which passes through the suprascapular notch and courses obliquely and laterally along the undersurface of the supraspinatus [8].

The infraspinatus originates in the infraspinous fossa. As opposed to the supraspinatus, which converges to a single dominant tendon, the infraspinatus has a multipennate configuration with the myotendinous junction having a somewhat fanlike configuration (Fig. 3). The infraspinatus is separated from the overlying deltoid by a fascial layer. The inferior margin of the infraspinatus blends with the joint capsule. The distal fibers of the suprascapular nerve, once they pass through a fibro-osseous tunnel at the spinoglenoid notch, innervate the infraspinatus muscle. These distal nerve fibers of the suprascapular nerve terminate within the infraspinatus. The infraspinatus is best evaluated in the coronal oblique and sagittal oblique planes. The teres minor originates along the upper two thirds of the lateral border of the scapula and blends into the posterior glenohumeral joint capsule more distally (see Fig. 3).

The teres minor forms the superior border of the quadrilateral space and the triangular space (Fig. 4). The quadrilateral space is bordered by the teres minor superiorly, the teres major inferiorly, the long head triceps medially, and the surgical neck of the humerus laterally. The quadrilateral space contains the axillary nerve and the posterior circumflex vessels. The triangular space is more medially located and is bordered by the teres minor superomedially, the teres major inferomedially, and the long head triceps laterally. The triangular space contains the circumflex scapular artery. Although the quadrilateral space and triangular space

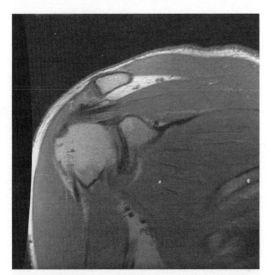

Fig. 2. Supraspinatus. Coronal oblique proton density image shows normal supraspinatus myotendinous junction.

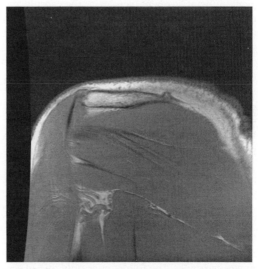

Fig. 3. Infraspinatus and teres minor. Coronal oblique proton density image shows normal infraspinatus and teres minor.

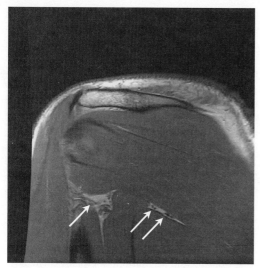

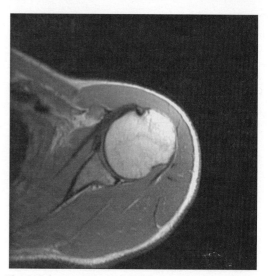

Fig. 4. Quadrilateral space and triangular space. Coronal oblique proton density image shows normal quadrilateral space (*arrow*) and triangular space (*double arrow*).

Fig. 5. Subscapularis. Axial oblique image shows normal subscapularis tendon.

are clearly delineated in the coronal oblique plane, the teres minor muscle is best evaluated in the axial and sagittal oblique planes.

The subscapularis muscle originates from the subscapular fossa along the anterior aspect of the scapula. Similar to the infraspinatus, the subscapularis has a multipennate configuration. The subscapularis recess, which communicates with the glenohumeral joint, separates the subscapularis muscle from the coracoid. The deep fibers of the subscapularis tendon blend with and reinforce the anterior capsule of the glenohumeral joint (Fig. 5). The mid and distal portions of the middle glenohumeral ligament blend with the capsule and deep fibers of the subscapularis before inserting into the lesser tuberosity [9]. The subscapularis is best evaluated in the axial and sagittal oblique planes.

The coracoacromial arch is composed of the undersurface of the acromion, the anterior portion of the coracoid, the coracoacromial ligament, the distal clavicle, and the undersurface of the acromioclavicular joint (Fig. 6). The supraspinatus, infraspinatus, long head biceps, and subacromial bursa pass under the coracoacromial arch. The coracoacromial arch is best evaluated in the sagittal oblique and coronal oblique planes.

Rotator cuff impingement

Rotator cuff impingement can take various forms, and attempts have been made to classify impingement syndromes. The following is only one of several methods of classifying rotator cuff impingement.

Primary extrinsic impingement includes subacromial and subcoracoid impingement. Subacromial impingement refers to impingement of the rotator cuff, typically the supraspinatus, as it passes under the coracoacromial arch. Potential etiologies of subacromial impingement include subacromial spurs, variations in acromial morphology or position, hypertrophic acromioclavicular joint abnormalities, an unstable os acromiale, subacromial-subdeltoid bursitis, and thickening of the coracoacromial ligament [10]. Subcoracoid impingement is associated with abnormalities of the coracoid process that result in a decrease in the distance between the coracoid and the anterior aspect of the humeral head.

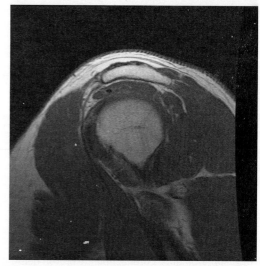

Fig. 6. Coracoacromial arch. Sagittal oblique T1-weighted image shows normal coracoacromial arch.

This abnormal relationship typically results in impingement of the subscapularis and the long head biceps brachii [11,12].

Secondary extrinsic impingement occurs in the setting of a normal coracoacromial arch [13]. In this setting, impingement results from abnormal glenohumeral or scapulothoracic motion secondary to instability.

Internal impingement refers to contact between the glenoid rim and the undersurface of the rotator cuff, particularly when the arm is in the late cocking phase of a throwing motion with the arm in 90 degrees of abduction and maximal external rotation [14]. Internal impingement also may result from narrowing of the coracoacromial outlet as a result of supraspinatus hypertrophy or abnormalities of the greater tuberosity [10].

Primary extrinsic impingement: subacromial

Subacromial impingement refers to a clinical syndrome in which the subacromial bursa and supraspinatus are entrapped underneath the coracoacromial arch. The etiology of this syndrome is variable, including subacromial spurs, undersurface acromioclavicular joint osteophytes, morphologic variations of the acromion, such as anterior down sloping, lateral down sloping, or low-lying acromion, an os acromiale, or a thickened coracoacromial ligament [3]. These anatomic abnormalities lead to a decrease in the space beneath the coracoacromial arch. As this space is reduced, repeated microtrauma to the subacromial bursa and supraspinatus tendon is thought to lead to bursitis and tendon injury. Although the anatomic abnormalities may be identified on MR imaging, they should only be considered a substrate for impingement as the diagnosis of impingement is based on clinical criteria. Provocative tests, such as full forward flexion and internal rotation (Neer's sign) or internal rotation of a 90-degree flexed arm (Hawkins' sign), which result in pain are considered positive clinical signs of subacromial impingement [15]. The former is thought to compress the greater tuberosity against the anterior acromion, whereas the latter is thought to compress the greater tuberosity against the leading edge of the coracoacromial ligament. Occasionally, a diagnostic injection of lidocaine within the subacromial region is employed to help differentiate an impingement syndrome from other etiologies of shoulder pain. If such a diagnostic injection has been performed, MR imaging should be delayed for at least 24 hours to avoid misinterpretation of subacromial fluid as evidence of bursitis or rotator cuff tear [16].

Although MR imaging provides excellent anatomic detail of the components of the rotator cuff and the coracoacromial arch, the patient is typically scanned with the arm at their side, a position that does not reflect the physiologic position of impingement [17]. Despite this limitation, MR imaging is useful in demonstrating potential substrates for impingement involving the coracoacromial arch and supraspinatus outlet. The supraspinatus, superior (anterior) 20% of the infraspinatus, and the subscapularis pass through the coracoacromial arch before their insertion onto the humerus [6].

The sagittal oblique plane is the optimal plane for evaluation of the coracoacromial ligament. The coracoacromial ligament, which has somewhat trapezoidal shape, extends from the coracoid to the undersurface of the acromion. The thickness of the coracoacromial ligament varies from 2 to 5.6 mm [18]. It may be difficult to distinguish a thickened acromial insertion of the coracoacromial ligament from an unossified subacromial spur as both may have low signal intensity on MR imaging. In addition, the deltoid ligament, which has an origin on the acromion along its inferomedial margin, may also be misinterpreted as a subacromial spur (see Fig. 6) [19]. Given these potential pitfalls, unless there is an ossified subacromial spur with intrinsic marrow signal, one must be cautious in ascribing subacromial low signal intensity to a subacromial spur (Fig. 7). Although a subacromial spur is thought to be a cause for subacromial impingement, it is not entirely clear whether coracoacromial ligament degeneration and subacromial spur formation are substrates for impingement or whether they represent sequelae of supraspinatus tendon degeneration [20,21].

Although not universally accepted, variations in the configuration of the acromion have been implicated in the pathogenesis of impingement

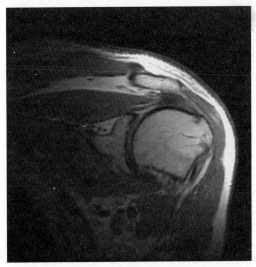

Fig. 7. Subacromial spur. Coronal oblique proton density image shows subacromial spur.

syndromes. Bigliani et al [22] described three acromial configurations. A type I acromion has a flat undersurface and is not thought to be implicated in subacromial impingement. A type II acromion has a concave undersurface and may have a moderate association with subacromial impingement. A type III acromion has a hooked anterior margin (Fig. 8). In a recent study of acromial morphology, type II was the most common (63%), and type III was the least common (14%) [23]. Some researchers believe that acromial morphology is developmental, as evidenced in one study by the lack of association between age, acromial type, and symmetry of acromial shape [24]. Type II and III acromia appear to be more strongly associated with subacromial spur formation. Thus, based on Neer's theory of impingement, which is not universally accepted, individuals with type II and III acromia should be at increased risk for rotator cuff pathology. In support of this theory, two studies demonstrated that 70% to 80% of cuff tears were associated with type III acromia [25,26]. Alternatively, some feel that subacromial spurs are a consequence of, and not a cause for, rotator cuff pathology [20,21]. As opposed to Neer's theory of impingement resulting in cuff abnormalities, some investigators feel that bursal surface cuff abnormalities result in subacromial spur formation. Along the same lines, some feel that the type III acromion is not truly a developmental configuration but actually represents an acquired enthesophyte or calcification/ossification at the coracoacromial attachment onto the anterior acromion [27,28]. Despite disagreement regarding pathogenesis of acromial morphology, oblique

sagittal MR images clearly demonstrate the shape of the acromion. However, there may be interobserver variability in assessing acromial morphology with MR imaging [29,30].

Other factors aside from acromial morphology may narrow the supraspinatus outlet and thus serve as a substrate for impingement. These include a laterally or anteriorly downsloping acromion, a low-lying acromion, and AC joint separation, or instability (Fig. 9) [18,31].

Coronal oblique and sagittal oblique MR imaging can be used to assess the shape of the acromion and its relationship to the distal clavicle and rotator cuff. The acromioclavicular joint, which is a fibrocartilaginous joint with a central disc, is somewhat immobile, with approximately 20 degrees of movement [6]. Acromioclavicular joint osteoarthritis is extremely common in asymptomatic individuals and is thus not specific for impingement [32]. However, undersurface osteophytes off the acromioclavicular joint can narrow the subacromial space and are thus potential substrates for impingement (Fig. 10). Specifically, the bursal surface of the supraspinatus tendon may be damaged as it moves under the acromioclavicular joint during glenohumeral joint abduction [10].

A normal variant of the acromion, the os acromiale, represents an unfused accessory ossification center of the anterior acromion (Fig. 11) [33]. The diagnosis can be made if there is failure of fusion by age 25. An os acromiale can be a substrate for impingement as a result of hypermobility/instability of the osseous fragment or osseous proliferation at the junction of the os acromiale with the

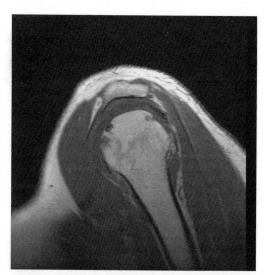

Fig. 8. Acromial morphology. Sagittal oblique T1-weighted images shows anterior acromial spur at insertion of coracoacromial ligament.

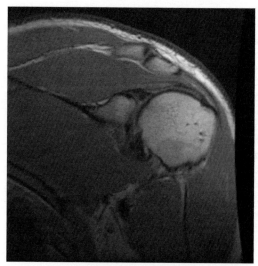

Fig. 9. Acromial position. Coronal oblique proton density image shows laterally downsloping acromion.

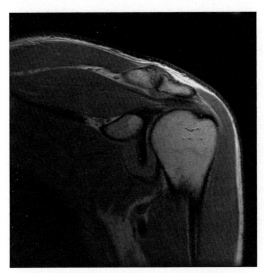

Fig. 10. Acromioclavicular joint. Coronal oblique proton density image shows acromioclavicular joint hypertrophic degenerative change with mass affect on supraspinatus.

remainder of the scapula [34]. The ossicle may be unstable as a result of attachment of the deltoid tendon into the inferior lateral aspect of the ossicle. An os acromiale is important to identify preoperatively as the synchondrosis may be weakened by a subacromial decompression and thus become more mobile. Alternatively, a standard subacromial decompression in the setting of an os acromiale may result in deltoid tendon detachment [35]. There are variable treatments for symptomatic os acromiale, from extended subacromial decompression to internal fixation of the synchondrosis [36].

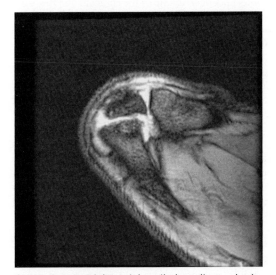

Fig. 11. Os acromiale. Axial spoiled gradient-echo image shows os acromiale.

Primary extrinsic impingement: subcoracoid

First described in 1985, subcoracoid impingement, also referred to as coracoid impingement, refers to impingement of the subscapular tendon between the coracoid process and the humerus, also known as the coracohumeral interval [11,12,37]. In addition, components of the rotator interval, such as the coracohumeral ligament and the long head biceps brachii tendon, may also become impinged in this location. Entrapment of these structures may lead to degeneration and tearing. The clinical signs of subcoracoid impingement include anterior shoulder pain, which is exacerbated by forward flexion, internal rotation, and cross-arm adduction [38]. Three general etiologies for architectural abnormalities of the coracoid that may lead to subcoracoid impingement have been described: (1) idiopathic enlargement, elongation, or downsloping of the coracoid process; (2) iatrogenic postsurgical deformities of the coracoid; and (3) posttraumatic deformities of the coracoid or lesser tuberosity. The common denominator in these three situations is narrowing of the coracohumeral space. The coracohumeral space, as measured on axial CT or MR imaging, is the distance between the tip of the coracoid process and the lesser tuberosity of the humerus with the arm in internal rotation. In one study, although there was overlap between symptomatic and asymptomatic individuals, the mean coracohumeral distance in patients with subcoracoid impingement was 5.5 mm, whereas that in asymptomatic patients was 11 mm, with none in the latter group having a distance of less than 4 mm [39]. Given these anatomic factors, when abnormalities of the subscapularis tendon and the rotator interval are identified, the coracohumeral space should be carefully evaluated for potential causes of subcoracoid impingement (Fig. 12). Subcoracoid impingement, which may be overlooked at initial evaluation of a patient with an impingement syndrome, may lead to persistent pain following routine rotator cuff surgery [40]. In such patients, treating the abnormalities of the coracoid with coracoplasty was shown to result in complete relief of pain in nine of nine patients who had previously failed prior anterior acromioplasty and rotator cuff repair [40].

Secondary extrinsic impingement

Secondary extrinsic impingement refers to rotator cuff impingement secondary to glenohumeral or, rarely, scapulothoracic instability [10,13]. This type of impingement is typically seen in athletes who participate in sports that require repetitive overhead or throwing motions. In these cases, the coracoacromial arch has a normal configuration

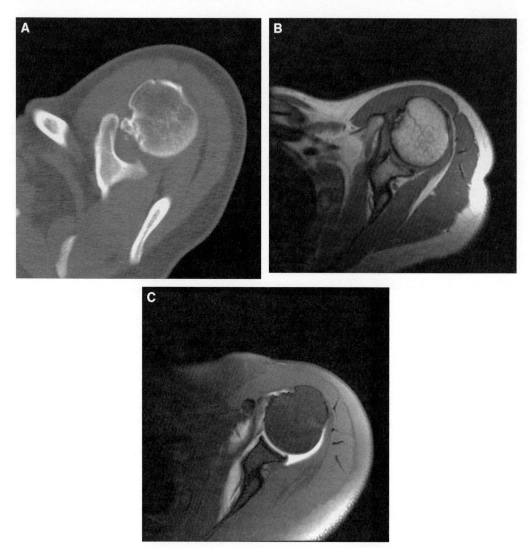

Fig. 12. Subcoracoid impingement. (*A*) axial CT scan shows contact between the tip of the coracoid and the lesser tuberosity, the latter of which is sclerotic and hypertrophied. (*B*) Axial proton density image shows decreased coracohumeral distance with partial tear of the subscapularis muscle as evidenced by expansion and high signal intensity. (*C*) Axial fat-suppressed T1-weighted image from MR arthrogram shows partial tear of the subscapularis tendon.

without any of the previously described abnormalities that may result in primary extrinsic subacromial impingement. On clinical exam, the signs of impingement may predominate and thus mask signs of underlying glenohumeral instability. Examination under anesthesia is helpful in such cases as it allows identification of glenohumeral instability. With instability, superior migration of the humeral head may lead to narrowing of the supraspinatus outlet. In these cases, chronic instability may be a result of weakening of the glenohumeral ligaments and anterior capsule [41]. As these static stabilizers are weakened, more load is placed on dynamic stabilizers, namely, the muscles of the rotator cuff.

Such a workload may result in fatigue of the cuff muscles, which thus allows superior migration of the humeral head resulting in a decreased acromiohumeral distance. This type of instability results in impingement of the rotator cuff, which may lead to degeneration and tear of the rotator cuff, particularly on its articular surface along the posterior rotator interval where the supraspinatus and infraspinatus tendons converge (**Fig. 13**) [42].

Internal impingement

Internal impingement may be classified as posterosuperior impingement or anterosuperior impingement. Posterosuperior impingement refers to

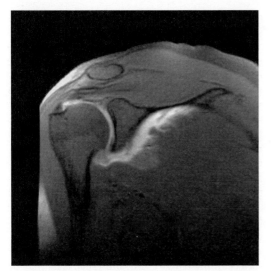

Fig. 13. Partial-thickness rotator cuff tear. Coronal oblique fat-suppressed image from MR arthrogram demonstrates partial-thickness undersurface tear at the junction of the supraspinatus and infraspinatus, a region referred to as the posterior interval.

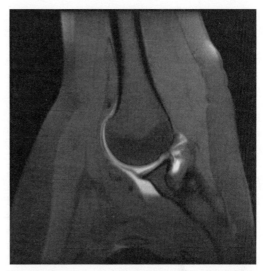

Fig. 14. Posterior superior impingement. MR arthrogram obtained in the ABER position shows posterior superior labral tear, undersurface tear of the supraspinatus, and small defect in humeral head in a patient with posterior superior impingement.

abnormalities caused by friction between the posterosuperior labrum and glenoid and the undersurface of the supraspinatus as the shoulder is moved through the abduction external rotation (ABER) position (Fig. 14) [14]. This type of impingement typically is seen in overhead and throwing athletes and may occur without or with glenohumeral instability. MR imaging demonstrates degeneration and tearing of the posterosuperior glenoid labrum, articular surface fraying, and partial-thickness tearing of the supraspinatus, occasionally as far posteriorly as its junction with the infraspinatus (posterior interval) [43]. Additional findings may include glenoid cysts and osteochondral impaction fractures of the greater tuberosity. Because of the location of these lesions, MR arthrography with the patient in the ABER position provides excellent visualization of the affected regions of the posterosuperior labrum, glenoid, and articular surface of the rotator cuff [44].

A second type of internal impingement has recently been described. Gerber and Sebesta [37] described an impingement of the articular surface fibers of the subscapularis tendon along the anterior superior glenoid rim. In their arthroscopic study, when the glenohumeral joint was flexed and internally rotated, anterior tissues were impinged along the anterior superior glenoid. If the arm was elevated greater than 90 degrees, the long head biceps and the common insertion of the superior glenohumeral ligament and coracohumeral ligament (biceps pulley) was impinged against the superior labrum. With less than 90 degrees elevation, the articular surface fibers of the subscapularis

tendon contacted the anterior superior labrum and glenoid rim. None of the patients had signs or symptoms of instability. In 10 of 13 patients with arthroscopically proven partial-thickness subscapularis tears, MR arthrography demonstrated partial articular surface tears of the subscapularis tendon. In another study using nonarthrographic MR imaging, only 20% of arthroscopically proven partial-thickness articular surface tears were identified on MR imaging in the setting of anterosuperior impingement [45].

Rotator cuff tendon abnormalities

Tendinopathy

Classically, rotator cuff tears occur in the insertional fibers of the cuff tendons in regions of preexisting tendinopathy [46]. The etiology of tendinopathy, or tendinosis, is likely multifactorial with contributions from aging, trauma, overuse, and metabolic conditions [10]. The typical MR appearance of tendinopathy is high signal on short TE sequences, such as proton density sequences, which does not become as high as fluid signal on long TE sequences, such as T2-weighted sequences [46]. The signal abnormalities may be seen in the setting of either normal tendon morphology or somewhat thickened tendons. One pitfall to assessing the cuff tendons with short TE imaging is that the magic angle phenomenon may result in artifactually increased signal in regions where the tendon courses at a 55-degree angle in relation to the main magnetic field. Magic angle artifact should resolve on T2-weighted (long TE) sequences, thus differentiating it from tendinopathy. Additionally, volume averaging between the tendon and adjacent tissues such as muscle, fascia, fat, and cartilage may result in high tendon signal on short TE imaging. Again, use of T2-weighted imaging and assessing tendons in at least two planes can increase confidence in differentiating artifact from true intratendinous signal abnormalities [19,47].

Partial-thickness tears

Partial-thickness rotator cuff tears can be described according to the surface of the tendon involved as well as the percentage of tendon involved. Tears may involve one of three regions of distal tendon fibers: articular surface (aka, undersurface), bursal surface, and intrasubstance. Articular surface tears are the most common type and are easily diagnosed with standard MR imaging when a joint effusion is present. Partial-thickness articular surface tears are characterized by a focal region of fiber discontinuity that is filled with fluid signal as demonstrated on T2-weighted imaging. Fat-suppressed T2-weighted imaging can increase lesion conspicuity by better demonstrating the fluid-filled tendon defect (Fig. 15) [2]. Aside from a focal tendon defect, additional findings may include surface fraying or changes in tendon caliber, such as attenuation or thickening [47]. Tendon retraction is uncommon but may occasionally be seen in high-grade partial-thickness tears. In the absence of a joint effusion, articular surface partial-thickness tears may be difficult to identify, particularly in the setting of

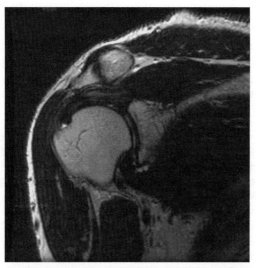

Fig. 15. Partial-thickness rotator cuff tear. Coronal T2-weighted image shows partial thickness articular surface tear of the supraspinatus.

granulation tissue or scarring. In one study, the sensitivity, specificity, and accuracy of standard MR imaging for partial tears were 35% to 44%, 85% to 97%, and 77% to 87%, respectively [48]. In these cases, MR arthrography without and with additional imaging in the ABER position has been shown to improve conspicuity of articular surface tears of the rotator cuff (Fig. 16) [44,49–51]. Two recent studies demonstrated MR arthrography to be 84% to 95% sensitive and 96% to 100% specific for partial-thickness articular surface tears of the rotator cuff [52,53]. Intrasubstance tears are characterized by intratendinous T2 fluid signal without extension to either the bursal or articular surface (Fig. 17). These lesions will not fill with gadolinium on MR arthrography because of lack of communication between the tear and the articular surface of the tendon. Intrasubstance tears may be occult on tendon visualization during arthroscopic or open surgery because of intact tendon surfaces. However, careful probing may demonstrate the focal tendon abnormality.

Partial-thickness bursal surface tears result in discontinuity of the tendon along its superior (bursal) surface with an extraarticular fluid-filled gap. The articular surface remains intact. When there is fluid in the subacromial bursa, the tears are well visualized, particularly on T2-weighted images. However, these tears may not be visible on T1-weighted MR arthrographic images as the intraarticular gadolinium will not enter the gap in the tendon because of intact articular surface fibers. In addition, the presence of bursal fluid may not be appreciated on T1-weighted imaging (Fig. 18). For these reasons, it is crucial to include at least one T2-weighted sequence on all MR arthrographic exams to assess for fluid-filled bursal surface tears. These T2-weighted images are also useful for assessing other periarticular fluid collections and cysts that may be occult on T1-weighted imaging. Although rarely performed, bursal injection of gadolinium for direct MR bursography can be performed to outline bursal surface partial-thickness rotator cuff tears [54].

Partial-thickness rotator cuff tears have been classified arthroscopically according to the degree of tendon involvement [55,56]. Grade 1 lesions involve less than 25% of the tendon thickness (less than 3 mm); grade 2 lesions involve 25% to 50% (3 to 6 mm); and grade 3 lesions involve greater than 50% of the tendon (greater than 6 mm). In the end, surgical treatment, including debridement versus actual cuff repair, depends on degree of tearing, tendon quality, and activity level of the patient [57].

Full-thickness tears

When a tear of the rotator cuff results in a discontinuity in the tendon that extends from the articular

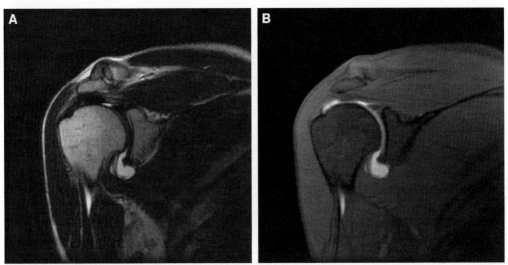

Fig. 16. Partial-thickness tear not visible on T2-weighted imaging. (*A*) Coronal oblique T2-weighted image shows thickening of the distal supraspinatus tendon without specific evidence for a rotator cuff tear. (*B*) Coronal oblique T1-weighted fat-suppressed image from MR arthrogram in the same patient shows partial-thickness articular surface tear not visible on T2-weighted imaging.

surface to the bursal surface, it is referred to as a full-thickness tear (Fig. 19). Full-thickness tears can be classified according to the size of the tear: small (less than 1 cm), medium (1 to 3 cm), large (3 to 5 cm), and massive (greater than 5 cm). Massive tears of the rotator cuff involve supraspinatus and infraspinatus and are usually associated with tendon retraction. Supraspinatus tears that are greater than 2.5 cm in anteroposterior dimension often extend into the infraspinatus or the subscapularis. The

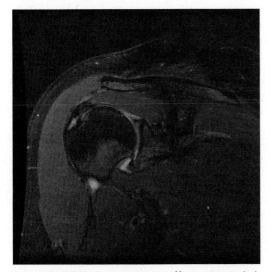

Fig. 17. Partial-thickness rotator cuff tear. Coronal oblique fat-suppressed T2-weighted image shows intra-substance tear of the supraspinatus with normal articular and bursal surfaces.

tear does not need to involve the entire tendon in an anteroposterior dimension to be considered a full-thickness tear. Conventional nonarthrographic MR imaging is an accurate test for depicting full-thickness tears of the rotator cuff. Although fat-suppressed imaging may increase sensitivity for full-thickness tears, there is no significant change in specificity [2]. The characteristic and most specific sign of a full-thickness rotator cuff tear is tendon discontinuity [58]. The presence of fluid in the subacromial-subdeltoid bursa, although not specific for a full-thickness tear, is considered by some authors to be the most sensitive sign [58]. In one study, the sensitivity, specificity, and accuracy of MR imaging for full-thickness rotator cuff tears were 84% to 96%, 94% to 98%, and 92% to 97%, respectively [48]. Recently, MR arthrography was shown to be 98% sensitive and 100% specific for partial-thickness articular surface rotator cuff tears, with 100% accuracy for full-thickness tears [52]. MR arthrography may demonstrate a small full-thickness component of a rotator cuff tear that may appear as being only a partial-thickness tear on standard MR imaging (Fig. 20). When evaluating rotator cuff tears, the anteroposterior and mediolateral (ie, tendon retraction) measurements as well as the quality of torn tendon margin should be described in the report as these factors are valuable to the surgeon when assessing prognosis and planning surgery (arthroscopic versus open) [59].

Although rotator cuff tears typically appear as areas of fluid signal intensity on T2-weighted images, in about 10% of tears, the region of tendon

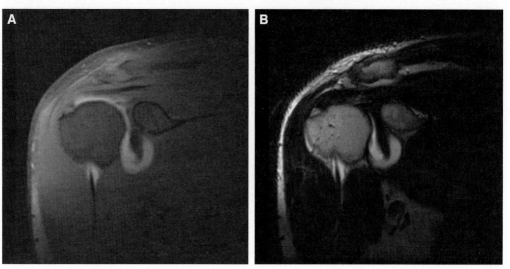

Fig. 18. Bursal surface tear not visible on T1-weighted images from MR arthrogram. (*A*) Coronal oblique fat-suppressed T1-weighted image shows a normal rotator cuff. (*B*) T2-weighted image at same level shows partial-thickness bursal surface tear of the supraspinatus.

discontinuity is low in signal on T2-weighted images, possibly because of chronic scarring (Fig. 21A) [47]. These tears may be visualized at MR arthrography because intraarticular contrast fills the tear (Fig. 21B). On conventional MR imaging, secondary signs of cuff tear, such as tendon retraction, may be the only indication of a full-thickness tear. The normal myotendinous junction should lie within a 15-degree arc of the 12 o'clock position of the humeral head on coronal oblique imaging [58]. Thus, if the myotendinous

junction is more than 15 degrees medial to the 12 o'clock position, there may be a full-thickness cuff tear. In addition, if there is superior translation of the humeral head with associated remodeling of the undersurface of the acromion, one should suspect a full-thickness tear with retraction, which resulted in acromiohumeral articulation (Fig. 22). Although muscle atrophy may be seen in the setting of rotator cuff tears and usually indicates chronicity, there may be other, although less common, causes for muscle atrophy in the setting of an intact cuff. Muscle atrophy represents an important component in managing rotator cuff tears as it may determine surgical approach (open versus arthroscopic) and may be a predictor of operative success (Fig. 23) [59]. Muscle atrophy is best depicted on T1 weighted, particularly in the sagittal oblique plane. MR imaging has been proposed as a method for quantifying degree of muscle atrophy [60]. Alternatively, preliminary work suggests that early metabolic changes associated with muscle atrophy may be detected by MR spectroscopy despite normal morphology of a muscle on MR imaging (M. Torriani, personal communication, September 2003).

Two types of periarticular cysts have been reported to be associated with rotator cuff tear [61,62]. An acromioclavicular joint cyst likely develops from leakage of fluid from the glenohumeral joint through a full-thickness rotator cuff tear into a degenerated acromioclavicular joint (Fig. 24). The presence of such a cyst, which communicates with the glenohumeral joint, a finding that can be confirmed by MR arthrography, may require distal

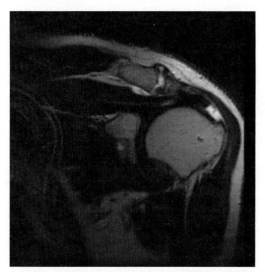

Fig. 19. Full-thickness rotator cuff tear. Coronal oblique T2-weighted image shows full-thickness supraspinatus tear with tendon retraction and a fluid-filled gap.

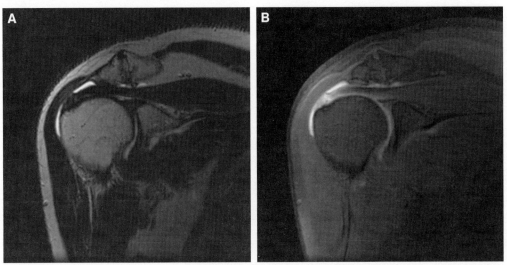

Fig. 20. Full-thickness rotator cuff tear not visible on T2-weighted image. (*A*) Coronal oblique T2-weighted image shows fluid in the subdeltoid bursa without evidence of full-thickness supraspinatus tear. (*B*) Coronal oblique fat-suppressed T1-weighted at same level shows gadolinium traversing full-thickness tear with gadolinium in the subdeltoid bursa.

clavicular resection in addition to acromioplasty at the time of rotator cuff repair to avoid cyst recurrence [61]. If no such communication exists with the glenohumeral joint on MR arthrography, the cyst is less likely to recur following local excision without distal clavicular resection. Intramuscular cysts, or ganglia, are formed as fluid from the glenohumeral joint dissects along the rotator cuff muscle either along the fascial sheath or within the substance of the muscle, typically along the myotendinous plane (Fig. 25). The presence of such an intramuscular fluid collection has been associated with small

full-thickness or articular surface partial-thickness tears of the rotator cuff and should thus prompt a meticulous search for rotator cuff tears [62].

In the setting of a chronic supraspinatus tear, the long head biceps brachii tendon may become impinged between the humeral head and the acromion [10]. Thus, tendinopathy or tears of the intracapsular portion of the long head biceps tendon may be seen associated with supraspinatus tears. If the rotator cuff tear extends to and involves the rotator interval and subscapularis, the biceps tendon may dislocate out of the bicipital groove

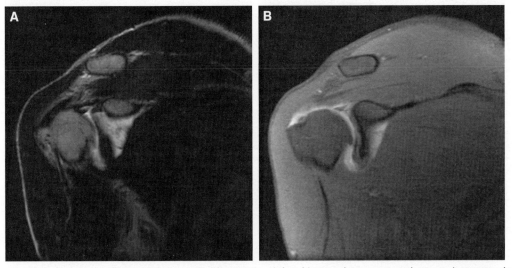

Fig. 21. T2 dark rotator cuff tear. (*A*) Coronal oblique T2-weighted image shows a normal supraspinatus tendon. (*B*) Coronal oblique fat-suppressed T1-weighted image shows near full-thickness tear of supraspinatus.

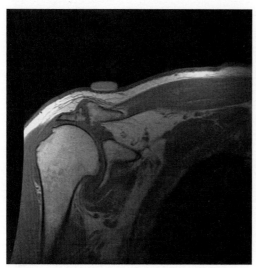

Fig. 22. Acromiohumeral articulation. Coronal oblique proton density image shows full-thickness supraspinatus tear with retraction and atrophy resulting in acromiohumeral articulation and remodeling of undersurface of acromion.

(see article on biceps/interval in this issue of MR clinics) [63].

Identification of subscapularis tear can be challenging clinically and surgically [64]. Imaging plays a crucial role in preoperative identification of such tears as their presence may affect surgical planning. Typically, traumatic subscapularis tears involve the cranial fibers with the caudal fibers being involved in extensive tears. Isolated tears of the caudal fibers of the subscapularis are rare [65]. Subscapularis

injuries typically follow one of three patterns: (1) isolated subscapularis tear; (2) subscapularis tear in the setting of a large rotator cuff tear; and (3) subscapularis tear in the setting of anterosuperior lesions of the rotator cuff. Isolated full-thickness subscapularis tears are uncommon and typically occur in the setting of acute trauma, often the result of forced external rotation of an adducted arm, forceful extreme abduction and external rotation, anterior dislocation, or recurrent anterior glenohumeral instability. A far more frequent situation is extension of a supraspinatus tear into the subscapularis [64]. Anterior superior lesions of the rotator cuff involve the most anterior fibers of the supraspinatus, the cranial fibers of the subscapularis, and the intervening components of the rotator interval, the coracohumeral and superior glenohumeral ligaments [66]. The diagnosis of subscapularis tear on MR imaging is based on the identification of tendon discontinuity, gadolinium filling a gap over the lesser tuberosity, atrophy of the subscapularis, or malposition of the tendon of the long head biceps brachii (Fig. 26) [64]. These findings are best seen on axial and oblique sagittal images. Aside from tendon discontinuity, the remaining signs are reported to be specific but not sensitive on MR arthrography for the diagnosis of subscapularis tears. In skeletally immature patients, an avulsion injury of the lesser tuberosity, often associated with a tear of the anterior band of the inferior glenohumeral ligament, may be seen (Fig. 27) [67,68]. As with most tendon injuries, subscapularis tears are treated differently depending on the extent of the lesion and the functional demand of the

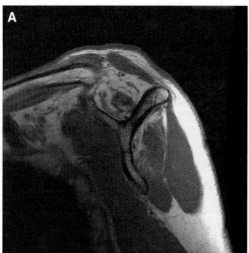
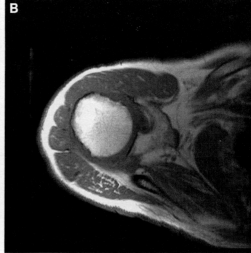

Fig. 23. Full-thickness tear with retraction and atrophy. (A) Sagittal oblique T1-weighted image shows atrophic supraspinatus muscle. (B) Axial T1-weighted image shows retraction of myotendinous junction medial to glenoid.

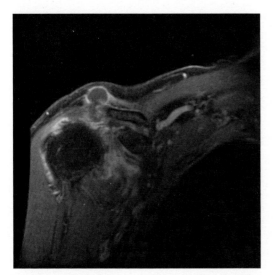

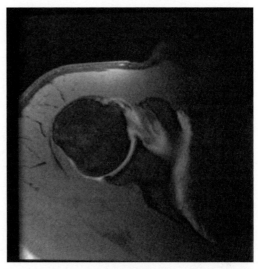

Fig. 24. Acromioclavicular joint cyst communicating with glenohumeral joint. Coronal oblique fat-suppressed T1-weighted image following administration of intravenous gadolinium demonstrates full-thickness rotator cuff tear with atrophy. There is communication between glenohumeral joint and large acromioclavicular cyst, which demonstrates peripheral enhancement.

Fig. 26. Biceps tendon dislocation. Axial fat-suppressed T1-weighted image from MR arthrogram shows a split tear of subscapularis with intratendinous dislocation long head biceps brachii tendon.

patient. In patients with low functional demand, physical therapy, pain control, and steroid injections may be sufficient. Small degenerative tears and large inoperable tears may be treated with arthroscopic debridement for symptomatic relief. Patients with high functional demand generally require reconstruction with arthroscopic or open surgery either by direct tendon repair or with a pectoralis major tendon transfer [69].

In approximately 8% to 10% of cases, a rotator cuff tear is caused by acute injury to an otherwise healthy tendon (Fig. 28) [70]. Patients under the age of 40 who have an acute traumatic event and are suspected of having an acute rotator cuff tear are at risk of having an undisplaced greater tuberosity fracture. Such fractures are often treated conservatively as the periosteum is thought to stabilize the fracture and thus aid in healing without the need for rotator cuff surgery [71]. In the same series, patients over 40 with a suspicion of acute rotator cuff injury had a high prevalence of subscapularis tears. Thus, in the setting of acute trauma, special attention should be paid to the greater tuberosity and the subscapularis tendon.

Rotator interval tears

The rotator interval lies between the anterior fibers of the supraspinatus and the cranial fibers of the subscapularis. Although the anatomy and pathophysiology of the rotator interval is discussed in detail elsewhere in this issue, one must be sure to evaluate the rotator interval in all cases of anterior supraspinatus tears, cranial subscapularis tears, biceps tendon abnormalities, and subcoracoid bursal effusions or bursitis [72]. The rotator interval is best evaluated on sagittal oblique images, particularly with MR arthrography.

Mimics of rotator cuff tears

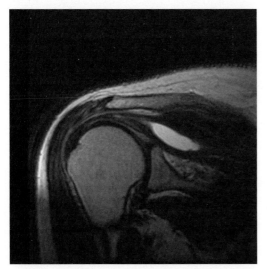

Fig. 25. Intramuscular cyst. Coronal oblique T2-weighted image shows intramuscular ganglion or cyst within the infraspinatus muscle.

Greater tuberosity fractures may mimic a rotator cuff tear. These fractures are often nondisplaced fractures that are radiographically occult (Fig. 29).

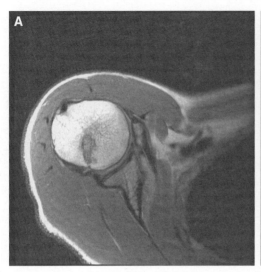
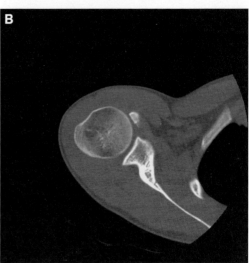

Fig. 27. Lesser tuberosity avulsion. (*A*) Axial proton density-weighted image in an adolescent shows flattening of lesser tuberosity and clearly defines relationship of the intact subscapularis tendon and the avulsed fragment of bone. (*B*) Axial CT scan shows ossific fragment anterior to humerus with some flattening of the lesser tuberosity.

The mechanism for these fractures is often either shoulder dislocation or impaction of the greater tuberosity and the acromion during forced abduction. Using the Neer classification, these are one-part fractures and usually do not need surgical treatment [73]. These patients are often referred to MR imaging for suspected rotator cuff tears. In one series that included MR imaging of 12 patients with acute traumatic radiographically occult greater tuberosity fractures, all 12 patients had either tendinosis or partial-thickness cuff tears without any full-thickness cuff component [74]. All patients were treated nonoperatively. The authors postulated that the greater tuberosity fracture precluded a full-thickness rotator cuff tear. If one is to treat a rotator cuff tear associated with a greater tuberosity fracture, one must postpone surgery to allow fracture healing to ensure subsequent successful cuff repair [71].

Distal clavicular osteolysis may be seen in acute injury or following repeated stress-related microtrauma to the acromioclavicular joint. The latter

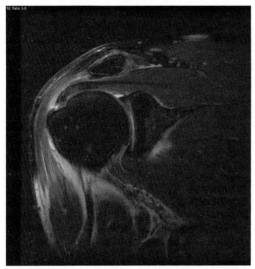

Fig. 28. Acute full-thickness rotator cuff tear. Coronal oblique fat-suppressed intermediate-weighted image show acute full-thickness supraspinatus tear with associated edema in surrounding tissues.

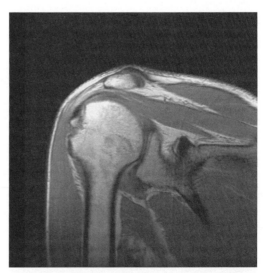

Fig. 29. Greater tuberosity fracture. Coronal oblique proton density image show avulsion of the greater tuberosity in a patient suspected of having rotator cuff tear.

may be related to athletic or work-related activities. Distal clavicular osteolysis manifests radiographically as resorption of the distal clavicle with loss of the distal clavicular cortical line and pseudo widening of the acromioclavicular joint [75]. The most common finding on MR imaging is edema, predominantly in the distal clavicle. As with most types of edema, this is best demonstrated on fat-suppressed T2 or inversion recovery imaging (Fig. 30). Additional features include acromioclavicular joint fluid, distention of the joint capsule, and cortical irregularity without or with fragmentation of the distal clavicle [75].

Muscle weakness secondary to denervation or neuritis may mimic rotator cuff tears. This typically occurs when the suprascapular nerve, which innervates the supraspinatus and infraspinatus, is affected. The suprascapular nerve may be compromised as a result of trauma, inflammation, or compression. In the setting of acute trauma, a scapular fracture may be associated with suprascapular nerve injury. Alternatively, the nerve may experience a stretch injury, often in the setting of a brachial plexus injury or other distraction type injury. One cadaveric study demonstrated stretching of the suprascapular nerve at the level of the spinoglenoid notch as the glenohumeral joint was moved into a cross-body adduction and internal rotation position [76]. Volleyball players, particularly those who use a "float" serve, may have selective infraspinatus atrophy caused by stretch injury of the suprascapular nerve at the level of the spinoglenoid notch [8]. This is thought to result from a strong eccentric contraction of the infraspinatus that is required to quickly retract the arm immediately following contact with the ball. In addition, a stretching injury of the axillary nerve in the setting of an anterior shoulder dislocation may result in selective teres minor atrophy [77]. Neuritis, or nerve inflammation, may have many etiologies, including postviral neuritis. Acute brachial neuritis, also known as Parsonage-Turner syndrome, may result in atraumatic shoulder pain and weakness, thereby mimicking a rotator cuff tear [78]. Although the pain may resolve in 1 to 3 weeks, weakness of the affected muscles may persist and result in atrophy. Although the supraspinatus and infraspinatus are typically affected, the deltoid and rhomboids may also be affected [79]. Finally, compression of the suprascapular nerve may result in denervation. Although this is typically caused by paralabral cysts, any strategically located space-occupying lesion may cause compression of the suprascapular nerve (Fig. 31). If the lesion is located along the course of the suprascapular nerve proximal to the spinoglenoid notch, both the supraspinatus and infraspinatus will be affected, whereas a lesion at or distal to the spinoglenoid notch will selectively affect the infraspinatus.

Regardless of the cause, neural compromise may result in interstitial denervation edema, which is well depicted on fluid-sensitive sequences, such as fat-suppressed T2 or inversion recovery [80]. At later stages, muscle atrophy may be present. In an experimental study, such edema was present on inversion recovery imaging at 24 hours following

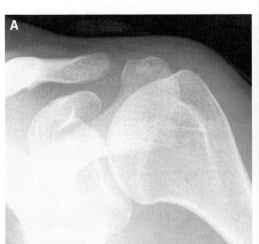
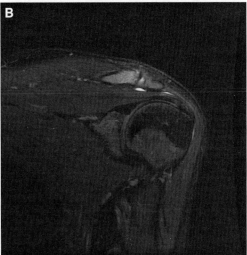

Fig. 30. Posttraumatic osteolysis of the distal clavicle. (*A*) Magnified view from shoulder radiograph 3 weeks following acute trauma shows subtle osteolysis of distal clavicle with loss of cortical line. Note normal acromial cortical line. (*B*) Coronal oblique fat-suppressed intermediate weighted image shows mild edema in the distal clavicle and indistinct cortical margin.

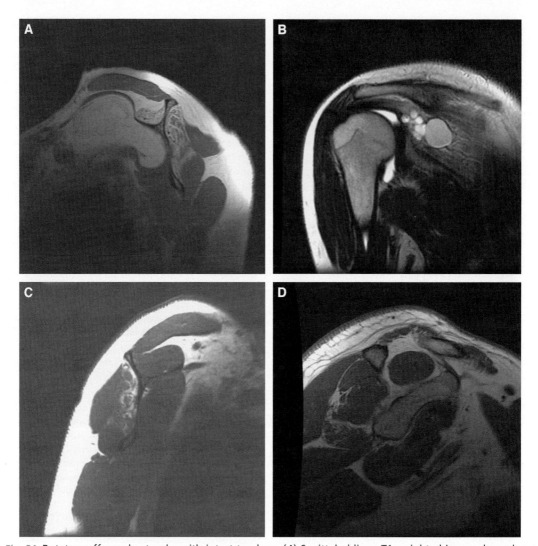

Fig. 31. Rotator cuff muscle atrophy with intact tendons. (*A*) Sagittal oblique T1-weighted image shows large lipoma compressing suprascapular nerve resulting in atrophy of the supraspinatus and infraspinatus. (*B*) Coronal oblique T2-weighted image shows multiloculated cyst in spinoglenoid notch resulting in selective infraspinatus atrophy. (*C*) Sagittal oblique T1-weighted image in same patient shows selective infraspinatus atrophy. (*D*) Sagittal oblique T1-weighted image in a different patient shows selective teres minor atrophy following anterior shoulder dislocation.

denervation, and atrophy was visible on T1-weighted images as early as 7 days following denervation [81]. Muscle atrophy in the absence of a rotator cuff tear should prompt a search for neural compromise.

MR arthrography can increase diagnostic accuracy in small partial-thickness articular surface tears. MR imaging helps to distinguish between many other causes of shoulder pain that may mimic rotator cuff tears.

Summary

MR imaging is an exquisite tool for delineating normal structures and abnormalities of the rotator cuff and for determining the location and extent of rotator cuff tears before surgery. Although standard MR imaging can accurately demonstrate full-thickness rotator cuff tears and some partial-thickness tears,

References

[1] Hawkins RJ, Hobeika PE. Impingement syndrome in the athletic shoulder. Clin Sports Med 1983;2(2):391–405.
[2] Reinus WR, Shady KL, Mirowitz SA, Totty WG. MR diagnosis of rotator cuff tears of the

shoulder: value of using T2-weighted fat-saturated images. AJR Am J Roentgenol 1995; 164(6):1451–5.

[3] Seeger LL, Gold RH, Bassett LW, Ellman H. Shoulder impingement syndrome: MR findings in 53 shoulders. AJR Am J Roentgenol 1988; 150(2):343–7.

[4] Tirman PF, Bost FW, Steinbach LS, Mall JC, Peterfy CG, Sampson TG, et al. MR arthrographic depiction of tears of the rotator cuff: benefit of abduction and external rotation of the arm. Radiology 1994;192(3):851–6.

[5] Hollingshead WH, Rosse C. Textbook of anatomy. Fourth edition. Philadelphia: Harper & Row; 1985. p. 199–201.

[6] Petersilge CA, Witte DH, Sewell BO, Bosch E, Resnick D. Normal regional anatomy of the shoulder. Magn Reson Imaging Clin N Am 1993;1(1):1–18.

[7] Neumann CH, Holt RG, Steinbach LS, Jahnke AH Jr, Petersen SA. MR imaging of the shoulder: appearance of the supraspinatus tendon in asymptomatic volunteers. AJR Am J Roentgenol 1992;158(6):1281–7.

[8] Ferretti A, De Carli A, Fontana M. Injury of the suprascapular nerve at the spinoglenoid notch. The natural history of infraspinatus atrophy in volleyball players. Am J Sports Med 1998; 26(6):759–63.

[9] Beltran J, Bencardino J, Padron M, Shankman S, Beltran L, Ozkarahan G. The middle glenohumeral ligament: normal anatomy, variants and pathology. Skeletal Radiol 2002;31(5):253–62.

[10] Steinbach LS. Rotator cuff disease. In: Steinbach LS, Tirman PFJ, Peterfy CG, Feller JF, editors. Shoulder magnetic resonance imaging. Philadelphia: Lippincott Williams & Wilkins; 1988. p. 99–133.

[11] Gerber C, Terrier F, Ganz R. The role of the coracoid process in the chronic impingement syndrome. J Bone Joint Surg Br 1985;67(5): 703–8.

[12] Ferrick MR. Coracoid impingement. A case report and review of the literature. Am J Sports Med 2000;28(1):117–9.

[13] Jobe FW, Kvitne RS, Giangarra CE. Shoulder pain in the overhand or throwing athlete. The relationship of anterior instability and rotator cuff impingement. Orthop Rev 1989;18(9): 963–75.

[14] Walch G, Liotard JP, Boileau P, Noel E. Posterosuperior glenoid impingement. Another shoulder impingement. Rev Chir Orthop Reparatrice Appar Mot 1991;77(8):571–4.

[15] Boenisch U, Lembcke O, Naumann T. Classification, clinical findings and operative treatment of degenerative and posttraumatic shoulder disease: what do we really need to know from an imaging report to establish a treatment strategy? Eur J Radiol 2000;35(2):103–18.

[16] Wright RW, Fritts HM, Tierney GS, Buss DD. MR imaging of the shoulder after an impingement test: how long to wait. AJR Am J Roentgenol 1998;171(3):769–73.

[17] Beaulieu CF, Hodge DK, Bergman AG, Butts K, Daniel BL, Napper CL, et al. Glenohumeral relationships during physiologic shoulder motion and stress testing: initial experience with open MR imaging and active imaging-plane registration. Radiology 1999;212(3):699–705.

[18] Gallino M, Battiston B, Annaratone G, Terragnoli F. Coracoacromial ligament: a comparative arthroscopic and anatomic study. Arthroscopy 1995;11(5):564–7.

[19] Kaplan PA, Bryans KC, Davick JP, Otte M, Stinson WW, Dussault RG. MR imaging of the normal shoulder: variants and pitfalls. Radiology 1992;184(2):519–24.

[20] Ogata S, Uhthoff HK. Acromial enthesopathy and rotator cuff tear. A radiologic and histologic postmortem investigation of the coracoacromial arch. Clin Orthop 1990;254:39–48.

[21] Ozaki J, Fujimoto S, Nakagawa Y, Masuhara K, Tamai S. Tears of the rotator cuff of the shoulder associated with pathological changes in the acromion. A study in cadavera. J Bone Joint Surg Am 1988;70(8):1224–30.

[22] Bigliani LU, Ticker JB, Flatow EL, Soslowsky LJ, Mow VC. The relationship of acromial architecture to rotator cuff disease. Clin Sports Med 1991;10(4):823–38.

[23] von Schroeder HP, Kuiper SD, Botte MJ. Osseous anatomy of the scapula. Clin Orthop 2001; 383:131–9.

[24] Getz JD, Recht MP, Piraino DW, Schils JP, Latimer BM, Jellema LM, et al. Acromial morphology: relation to sex, age, symmetry, and subacromial enthesophytes. Radiology 1996; 199(3):737–42.

[25] Morrison DS, Bigliani LU. The clinical significance of variation in acromial morphology. Orthop Trans 1986;11:234.

[26] Bigliani LU, Morrison DS, April EW. The morphology of the acromion and its relationship to rotator cuff tears. Orthop Trans 1986; 10:228.

[27] Edelson JG. The 'hooked' acromion revisited. J Bone Joint Surg Br 1995;77(2):284–7.

[28] Shah NN, Bayliss NC, Malcolm A. Shape of the acromion: congenital or acquired—a macroscopic, radiographic, and microscopic study of acromion. J Shoulder Elbow Surg 2001; 10(4):309–16.

[29] Haygood TM, Langlotz CP, Kneeland JB, Iannotti JP, Williams GR Jr, Dalinka MK. Categorization of acromial shape: interobserver variability with MR imaging and conventional radiography. AJR Am J Roentgenol 1994; 162(6):1377–82.

[30] Peh WC, Farmer TH, Totty WG. Acromial arch shape: assessment with MR imaging. Radiology 1995;195(2):501–5.

[31] Banas MP, Miller RJ, Totterman S. Relationship between the lateral acromion angle and rotator

cuff disease. J Shoulder Elbow Surg 1995; 4(6):454–61.

[32] Needell SD, Zlatkin MB, Sher JS, Murphy BJ, Uribe JW. MR imaging of the rotator cuff: peritendinous and bone abnormalities in an asymptomatic population. AJR Am J Roentgenol 1996; 166(4):863–7.

[33] Sammarco VJ. Os acromiale: frequency, anatomy, and clinical implications. J Bone Joint Surg Am 2000;82(3):394–400.

[34] Sterling JC, Meyers MC, Chesshir W, Calvo RD. Os acromiale in a baseball catcher. Med Sci Sports Exerc 1995;27(6):795–9.

[35] Wright RW, Heller MA, Quick DC, Buss DD. Arthroscopic decompression for impingement syndrome secondary to an unstable os acromiale. Arthroscopy 2000;16(6):595–9.

[36] Ryu RK, Fan RS, Dunbar WH 5th. The treatment of symptomatic os acromiale. Orthopedics 1999; 22(3):325–8.

[37] Gerber C, Sebesta A. Impingement of the deep surface of the subscapularis tendon and the reflection pulley on the anterosuperior glenoid rim: a preliminary report. J Shoulder Elbow Surg 2000;9(6):483–90.

[38] Bigliani LU, Levine WN. Subcoracoid impingement syndrome [current concepts review]. J Bone Joint Surg Am 1997;79:1854–68.

[39] Friedman RJ, Bonutti PM, Genez B. Cine magnetic resonance imaging of the subcoracoid region. Orthopedics 1998;21(5):545–8.

[40] Suenaga N, Minami A, Kaneda K. Postoperative subcoracoid impingement syndrome in patients with rotator cuff tear. J Shoulder Elbow Surg 2000;9(4):275–8.

[41] Warner JJ, Micheli LJ, Arslanian LE, Kennedy J, Kennedy R. Patterns of flexibility, laxity, and strength in normal shoulders and shoulders with instability and impingement. Am J Sports Med 1990;18(4):366–75.

[42] Nakagawa S, Yoneda M, Hayashida K, et al. The posterior rotator interval may be the initial site of rotator cuff tears in baseball players. J Shoulder Elbow Surg 1997;6:S246.

[43] Paley KJ, Jobe FW, Pink MM, Kvitne RS, ElAttrache NS. Arthroscopic findings in the overhand throwing athlete: evidence for posterior internal impingement of the rotator cuff. Arthroscopy 2000;16(1):35–40.

[44] Tirman PF, Bost FW, Garvin GJ, Peterfy CG, Mall JC, Steinbach LS, et al. Posterosuperior glenoid impingement of the shoulder: findings at MR imaging and MR arthrography with arthroscopic correlation. Radiology 1994;193(2): 431–6.

[45] Struhl S. Anterior internal impingement. An arthroscopic observation. Arthroscopy 2002; 18(1):2–7.

[46] Kjellin I, Ho CP, Cervilla V, Haghighi P, Kerr R, Vangness CT, et al. Alterations in the supraspinatus tendon at MR imaging: correlation with histopathologic findings in cadavers. Radiology 1991;181(3):837–41.

[47] Rafii M, Firooznia H, Sherman O, Minkoff J, Weinreb J, Golimbu C, et al. Rotator cuff lesions: signal patterns at MR imaging. Radiology 1990; 177(3):817–23.

[48] Balich SM, Sheley RC, Brown TR, Sauser DD, Quinn SF. MR imaging of the rotator cuff tendon: interobserver agreement and analysis of interpretive errors. Radiology 1997;204(1):191–4.

[49] Hodler J, Kursunoglu-Brahme S, Snyder SJ, Cervilla V, Karzel RP, Schweitzer ME, et al. Rotator cuff disease: assessment with MR arthrography versus standard MR imaging in 36 patients with arthroscopic confirmation. Radiology 1992; 182(2):431–6.

[50] Flannigan B, Kursunoglu-Brahme S, Snyder S, Karzel R, Del Pizzo W, Resnick D. MR arthrography of the shoulder: comparison with conventional MR imaging. AJR Am J Roentgenol 1990; 155(4):829–32.

[51] Palmer WE, Brown JH, Rosenthal DI. Rotator cuff: evaluation with fat-suppressed MR arthrography. Radiology 1993;188(3):683–7.

[52] Ferrari FS, Governi S, Burresi F, Vigni F, Stefani P. Supraspinatus tendon tears: comparison of US and MR arthrography with surgical correlation. Eur Radiol 2002;12(5):1211–7.

[53] Meister K, Thesing J, Montgomery WJ, Indelicato PA, Walczak S, Fontenot W. MR arthrography of partial thickness tears of the undersurface of the rotator cuff: an arthroscopic correlation. Skeletal Radiol 2003;26.

[54] Yamazaki Y, Moro K. MRI by infusing xylocaine and Gd-DTPA into the subacromial bursa. J Shoulder Elbow Surg 1995;4:S87.

[55] Gartsman GM. Combined arthroscopic and open treatment of tears of the rotator cuff. J Bone Joint Surg Am 1997;79(5):776–83.

[56] Ellman H. Diagnosis and treatment of incomplete rotator cuff tears. Clin Orthop 1990; 254:64–74.

[57] McConville OR, Iannotti JP. Partial-thickness tears of the rotator cuff: evaluation and management. J Am Acad Orthop Surg 1999;7(1): 32–43.

[58] Farley TE, Neumann CH, Steinbach LS, Jahnke AJ, Petersen SS. Full-thickness tears of the rotator cuff of the shoulder: diagnosis with MR imaging. AJR Am J Roentgenol 1992; 158(2):347–51.

[59] Warner JJ, Goitz RJ, Irrgang JJ, Groff YJ. Arthroscopic-assisted rotator cuff repair: patient selection and treatment outcome. J Shoulder Elbow Surg 1997;6(5):463–72.

[60] Zanetti M, Gerber C, Hodler J. Quantitative assessment of the muscles of the rotator cuff with magnetic resonance imaging. Invest Radiol 1998 Mar;33(3):163–70.

[61] Cvitanic O, Schimandle J, Cruse A, Minter J. The acromioclavicular joint cyst: glenohumeral joint

communication revealed by MR arthrography. J Comput Assist Tomogr 1999;23(1):141–3.

[62] Sanders TG, Tirman PF, Feller JF, Genant HK. Association of intramuscular cysts of the rotator cuff with tears of the rotator cuff: magnetic resonance imaging findings and clinical significance. Arthroscopy 2000;16(3):230–5.

[63] Patten RM. Tears of the anterior portion of the rotator cuff (the subscapularis tendon): MR imaging findings. AJR Am J Roentgenol 1994; 162(2):351–4.

[64] Pfirrmann CW, Zanetti M, Weishaupt D, Gerber C, Hodler J. Subscapularis tendon tears: detection and grading at MR arthrography. Radiology 1999;213(3):709–14.

[65] Nove-Jesserand L, Gereber C, Walch G. Lesions of the anterior-superior rotator cuff. In: Warner JJP, Iannotti JP, Gerber C, editors. Complex and revision problems in shoulder surgery. Philadelphia: Lippincott-Raven; 1997. p. 165–76.

[66] Beall DP, Williamson EE, Ly JQ, Adkins MC, Emery RL, Jones TP, et al. Association of biceps tendon tears with rotator cuff abnormalities: degree of correlation with tears of the anterior and superior portions of the rotator cuff. AJR Am J Roentgenol 2003;180(3):633–9.

[67] Earwaker J. Isolated avulsion fracture of the lesser tuberosity of the humerus. Skeletal Radiol 1990;19(2):121–5.

[68] Coates MH, Breidahl W. Humeral avulsion of the anterior band of the inferior glenohumeral ligament with associated subscapularis bony avulsion in skeletally immature patients. Skeletal Radiol 2001;30(12):661–6.

[69] Bennett WF. Arthroscopic repair of isolated subscapularis tears: a prospective cohort with 2- to 4-year follow-up. Arthroscopy 2003;19(2): 131–43.

[70] Bassett RW, Cofield RH. Acute tears of the rotator cuff. The timing of surgical repair. Clin Orthop 1983;175:18–24.

[71] Zanetti M, Weishaupt D, Jost B, Gerber C, Hodler J. MR imaging for traumatic tears of the rotator cuff: high prevalence of greater tuberosity fractures and subscapularis tendon tears. AJR Am J Roentgenol 1999;172(2):463–7.

[72] Grainger AJ, Tirman PF, Elliott JM, Kingzett-Taylor A, Steinbach LS, Genant HK. MR anatomy of the subcoracoid bursa and the association of subcoracoid effusion with tears of the anterior rotator cuff and the rotator interval. AJR Am J Roentgenol 2000;174(5): 1377–80.

[73] Neer CS II. Displaced proximal humeral fractures: I. Classification and evaluation. J Bone Joint Surg Am 1970;52(6):1077–89.

[74] Mason BJ, Kier R, Bindleglass DF. Occult fractures of the greater tuberosity of the humerus: radiographic and MR imaging findings. AJR Am J Roentgenol 1999;172(2):469–73.

[75] de la Puente R, Boutin RD, Theodorou DJ, Hooper A, Schweitzer M, Resnick D. Post-traumatic and stress-induced osteolysis of the distal clavicle: MR imaging findings in 17 patients. Skeletal Radiol 1999;28(4):202–8.

[76] Demirhan M, Imhoff AB, Debski RE, Patel PR, Fu FH, Woo SL. The spinoglenoid ligament and its relationship to the suprascapular nerve. J Shoulder Elbow Surg 1998;7(3):238–43.

[77] Pasila M, Jaroma H, Kiviluoto O, Sundholm A. Early complications of primary shoulder dislocations. Acta Orthop Scand 1978;49(3):260–3.

[78] Turner JW, Parsonage MJ. Neuralgic amyotrophy (paralytic brachial neuritis); with special reference to prognosis. Lancet 1957;273(6988):209–12.

[79] Fink GR, Haupt WF. Neuralgic amyotrophy (Parsonage-Turner syndrome) following streptokinase thrombolytic therapy. [in German]. Dtsch Med Wochenschr 1995;120(27):959–92.

[80] Fleckenstein JL, Watumull D, Conner KE, Ezaki M, Greenlee RG Jr, Bryan WW, et al. Denervated human skeletal muscle: MR imaging evaluation. Radiology 1993;187(1):213–8.

[81] Bendszus M, Koltzenburg M, Wessig C, Solymosi L. Sequential MR imaging of denervated muscle: experimental study. AJNR Am J Neuroradiol 2002;23(8):1427–31.

ELSEVIER
SAUNDERS

RADIOLOGIC
CLINICS
OF NORTH AMERICA

Radiol Clin N Am 44 (2006) 525–536

MR Imaging of the Rotator Cuff Interval

Brian J. Bigoni, MD[a,b], Christine B. Chung, MD[c],*

- Technique
- Anatomy
- Role in stability
- Pathology
- Synovial inflammatory processes
  - *Adhesive capsulitis*
  - *Rheumatologic disorders*
  - *Septic arthritis*
- Rotator cuff interval tear
- Biceps tendon dislocation/pathology
- Superior labrum anterior to posterior (SLAP) pathology
- Ganglion cyst/paralabral cyst
- Summary
- References

The rotator cuff interval (RCI) is defined as the space between the anterior aspect of the supraspinatus tendon (SST) and superior aspect of the subscapularis tendon (SCT). The space is bounded by the joint capsule anteriorly and the humeral head medially. It is the result of the imposed discontinuity of the rotator cuff caused by the interposition of the coracoid process between the supraspinatus and subscapularis muscles, and as such represents a region of capsule that is not reinforced by overlying rotator cuff tendon.

The glenohumeral joint (GHJ) has the greatest range of motion of any articulation in the human body facilitated by the relative disparity of the surface area of the articulating portions of the humeral head and the glenoid. This, in conjunction with the spherical morphology of the humeral head in relation to the shallow, concave articular surface of the glenoid, the GHJ often is compared to a golf ball on a tee. This degree of mobility needed to maintain

functionality demands compensatory stabilization. The stabilizers of the GHJ have been subdivided into two categories, static and dynamic. The dynamic stabilizers are the tendons of the rotator cuff and the long head of the biceps tendon; static stabilizers include the negative pressure of the glenohumeral joint, the capsulolabral structures, including the labrum, glenohumeral ligaments, RCI, and axillary pouch. Joint stability is orchestrated by the complex interplay of these structures, the relative contribution of each determined not only by structural integrity but by arm position.

The RCI, because of its capsular composition and lack of superficial reinforcing tendon, is an inherently weak area of the GHJ and one that manifests synovial disorders. Structural insufficiency of the components of the RCI and its overlying capsule caused by trauma can result in instability. The structures of the rotator cuff interval are capsular and readily manifest the imaging findings of synovial

This article was previously published in *Magnetic Resonance Imaging Clinics of North America* 2004;12:61–73.
[a] Department of Radiologic Sciences, University of California–Los Angeles, 10833 LeConte Avenue, Los Angeles, CA, 90024, USA
[b] Department of Radiology, Naval Hospital, Post Office Box 555191, Camp Pendleton, CA 92055-5191, USA
[c] Department of Radiology, University of California–San Diego, 3350 La Jolla Village Drive, La Jolla, CA 92161, USA
* Corresponding author.
E-mail address: cbchung@ucsd.edu (C.B. Chung).

doi:10.1016/j.rcl.2006.04.001

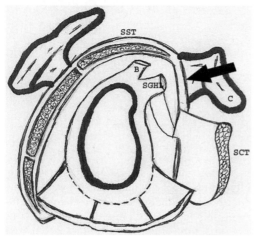

Fig. 1. Schematic sagittal view of the RCI. The RCI is defined as the space between the supraspinatus tendon (SST) and subscapularis tendon (SCT) that results from the interposition of the coracoid process (C) between these two tendons. The anchor for the long head of the biceps tendon (B), the superior glenohumoral ligament (SGHL), and the rotator interval capsule (*arrow*) are depicted.

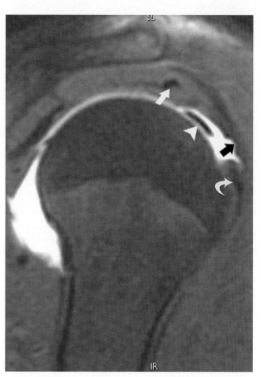

Fig. 3. Anatomy of the rotator cuff interval. Sagittal T1-weighted fat-suppressed MR arthrogram image shows the rotator cuff interval, defined by the borders of the supraspinatus tendon (*white arrow*) and subscapularis tendon (*white curved arrow*). The rotator interval capsule (*black arrow*) and long head of the biceps tendon (*arrowhead*) are well demonstrated.

inflammatory processes along with the axillary recess, allowing areas of decompression from the otherwise reinforced capsule. Masses around the shoulder joint may project into, or arise from, the RCI. This article reviews the basic normal anatomy of the RCI, the imaging considerations unique to this area, and commonly encountered pathology.

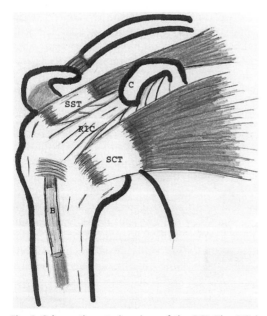

Fig. 2. Schematic anterior view of the RCI. The RCI is bordered superiorly by the supraspinatus tendon (SST) and inferiorly by the subscapularis tendon (SCT). The bursal side of the rotator cuff interval capsule (RIC) is formed by the coracohumeral ligament, which attaches at the coracoid process (C) and in the region of the intertubercular sulcus. The long head of the biceps tendon (B) also is shown.

Technique

MR imaging is the ideal imaging method to evaluate pathology of the shoulder joint because of its excellent soft tissue contrast and multiplanar imaging capabilities. In the absence of detailed clinical history, standard MR imaging protocols should be adequate for the initial detection of RCI pathology. All standard protocols should include fluid-sensitive sequences in each imaging plane that provide an optimal balance of resolution and fluid sensitivity. It is the bias of the authors that T2 fast spin-echo imaging sequences, if used, should always be coupled with fat-suppression to optimize the latter.

If the clinical history of synovial inflammation has been provided, standard MR imaging followed by T1-weighted fat-suppressed images after the intravenous administration of a gadoloinium-based contrast agent is suggested. In the case of trauma, detection of RCI ligament integrity or capsule tear is best profiled by MR arthrography, allowing direct visualization of structural insufficiency and an abnormal distribution of articular fluid. Specific comments regarding the technique for MR arthrography of the glenohumeral joint are outside the scope of this article. As a general rule, however, a fluid-sensitive sequence should always accompany the standard T1-weighted fat-suppressed sequences performed. In addition, the arthrographer should pay attention to the ease of injection and amount of contrast placed into the articulation.

Indirect arthrography may be useful in the appropriate clinical setting. For this technique, contrast is injected intravenously, and images are obtained after passive or active joint exercise. Contrast then diffuses into the joint space and enhances vascular structures and areas of hyperemia. Pathology can be demonstrated either by enhancement, which indicates hyperemia, or outlined by the contrast that accumulates in the joint. However, this technique, when compared with direct arthrography, does not result in distended joint unless a substantial joint effusion is present. Therefore, this is not an ideal method for evaluating the integrity of the intracapsular structures [1,2]. The authors have little experience with this technique, and will defer further commentary.

Anatomy

The rotator cuff interval is defined as the discontinuity of the rotator cuff that occurs between the superior border of the subscapularis tendon and the anterior border of the supraspinatus tendon. It results from the perforation of the rotator cuff by the coracoid process. Three dimensionally, this space has been described as having a triangular configuration with its base at the coracoid process and its apex at the intertubercular sulcus [3]. In the sagittal imaging plane, the space is quadrilateral in configuration, bordered anterosuperiorly by the rotator cuff interval capsule, anteroinferiorly by the

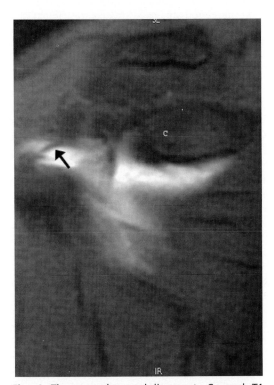

Fig. 4. The coracohumoral ligament. Coronal T1-weighted fat-suppressed MR arthrogram image through the anterior aspect of the joint shows the coracohumoral ligament (*arrow*). The coracoid process (C) is labeled.

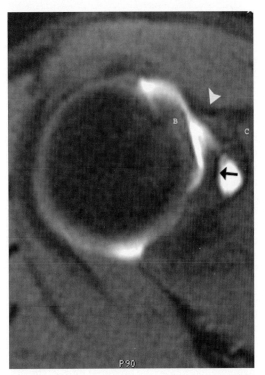

Fig. 5. The superior glenohumoral ligament. Axial T1-weighted fat-suppressed MR arthrogram image of the superior glenohumoral joint at the level of the coracoid process (C) shows the course of the superior glenohumoral ligament (*black arrow*) paralleling the coracoid concavity, moving toward the coracohumeral ligament (*arrowhead*). Note the intraarticular course of the long head of the biceps tendon (B).

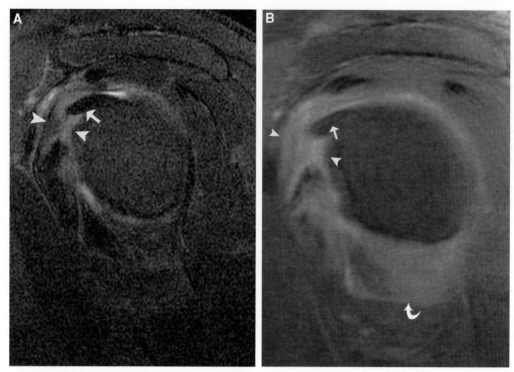

Fig. 6. Adhesive capsulitis. (A) Sagittal T2-weighted fat-suppressed MR image demonstrates increased signal in the rotator interval (*between the arrowheads*), consistent with adhesive capsulitis. Note the traversing long head of the biceps tendon (*arrow*). (B) Sagittal T1-weighted fat-suppressed MR image after contrast administration shows diffuse enhancement of the joint capsule including the rotator cuff interval (*between the white arrowheads*) and the axillary recess (*curved arrow*). Note the traversing long head of the biceps tendon (*arrow*).

subscapularis tendon, medially by the humeral head, and posterosuperiorly by the supraspinatus tendon (Figs. 1 and 2). This imaging plane offers an excellent vantage point for a global assessment of the RCI and its overlying capsule. This can be ideally demonstrated when the joint is distended by fluid, either by joint effusion or by direct arthrography (Fig. 3). An understanding of the anatomy of the structures comprising the rotator cuff interval and its capsule, as well as the structures crossing it, is integral in the assessment of pathology that affects this region of the glenohumeral joint.

The two primary ligaments that comprise the rotator cuff interval capsule are the coracohumeral ligament and the superior glenohumeral ligament forming the bursal and articular sides of this region of the capsule respectively. The coracohumeral ligament originates from the proximal third of the dorsolateral aspect of the coracoid process, with superficial fibers inserting at the greater and lesser tuberosities. The deep fibers insert on the greater and lesser tuberosity and surround the tendon of the long head of the biceps as it exits the intertubercular sulcus to enter the articulation. The CHL is best visualized in the coronal and axial planes

(Figs. 4 and 5). The superior glenohumeral ligament originates at the supraglenoid tubercle along with the long head of the biceps. The SGHL is best identified in the axial imaging plane (see Fig. 5). It follows the coracoid concavity in its midsubstance and inserts proximally at the lesser tuberosity where it fuses with the coracohumeral ligament to surround the long head of the biceps tendon as previously described. This reinforcement of the long head of the biceps tendon by the combined fibers of the coracohumeral and superior glenohumeral ligaments at the junction of the extra- and intraarticular biceps tendon has been referred to as the biceps tendon pulley. This insertion site is shown to best advantage in the sagittal imaging plane. The long head of the biceps tendon is seen on all imaging planes, optimally identified with contrast or fluid within the articulation (see Figs. 3 and 5).

Taking into consideration the anatomy of its constituents, Jost et al [4] described the rotator cuff interval capsule in great detail, documenting a lateral and medial portion. The former was designated as that capsule lateral to the cartilage bone transition of the humeral head and consisted of four layers from superficial to deep, including the superficial fibers of the coracohumeral ligament, fibers of the suprasinatus and subscapularis tendons, deep fibers of the coracohumeral ligament, and the superior glenohumeral ligament. The medial rotator cuff interval covered the cartilaginous humeral head and consisted of only the coracohumeral ligament superficially, and the superior glenohumeral ligament at the articular side. Throughout its course the normal rotator cuff interval capsule should have a smooth contour with a thickness of approximately 2 mm as measured on sagittal images just lateral to the coracoid process (see Fig. 3) [3].

The long head of the biceps tendon originates in the region of the supraglenoid tubercle, crosses the articulation obliquely over the humeral articular surface, and enters the bicipital groove or intertubercular sulcus where it becomes extraarticular. The tendon effectively crosses the rotator cuff interval and its capsule.

Role in stability

Glenohumeral joint stability is defined as the maintenance of central positioning of the humeral head within the glenoid fossa throughout its range of motion. Glenohumeral joint stability and the structures implicated in stability are controversial in the literature and complex in practice, largely because of the delicate balance of structural activation required with every change in arm position, no matter how small or large the movement. This is further compounded by the vast range of motion of the GHJ and the wide spectrum of pathology affecting it, ranging from single acute traumatic episodes to chronic repetitive microtrauma.

The rotator interval capsule and its components, the CHL and the SGHL, have been shown to play a role in GHJ stability, though the exact nature of that role has not been elucidated. The course and attachment site of the CHL and SGHL, both of which reside primarily in an axial plane at the superior aspect of the GHJ, supports studies that emphasize the role of the these structures in restriction of external rotation of the humerus [5]. This is further supported by studies in which closure of the RCI capsule showed a statistically significant reduction in external rotation of the GHJ [6]. Harryman et al [5] demonstrated that sectioning of the rotator interval capsule in cadavers, resulted increase in translation in the anterior, posterior, and inferior directions. Cadaveric studies have also demonstrated the CHL to be a stabilizer in superior-inferior directions with the arm in external rotation [7].

Clinical studies of patients that have indicated rotator interval lesions present most commonly with anterior and inferior instability, and that isolated

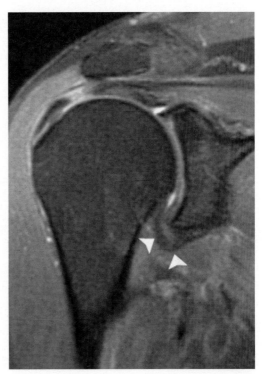

Fig. 7. Adhesive capsulitis on routine MR imaging. Coronal T2-weighted fat-suppressed MR image shows thickening of the inferior glenohumeral ligament (*arrowheads*) suggestive of adhesive capsulitis. The normal thickness of the IGHL is less than 4 mm.

closure of the RCI defects improves stability [8]. Finally, release of the RCI and its capsule, specifically the CHL, may be a useful treatment for recalcitrant adhesive capsulitis, the clinical manifestation of which proves to be pain in conjunction with a markedly restricted range of motion [9].

Though these findings do not present a unified hypothesis as to the exact stabilizing role of the RCI and its capsule, the underlying message communicates that the RCI and its capsule play a part in joint stability. Insufficiency of the structures can result in clinical instability, and surgical manipulation of these structures can result in an overall change in joint laxity.

Pathology

Pathology that commonly affects the RCI and its structures can be subdivided into three main categories of disease: synovial inflammatory processes, including adhesive capsulitis, inflammatory arthritides, such as rheumatoid arthritis, and infectious processes, including septic arthritis; posttraumatic lesions, such as rotator cuff interval tear or superior labrum anterior to posterior (SLAP) pathology; and

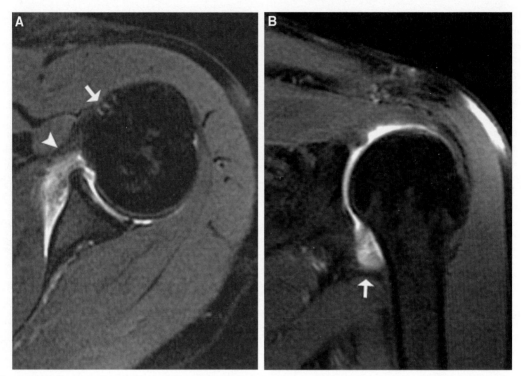

Fig. 8. MR arthrogram images in a patient with clinical symptoms of adhesive capsulitis. A total of 10 mL of contrast was placed in the joint with difficulty. (*A*) Axial T1-weighted fat-suppressed MR arthrogram image shows non-filling of the bicipital groove with intraarticular contrast (*arrow*) and thickening of the anterior capsule (*arrowhead*). (*B*) Coronal T1-weighted fat-suppressed MR arthrogram image show thickening of the inferior glenohumoral ligament (*arrow*).

benign soft tissue masses centered about the RCI, such as ganglion cysts.

Synovial inflammatory processes

Adhesive capsulitis

Adhesive capsulitis, the clinical entity of "frozen shoulder," is a synovial inflammatory condition of the shoulder that may be associated with trauma, osteoarthritis, or rheumatic disorders. Idiopathic cases have been reported [10]. It is a disease process most commonly encountered in females from 40 to 60 years of age. The clinical findings of decreased range of motion may be suggestive of this diagnosis, but are nonspecific and may overlap with other pathology of the shoulder, such as tendinosis, rotator cuff tear, or impingement. Histologically, the disease demonstrates inflammation of the joint capsule (particularly the synovium of the inferior capsule), capsular ligaments of the rotator interval, periarticular bursa (particularly the subscapularis bursa), and tendons (the biceps and subscapularis tendons) [10]. Though arthroscopy can directly evaluate for these changes, and typically demonstrates inflammation in the joint capsule with focal

change in the subscapularis bursa, rotator interval, axillary pouch, and in the bicipital groove. Arthroscopy is impractical because of its invasive nature, cost, and most importantly the ease and availability of an accurate noninvasive means for diagnosis. MR imaging is the most common method for evaluating the shoulder for various disease processes that may present with clinical findings similar to adhesive capsulitis.

The MR imaging findings mirror the findings of arthroscopy for the diagnosis of adhesive capsulitis. The changes encountered occur in regions of the capsule not reinforced by tendons. In a study by Connell et al [11], MR imaging findings were described in patients who underwent surgery for adhesive capsulitis. Surgical findings included fibrovascular scar tissue in the rotator interval, around the biceps anchor, and within the glenohumeral capsule. MR imaging findings include abnormal soft tissue in the rotator interval (Fig. 6A), which may encase the superior glenohumeral ligament or the coracohumeral ligament, and may extend to contact the undersurface of the biceps anchor. Ancillary findings outside the rotator interval include thickening of the axillary pouch greater than 4 mm (Fig. 7). Finally, images after intravenous administration of gadolinium may demonstrate enhancement of the rotator interval or axillary recess (Fig. 6B). Carrillon et al [12] compared patients with adhesive capsulitis to patients with rotator cuff tear. In that study, enhancement of the rotator interval capsule and axillary recess after the intravenous administration of a gadolinium-based contrast agent proved specific for adhesive capsulitis, whereas enhancement of the rotator cuff tendons, subacromial bursa, and acromioclavicular joint was demonstrated in both groups.

Before the advent of MR imaging, imaging strategies for diagnosis of adhesive capsulitis included arthrography, which demonstrated decreased joint volume with obliteration of the axillary pouch [13]. MR arthrography with intraarticular contrast has also been considered for the diagnosis of adhesive capsulitis. Findings associated with adhesive capsulitis include decreased joint volume (less than 10 cc), decreased fluid volume in the biceps tendon sheath and axillary recess, corrugation of the capsule, capsule thickening, and abnormalities of the rotator cuff interval (Fig. 8). However, a recent study comparing MR arthrography findings in a control group with a group of patients in which

the diagnosis of adhesive capsulitis was established by clinical presentation and standard arthrography demonstrated no specific and reproducible MR arthrographic sign for adhesive capsulitis [14]. Additional studies have supported the finding that the volume of injected joint fluid is not diminished with adhesive capsulitis, making its use for the diagnosis of this entity questionable [15].

The diagnosis of adhesive capsulitis can be suggested with standard MR imaging. When standard MR imaging is coupled with the intravenous administration of a gadolinium-based contrast agent, the diagnosis can be confirmed. There is probably not a role for MR arthrography in the diagnosis of adhesive capsulitis. In the MR imaging evaluation of this entity, attention should be focused on the rotator cuff interval capsule and the capsule within the axillary recess.

Rheumatologic disorders

As the RCI is primarily capsular in nature, processes that present with inflamed synovium often demonstrate focal inflammation in the RCI. These processes include inflammatory arthritides, such as rheumatoid arthritis; seronegative arthritides, such as ankylosing spondylitis; nonseptic monoarthritis,

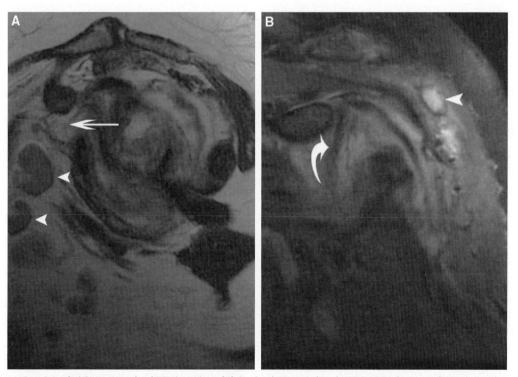

Fig. 9. Septic arthritis on standard MR imaging. (*A*) Sagittal T2-weighted MR image shows T2 hyperintensity extending into the rotator interval (*arrow*) representing inflamed synovium. Note the associated lymphadenopathy (*arrowheads*). (*B*) Coronal T2-weighted fat-suppressed MR image shows edema extending into the rotator interval (*curved arrow*). Note the edema involving the adjacent musculature and soft tissues with associated loculated abscess in the deltoid muscle (*arrowhead*).

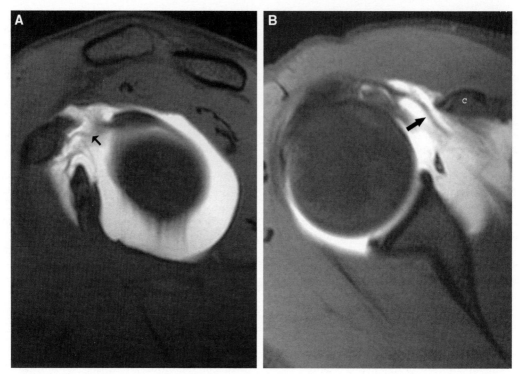

Fig. 10. Rotator cuff interval tear. (*A*) Sagittal T1-weighted fat-suppressed MR arthrogram image shows irregularity and thickening (*arrow*) of the rotator cuff interval capsule with contrast extending along its extraarticular border. (*B*) Axial T1-weighted fat-suppressed MR arthrogram image shows contrast crossing the rotator interval with discontinuity of the coracohumeral ligament (*arrow*) from the coracoid (C) process.

such as Milwaukee shoulder; rapidly destructive articular disease; amyloid arthropathy; hemophilic arthropathy; primary synovial osteochondromatosis; pigmented villonodular synovitis (PVNS); neuropathic arthropathy; and foreign body synovitis. These processes may all involve the shoulder joint and can have similar imaging findings, including joint effusions, synovial proliferation, articular and cartilage abnormalities, and edema in the juxtaarticular soft tissues, muscles, and ligaments [16]. Although specific imaging findings and correlation with the patient's clinical history can help to differentiate these entities, synovial proliferation is a prominent component of the pathology and therefore focal inflammation within the rotator interval may be seen on MR imaging examination.

Septic arthritis

Infectious process, such as septic joint, may demonstrate focal inflammation in the RCI, an area of decompression, along with the axillary recess, for synovial inflammatory processes (Fig. 9). Early MR imaging findings include joint effusion, synovial hypertrophy, and increased signal in the adjacent soft tissues and bones. More advanced disease may demonstrate articular cartilage erosions

and bony destruction. As with adhesive capsulitis, this would be best demonstrated with sagittal T2-weighted and postcontrast images of the shoulder joint. Clinical history of acute onset of symptomatology, laboratory findings, and joint aspiration might make this diagnosis obvious, but if inflammation of the RCI is observed in the correct clinical setting, this diagnosis should be given consideration.

Rotator cuff interval tear

The rotator cuff interval, like the tendons of the rotator cuff, may be torn either from a distinct traumatic event, which may result in dislocation, or more commonly with no known history of trauma, and therefore may be congenital or be secondary to recurrent repetitive microtrauma [6]. A congenital rotator interval defect in the capsule may be common, being demonstrated in 28 of 37 fetuses and 6 of 8 shoulder specimens from adult cadavers [17].

Clinically, tears of the rotator cuff interval present with instability, pain, or a combination of the two. Because clinical and pathological studies have demonstrated RCI tears to be associated with shoulder instability, diagnosis of a rotator interval tear with appropriate clinical pathology may be improved

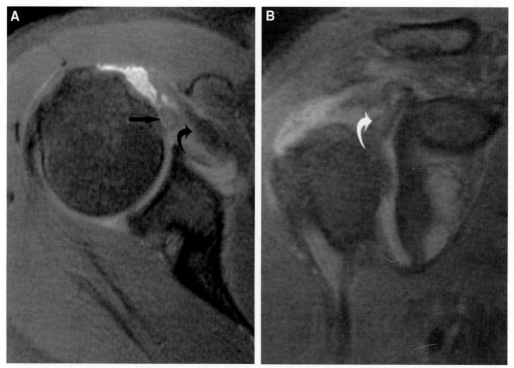

Fig. 11. Dislocation of the biceps tendon on MR arthrography. Intraarticular dislocation of the long head of the biceps tendon occurs with tears of the medial band of the CHL, the SGHL, and the subscapularis tendon at their insertion into the humerus. (*A*) Axial T1-weighted fat-suppressed MR arthrography image shows medial dislocation of the long head of biceps tendon (*arrow*) with a full thickness tear and retracted subscapularis tendon (*curved arrow*). (*B*) Coronal T1-weighted fat-suppressed MR arthrography image further demonstrates the dislocated long head of biceps tendon.

with surgical closure of the rotator interval defect. In a study by Field [8], closure of defects in the rotator interval in 15 symptomatic patients resulted in significant improvement in pain, stability, and function, with all patients reporting good to excellent results. More recent studies have confirmed that surgical tightening of the rotator interval in patients with laxity in this region and symptomatic instability can improve these symptoms [18]. Originally, surgery for repair of the rotator interval capsule was performed with an open technique, but the commonplace nature of the lesion and an increase in the skill of arthroscopists has led to the development of facile and effective arthroscopic techniques for repair [19].

The gold standard for evaluation for rotator cuff interval tears is arthroscopy, which is invasive. Non-invasive studies, MR imaging and MR arthrography, can also demonstrate this pathology. Unlike full-thickness tears of the rotator cuff, however, tear of the RCI typically does not appear as complete disruption of the fibers of the components of the RCI but as thinning, irregularity, or focal discontinuity of the rotator interval capsule. Therefore, an isolated rotator cuff interval tear, without corresponding

tears of the SST or SCT, is unlikely to be demonstrated with routine MR imaging of the shoulder. Sagittal T2-weighted images may demonstrate fluid signal crossing the rotator cuff interval, especially if there is a significant shoulder joint effusion. However, if a rotator cuff interval tear is a clinical consideration, optimal evaluation is achieved by MR arthrography. There may be free communication of the glenohumeral intraarticular contrast agent to the subacromial/subdeltoid bursa through the rotator cuff interval, in the absence of a full-thickness tear of the tendons of the rotator cuff. Less obvious signs of injury require close scrutiny of the RCI, as rotator interval lesions may present with thinning or discontinuity of the rotator interval capsule without communication with the subacromial/subdeltoid bursa (Fig. 10) [20]. A rotator interval tear may be isolated or may be associated with tears of the SST or SCT, specifically those regions of the tendons bordering the RCI (anterior fibers of SST and superior fibers of SCT). As the structures of the RCI serve to stabilize the biceps tendon as it moves from its extra- to intraarticular position in the form of the biceps tendon pulley, injuries of these structures may result in subluxation of the long head of the biceps tendon.

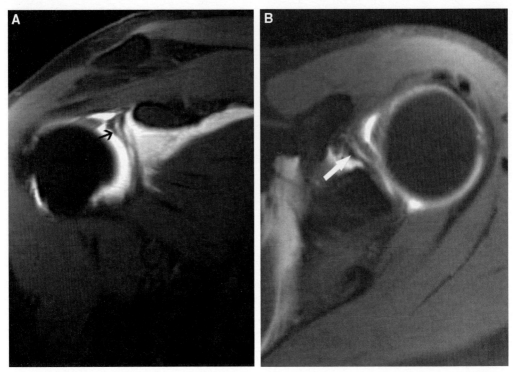

Fig. 12. SLAP (superior labrum anterior to posterior) tear extending to the superior glenohumoral ligament on MR arthrography. (*A*) Coronal T1-weighted fat-suppressed MR arthrography image shows contrast extending to the anterior superior labrum (*arrow*), consistent with a SLAP tear. (*B*) Axial T1-weighted fat-suppressed MR arthrography image shows that the tear extends into the substance of the superior glenohumoral ligament (*arrow*).

Tears of the rotator cuff interval are often overlooked on MR imaging of the shoulder, and unlikely to be diagnosed without intraarticular contrast administration with specific attention to the rotator interval. Therefore, in patients with no findings on routine MR imaging and complaints of shoulder pain or instability, an MR imaging arthrogram may be useful to specifically evaluate for rotator cuff interval tear.

Biceps tendon dislocation/pathology

Along with the subscapularis tendon, the stabilizers of the rotator cuff interval, the CHL and SGHL complex form the biceps tendon pulley. Lesions of these structures can result in subluxation of the biceps tendon. Injury of the humeral insertion of these two structures may or may not be associated with partial- or full-thickness tears of the rotator cuff, most commonly the SCT. The particular combination of tears of these structures can determine the direction of subluxation of the biceps tendon. If the medial band of the CHL, the SGL, and the subscapularis tendons are torn at their insertion into the humerus, the biceps tendon can sublux intraarticularly (Fig. 11). If the SCT is torn with an intact CHL/SGHL, the biceps

tendon may be lax, but will not truly sublux. If the CHL/SGHL is torn with intact SCT, the biceps tendon may sublux between the CHL and the SCT. Finally, a tear of the lateral band of the CHL may result in subluxation superficial to the CHL [21,22]. The CHL and SGHL play an integral role in biceps tendon stability in the bicipital groove.

As the biceps tendon traverses the RCI, most of its course can be easily followed through inspection of sequential images in all imaging planes. This task is made easier with the presence of intraarticular fluid in the form of native effusion or contrast agent. Nonvisualization of the biceps tendon in the RCI implies complete tear of the long head of the biceps tendon. Longitudinal or partial tears of the biceps tendon may also be present. Finally, tendinosis of the biceps tendon can also be observed. As pathology of the long head of the biceps tendon is well demonstrated in the RCI on MR imaging, this pathology needs to be actively sought.

Superior labrum anterior to posterior (SLAP) pathology

Superior labral tears, anterior to posterior (the so-called SLAP tear), represent a common pathology

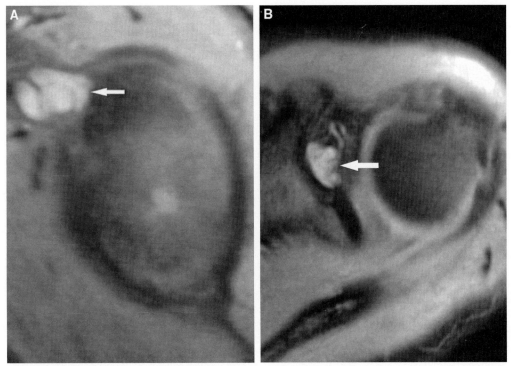

Fig. 13. Gangion cyst in the rotator interval in two patients on standard MR imaging. (*A*) Sagittal T2-weighted MR image shows a loculated fluid collection in the rotator interval (*arrow*), consistent with a ganglion cyst. No labral pathology was present. (*B*) Axial T2-weighted MR image shows a lobulated fluid collection (*arrow*) adjacent to the superior glenohumeral ligament. No labral pathology was present.

encountered on MR imaging of the shoulder. The SLAP lesion is a tear of the superior labrum from anterior to posterior including the anchor of the biceps tendon. Clinically, patients with these injuries present with pain, worse with overhead activity, or clicking. Common causes for injury include a fall on outstretched hand, direct compression force on the shoulder, or traction on the long head of the biceps tendon. Intraarticular contrast agent may help in differentiating pathology (SLAP) from normal anatomic variants, such as the sublabral foramen or hole, the sublabral recess or sulcus, and the Buford complex. Originally, Snyder [23] described four subtypes of SLAP tears, but recent classification systems include 10 subtypes. The SLAP X lesion is defined as SLAP tears that extend to involve the structures of the rotator interval, including the superior glenohumeral ligament (Fig. 12). Presumably, these tears would present with symptoms similar to the commonly encountered SLAP lesions (pain and clicking) with additional possible instability. As previously discussed, tears of the rotator cuff interval are likely only demonstrated with MR arthrography, and therefore full evaluation for SLAP pathology should include MR arthrography with close inspection of the RCI for involvement of these structures.

Ganglion cyst/paralabral cyst

Focal fluid collections can occur about the shoulder, as in other articulations, and can be associated with idiopathic ganglia formation, or ganglia formation from a preceding posttraumatic event involving the RCI or its capsule.

Glenohumeral joint fluid may extend from the glenohumeral joint through glenoid labral tears, presumably from a ball valve-type mechanism resulting in focal fluid-filled synovial-lined cavity, a paralabral cyst. When a paralabral cyst is observed, there is a high correlation with coexistent labral tear from the previously described mechanism. The labral tear may not be visualized on conventional MR imaging. Intraarticular contrast often demonstrates the labral tear, displaying communication between the paralabral cyst and the glenohumeral joint through the labral tear. These paralabral cysts most commonly extend posteriorly, but may occur throughout the course of the labrum and be present anterosuperiorly and extend to the rotator cuff interval. If a cyst is confirmed in the RCI, close inspection should be made to the adjacent anterior-superior labrum (Fig. 13).

An additional consideration for focal fluid collections in the region of the RCI is the presence of fluid in either the subcoracoid bursa or fluid preferentially residing in the subscapularis recess. The former is a normal bursa located beneath the coracoid process anterior to the subscapularis muscle. It communicates with the subacromial and subdeltoid bursa in up to 40% of the population, but has no normal communication with the articulation. The subscapular recess, on the contrary, is a bursa that communicates with the articulation in greater than 95% of the population and is located between the subscapular muscle and the neck of the scapula.

Summary

Pathology of the RCI is common and can be complex in nature. Knowledge of the anatomy, an understanding of commonly encountered pathology, and an approach for the systematic inspection of the rotator cuff interval on MR imaging examinations is crucial for the accurate characterization and diagnosis of RCI pathology.

References

[1] Maurer J, Rudolph J, Lorenz M, et al. A prospective study on the detection of lesion of the labrum glenoidale by indirect arthrography of the shoulder. Rofo Fortschr Geb Rontgenstr Neuen Bilbgeb Verfahr 1999;14:307–12.

[2] Steinbach LS, Palmer WE, Schweitzer ME. Plenary session/special focus session MR arthrography. Radiographics 2002;22:1223–46.

[3] Chung CB, Dwek JR, Cho GJ, et al. Rotator cuff interval: evaluation with MR imaging and MR arthrography of the shoulder in 32 cadavers. J Comput Assist Tomogr 2000;24(5):738–43.

[4] Jost B, Koch PP, Gerber C. Anatomy and functional aspects of the rotator interval. J Shoulder Elbow Surg 2000;9(4):336–41.

[5] Harryman DT II, Sidles JA, Harris SL, Matsen FA III. The role of the rotator interval capsule in passive motion and stability on the shoulder. J Bone Joint Surg Am 1992;74:53–66.

[6] Van der Reis W, Wolf EM. Arthroscopic rotator cuff interval capsular closure. Orthopedics 2001;24(7):657–61.

[7] Itoi E, Berglund LJ, Grabowski JJ, et al. Superior-inferior stability of the shoulder: role of the coracohumeral ligament and the rotator interval capsule. Mayo Clin Proc 1998;73:508–15.

[8] Field LD, Warren RF, O'Brien SJ, et al. Isolated closure of rotator interval defects for shoulder instability. Am J Sports Med 1995;23(5):557–63.

[9] Tetro AM, Bauer G, Hollstien SB, Yamaguchi K. Arthroscopic release of the rotator interval and coracohumeral ligament: an anatomic study in cadavers. Arthroscopy 2002;18(2):145–50.

[10] Hannafin JA, Chiaia TA. Adhesive capsulitis. A treatment approach. Clin Orthop 2000;372: 95–109.

[11] Connell D, Padmanabhan R, Buchbinder R. Adhesive capsulitis: role of MR imaging in differential diagnosis. Eur Radiol 2002;12:2100–6.

[12] Carrillon Y, Noel E, Fantino O, et al. Magnetic resonance imaging findings in idiopathic adhesive capsulitis of the shoulder. Rev Rhum Engl Ed 1999;66(4):201–6.

[13] Iannotti JP. Evaluation of the painful shoulder. J Hand Ther 1994;7(2):77–83.

[14] Manton GL, Schweitzer ME, Weishaupt D, Karasick D. Utility of MR arthrography in the diagnosis of adhesive capsulitis. Skeletal Radiol 2001;30:326–30.

[15] Emig EW, Schweitzer ME, Karasick D, Lubowitz J. Adhesive capsulitis of the shoulder: MR diagnosis. AJR Am J Roentgenol 1995; 164(6):1457–9.

[16] Llauger J, Palmer J, Roson N, et al. Multiregional pathologic processes nonseptic monoarthritis: imaging features with clinical and histopathologic correlation. Radiographics 2000; 20:S263–78.

[17] Cole BJ, Rodeo SA, O'Brien SJ, et al. The anatomy and histology of the rotator interval capsule of the shoulder. Clin Orthop 2001;390:129–37.

[18] Treacy SH, Field LD, Savoie FH. Rotator interval capsule closure: an arthroscopic technique. Arthroscopy 1997;13(1):103–6.

[19] Karas SG. Arthroscopic rotator interval repair and anterior portal closure: an alternative technique. Arthroscopy 2002;18(4):436–9.

[20] Seeger LL, Lubowitz J, Thomas BJ. Case report 815: tear of the rotator interval. Skeletal Radiol 1993;22(8):615–7.

[21] Bennett WF. Subscapularis, medial, and lateral head coracohumeral ligament insertion anatomy: arthroscopic appearance and incidence of "hidden" rotator interval lesions. Arthroscopy 2001;17(2):173–80.

[22] Bennett WF. Visualization of the anatomy of the rotator interval and bicipital sheath. Arthroscopy 2001;17(1):107–11.

[23] Snyder SJ, Karzel RB, Del Pizzo W, et al. SLAP lesions of the shoulder. Arthroscopy 1990; 6:274–9.

RADIOLOGIC
CLINICS
OF NORTH AMERICA

Radiol Clin N Am 44 (2006) 537–551

MR Imaging of the Shoulder after Surgery

Marco Zanetti, MD*, Juerg Hodler, MD, MBA

Postoperative MR imaging of the shoulder is challenging. In 1993, Haygood et al [1] stated that "in 2003 no doubt far more definitive pronouncements would be possible concerning the utility of MR imaging in evaluation of the shoulder after surgery." Although Haygood's 2003 [1] deadline has passed, many aspects of postoperative imaging are not yet covered by published data, though there may be personal experience available. Many imaging "abnormalities," such as irregular supraspinatus tendons, minor contrast leakage through the rotator cuff, rounded labrum, and fluid-like signal in the subacromial bursa, may be clinically irrelevant.

This article describes postoperative MR findings relating to surgery in shoulder impingement syndrome, including rotator cuff lesions, shoulder instability, and arthroplasty. Potentially misleading postoperative findings are emphasized. Because standard MR imaging may not always be the method of choice for postoperative imaging, alternative imaging techniques have been included (MR arthrography, CT arthrography, and sonography).

Imaging technique

A dedicated shoulder coil (commonly a phase-array coil) should be employed for imaging. MR protocols used after surgery are usually based on the standard protocols used for initial evaluation (Table 1). The protocol used at the authors' institution

This article was previously published in *Magnetic Resonance Imaging Clinics of North America* 2004; 12:169–183.
Department of Radiology, Orthopedic University Hospital Balgrist, Forchstrasse 340 CH-8008 Zurich, Switzerland
* Corresponding author.
E-mail address: marco.zanetti@balgrist.ch (M. Zanetti).

doi:10.1016/j.rcl.2006.04.003

Table 1:   MR standard protocols for postoperative shoulder

Sequence	TR/TE	FOV	Matrix	TA
Paracoronal pd weighted fat sat	2350/13	160 mm	256×512	2.09 min
Paracoronal STIR	5070/28/160	160 mm	256×512	3.14 min
Parasagittal SE T1 weighted	500/12	160 mm	256×512	3.48 min
Axial TSE T2 weighted	3500/91	160 mm	256×512	3.18 min
Sagittal STIR	5070/28/160	160 mm	256×512	3.14 min

Standard MR imaging on 1.5 T scanner. Section thickness = 4 mm for all sequences.
Abbreviations: SE, spin echo; STIR, short tau inversion recovery; TA, time of acquisition; TR/TE, repetition time/echo time; TSE, turbo spin echo.

includes images obtained in the angled coronal, angled sagittal, and the axial planes, with a slice thickness of 3 to 4 mm, an FOV of 16 × 16 cm, and a 256 × 512 matrix. Other imaging protocols have been published by other groups [2,3]. The sagittal T1-weighted spin-echo images routinely obtained at the authors' institution appear to be unusual at first glance. Their purpose is to assess the extent of fatty degeneration.

In suspected infection, intravenous gadopentetate injection is performed in addition to standard images. T1-weighted spin-echo images with fat suppression are typically obtained in the angled coronal plane. Direct MR arthrography after the injection of 10 to 12 mL 2 mmol/l gadopentetate may be indicated in certain abnormalities, mainly relating to recurrent instability. The MR arthrography imaging protocol employed at the authors' institution is provided in Table 2. Joint injections in the postoperative situation have a higher risk of infection than before surgery. In addition, at least for rotator cuff abnormalities, the role of intraarticular contrast is not as important postoperatively as before surgery. Small defects of the rotator cuff, which may be relevant before surgery, are commonly irrelevant clinically after surgery. Therefore, the indication for MR arthrography should be carefully discussed in individual patients.

Susceptibility artifacts represent a major problem in postoperative MR imaging. They are most pronounced in the presence of screws, staples, and,

most prominently, in shoulder prosthesis. Artifacts also may be caused by minor particles originating from surgery. They may be pronounced after acromioplasty.

Minimizing artifacts

Susceptibility artifacts can be reduced by employing one or several of the following suggestions: Gradient-echo sequences should be replaced by spin-echo sequences. Fast or turbo spin-echo sequences are superior to conventional spin-echo sequences in this regard, especially if long echo train lengths and short interecho spacing are employed. The artifacts are most pronounced in the frequency-encoding direction, which should be orientated in the direction least disturbing findings are expected (eg, long axis of humeral components after prosthesis when abscess formation is suspected, perpendicular to the long axis of the component when the supraspinatus is most relevant). In addition, artifacts are less pronounced in low field scanners when compared with 1.0 or 1.5 T magnets. They also depend on the direction of the main magnetic field B_0. This effect cannot easily be used in classical, closed magnets, however, for obvious reasons [4].

Increased sampling bandwidth also reduces artifacts. When fat-suppression sequences are employed, short tau inversion recovery sequences perform more favorably than frequency-selective fat-suppression techniques (Fig. 1) [5]. Water

Table 2:   Standard MR arthrography protocol for postoperative shoulders

Sequence	TR/TE	FOV	Matrix	TA
Paracoronal pd weighted fat sat	2350/13	160 mm	256×512	2.09 min
Paracoronal TSE T2 weighted fat sat	3000/91	160 mm	256×512	2.45 min
Paracoronal TSET1 weighted fat sat	792/12	160 mm	256×512	5.08 min
Parasagittal SE T1 weighted	500/12	160 mm	256×512	3.48 min
Axial SE T1 weighted	500/12	160 mm	256×512	3.18 min

Standard MR arthrography on 1.5 T scanner. Section thickness = 4 mm for all sequences, except T1 weighted fat suppressed = 3 mm.
Abbreviations: SE, spin echo; TSE, turbo spin echo; TA, time of acquisition; TR/TE, repetition time/echo time.

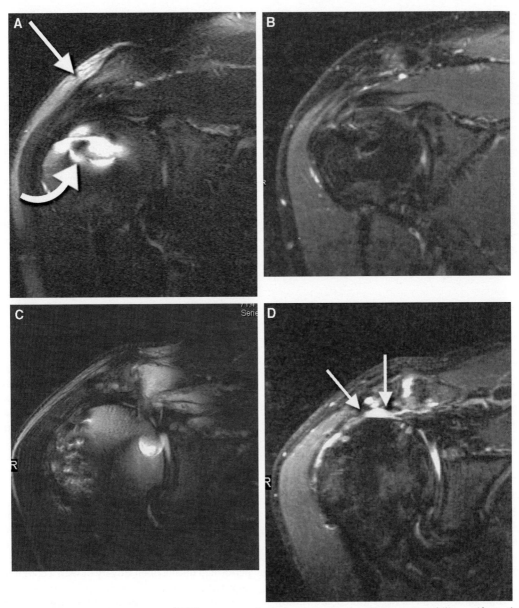

Fig. 1. Short tau inversion recovery (STIR) sequences in general are less prone to susceptibility artifacts than frequency-selective fat-suppression techniques. (*A*) Susceptibility artifacts (*curved arrow*) in the position of transosseous sutures and increased signal in the subcutaneous fat (*straight arrow*) caused by inhomogeneous fat saturation are conspicuous on the T2-weighted fat-suppressed sequence but nearly absent on the corresponding angled coronal STIR sequence (*B*). (*C*) On the T2-weighted fat-suppressed sequence a thin fibrous supraspinatous tendon appears to be present. (*D, E*) On STIR sequences (corresponding paracoronal and parasagittal), the recurrent tear of the supraspinatus tendon is obvious (*arrows*).

excitation sequences using section-selective spectral spatial pulses have also shown promise in reducing artifacts [6]. With this technique, only water is excited by using section-selective spectral spatial pulses, while lipid spins are left in equilibrium, thus not contributing to overall signal. Such sequences are potentially faster than conventional fat-saturation techniques and may produce images of better quality. Potential disadvantages of these artifact-reducing aspects are demonstrated in Table 3.

MR imaging after rotator cuff surgery

Clinical considerations

There are three major groups of surgery in shoulder impingement syndrome and rotator cuff lesions.

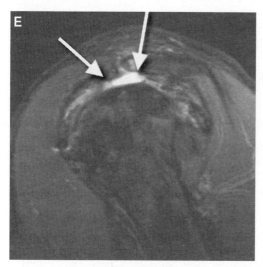

Fig. 1 (continued)

The first group includes patients with an intact rotator cuff. They commonly have acromioplasty. The second group includes patients with rotator cuff tear not associated with muscle atrophy or degeneration. This group commonly has rotator cuff repair by open surgery or arthroscopy. The third group includes patients with large rotator cuff tears associated with muscle atrophy and fatty muscle degeneration. In these patients, muscle transfers, such as latissimus dorsi transfer, are performed.

Acromioplasty and subacromial decompression

Subacromial decompression may be accomplished arthroscopically or during open surgery. Subacromial decompression includes the removal of the subacromial bursa and the anterior and inferior edge of the acromion [7–9]. The coracoacromial ligament is often partially removed. The acromioclavicular joint may be excised if there are clinical and imaging signs of osteoarthritis. The distal

clavicle may also be removed in the presence of large osteophytes.

Persistent symptoms after acromioplasty and subacromial decompression

Symptoms persisting after subacromial decompression are most commonly caused by abnormalities unrelated to the rotator cuff that may still mimic impingement syndrome clinically [10,11]. Anterior glenohumeral instability and acromioclavicular joint osteoarthritis may cause this problem. The second most common reason is residual impingement after incomplete removal of the responsible structures. Despite technically correct acromioplasty, symptoms may persist after surgery as the result of coexisting rotator cuff tears.

Rotator cuff repair

A large number of different surgical techniques have been described for rotator cuff repair. The technique should be chosen according to the size and location of the rotator cuff tear, the extent of rotator cuff muscle degeneration, and the presence of absence of osteoarthritis and biceps tendon abnormalities. The indications depend on the overall disability of the patients and whether pain or functional difficulties are the most relevant problems [12]. The applied surgical technique influences the postoperative appearance on MR images [13].

In patients with partial-thickness tears, treatment may vary from debridement of frayed tissue in superficial tears to complete excision of the area of the partial defect, followed by a repair technique similar to the one applied in full-thickness tears. Subacromial decompression is commonly performed. Both procedures are performed arthroscopically, although both are also commonly performed during open surgery or with a combined approach [14].

Full-thickness tears are treated with subacromial decompression and tendon repair after rotator cuff

Table 3: Reduction of magnetic susceptibility artifacts	
Options	**Potential drawbacks**
Spin-echo sequence instead of gradient-echo sequence	Loss of potentially relevant image information (such as cartilage)
Fast instead of conventional spin-echo sequences	Blurring, changed T2 characteristics
Water excitation	Not universally available
Reduced slice thickness (2 to 3 mm)	Reduced signal, reduced coverage
Increased echo train length (11 to 18)	Blurring
Shortened interecho spacing	Blurring
Orientation of frequency-encoding direction	Unwanted loss of information in the phase encoding direction
Increased sampling bandwidth	Blurring

mobilization. In small full-thickness tears, a tendon-to-tendon suturing technique is commonly employed. In distal lesion, a tendon-to-bone repair is performed. Defects larger than 3 cm commonly require mobilization of the remaining tendon in the supraspinatus fossa before repair. Muscle transfer is performed in the presence of large tendon defects accompanied by moderate to severe muscle atrophy (Goutallier III or IV) [15]. The Goutallier classification is commonly used for the assessment muscle degeneration: grade 0 indicates no intramuscular fat, grade 1 some fatty streaks, grade 2 fat is evident but less fat than muscle tissue, grade 3 fat equals muscle tissue, and in grade 4 more fat is present than muscle tissue [16]. The original description is based on CT; however, it also can be used on MR images [17].

Persistent symptoms after rotator cuff surgery
There are several reasons for pain persistence and reduced function following rotator cuff repair. Fixation failures (anchor pull-out, suture failure, or suture pull-out) may lead to a retear of the rotator cuff. Incomplete subacromial decompression can cause continued bony impingement. A further complication associated with open surgery is a defect of the anterior portion of the deltoid muscle. In arthroscopy, a rotator cuff tear may be created during placement of the arthroscope. Such tears are most commonly located in the infraspinatus and subscapularis but rarely in the supraspinatus [18].

Concomitant abnormalities of structures other than the rotator cuff may not be recognized before surgery. Their persistence can lead to an unfavorable outcome. Such conditions include frozen shoulder, suprascapular or axillary nerve lesion, unstable os acromiale, biceps tendon lesions, acromioclavicular joint disease, and superior labrum with anterior and posterior (SLAP) lesion [19]. These associated abnormalities can commonly be diagnosed on preoperative MR images [20–22].

Preoperative underestimation of the extent of rotator cuff tears represents another problem. In supraspinatus, tears involving the rotator interval and the subscapularis tendon may be missed clinically and radiologically. The so-called pulley lesion (lesion of the fibrous sling guiding the long biceps at the entrance of the intertubercular groove) can be missed during surgery. MR imaging allows for preoperative assessment even of hidden structures in the rotator cuff interval including the reflection pulley [23,24].

Even after initially successful subacromial decompression, new tears may develop as the result of persistent impingement or poor tendon quality. Loss of function persisting after technically correct rotator cuff repair may be caused by fatty muscle degeneration. This is an irreversible abnormality. If not diagnosed before surgery, technically correct tendon sutures may restore the continuity of the rotator cuff but will not improve shoulder function. Fatty degeneration may be overlooked in MR protocols not sufficiently covering the rotator cuff muscles or when predominantly fat-suppressed sequences are used on which fatty streaks within the rotator cuff muscles are easily overlooked.

Muscle transfer

Irreparable rotator cuff tears are not uncommon. Tears are irreparable when they are large and when they are accompanied by fatty degeneration of the rotator cuff muscles. Referrals to subspecialized shoulder surgeons may include up to 30% of such advanced rotator cuff tears. In irreparable subscapularis tendon tears, pain relief and stability appear to be reliably achieved by a split pectoralis major transfer. In the case of an irreparable posterosuperior rotator cuff tear, failed rotator cuff surgery, or massive tears (greater than 5 cm), a latissimus dorsi tendon transfer may be successfully performed [15].

MR findings in asymptomatic patients

Acromioplasty

After acromioplasty, characteristic MR findings (Fig. 2) include a flattened acromial undersurface, shortening of the anterior acromion, and decreased bone marrow signal in the remaining distal acromion as a result of marrow fibrosis [2]. Low-signal artifacts originating from minor metallic fragments related to the surgical access are common. Removal of the subacromial bursa results in the replacement of the bursa by granulation tissue, which later transforms to scar tissue. Bursitis-like signal abnormalities (Fig. 3) at the bursal surface of the rotator cuff are common (prevalence of up to 100%). These changes may persist for a long time after surgery. In

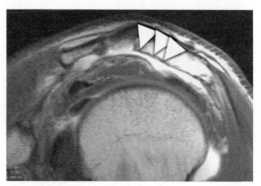

Fig. 2. Expected MR appearance of acromion after acromioplasty. A flattened acromial undersurface (*arrowheads*) is shown.

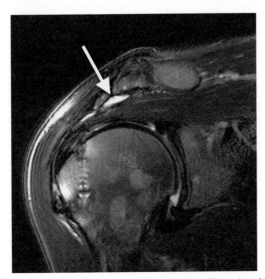

Fig. 3. Normal postoperative bursitis-like signal abnormalities at the bursal surface of the rotator cuff in a 55-year-old asymptomatic patient 3 years after supraspinatus reconstruction. Paracoronal T2-weighted fat-suppressed image demonstrates high signal abnormality in the region of subdeltoid bursa mimicking bursitis (*arrow*).

a group of asymptomatic patients with rotator cuff repair and a mean follow-up period of 40 months (range: 24 to 49 months), the prevalence of bursitis-like abnormalities was 100% (14 patients) [25]. Therefore, after surgery, the MR diagnosis of bursitis should not be made based on bursal signal abnormalities alone.

Rotator cuff repair

MR imaging findings after rotator cuff repair include nonvisualization of the subdeltoid fat and the presence of subacromial fluid. Minor to moderate joint effusions may be seen in successfully repaired rotator cuffs [26]. Mild edema-like bone marrow abnormalities (Fig. 4) may be seen in the humeral head up to several years after surgery (43%) [26]. Susceptibility artifacts are common, especially in the presence of anchors. A linear low-signal abnormality in the humeral head may be found when tendon-to-bone repair has been performed (Fig. 5). Granulation tissue around the sutures may result in high signal abnormality mimicking aretear on T2-weighted images or on T1-weighted images obtained after intravenous injection of gadopentetate.

Muscle atrophy [27] and fatty degeneration [17] is not reversible after rotator cuff repair. However, the remaining muscle belly may be pulled laterally during surgical reconstruction. Accordingly, the diameter of the muscle may appear erroneously larger than before surgery on parasagittal MR obtained at the same position as the preoperative ones.

Muscle transfers

Susceptibility artifacts are common after this extensive type of surgery. The humeral head is covered (although commonly not completely) by a thin layer of fibrous tissue, which is commonly irregular in signal intensity and thickness (Fig. 6). In the Delta flap-type of surgery the deltoid muscle has a characteristic appearance with signal alterations within the acromial part of the deltoid.

MR findings in symptomatic patients

Tendons

After surgery, a full-thickness retear is diagnosed in the presence of fluid-like signal intensity on

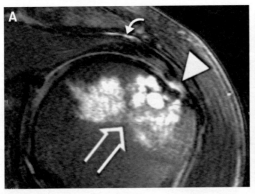
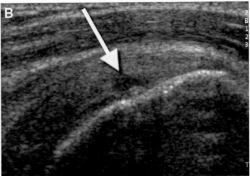

Fig. 4. A 60-year old asymptomatic patient 2 years after reconstruction of the supraspinatus tendon. (*A*) T2-weighted paracoronal fat-suppressed sequence demonstrates bone marrow abnormalities (*open arrow*) of the humeral head, partial tear of the supraspinatus tendon (*arrowhead*), and bursitis-like changes (*curved arrow*) in subcromial bursa. Partial tear of the tendon as demonstrated in this asymptomatic patient may represent normal postoperative findings. (*B*) Corresponding ultrasound image demonstrates partial tear (*arrow*) at undersurface of the supraspinatus tendon.

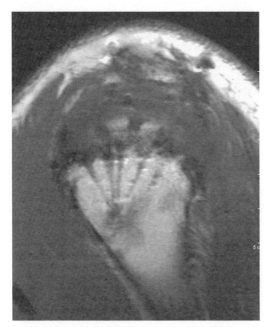

Fig. 5. Humeral head after tendon to bone repair. Parasagittal T1-weighted MR image demonstrates suture-related artifacts with linear low signal abnormality within the humeral head.

T2-weighted images that extends throughout the entire tendon substance and when there is nonvisualization of a portion of the rotator cuff (Fig. 7). These criteria are the same as the ones used in nonrepaired shoulders. Two previously published studies in patients with persistent symptoms after rotator cuff surgery had a diagnostic value comparable to MR images obtained before surgery [2,3]. Owen et al [2] reported 86% sensitivity and 92% specificity in diagnosing a retear. Gaenslen et al [3] used MR imaging with 84% sensitivity and 92% specificity. Ultrasound can be alternatively used for the assessment of full-thickness retears. Pricket el al [28] used ultrasound in shoulders that were painful postoperatively. They described 91% sensitivity and 86% specificity in diagnosing abnormalities of the rotator cuff. They classified minor partial-thickness tears requiring debridement only as intact, and large partial-thickness tears requiring as full-thickness tears.

The MR diagnosis of partial-thickness retears after surgery is far more debated than that of full-thickness tears. Owen et al [2] found that partial-thickness tears were indistinguishable from intact repaired tendons. They had included five partial-thickness retears in their series at the time of repeat surgery. All rotator cuffs were prospectively interpreted as intact. The retrospective review of these five MR examinations demonstrated minimal signal abnormality on proton density images in two shoulders and increased signal intensity within the rotator cuff on T2-weighted spin-echo images in the remaining three cases. In these three cases, however, the abnormal signal on the T2-weighted

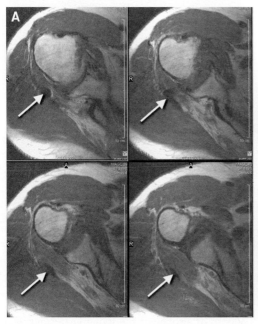

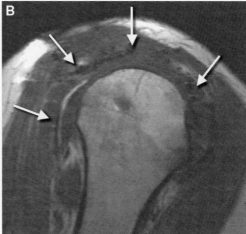

Fig. 6. Asymptomatic patient after latissimus dorsi transfer. (*A*) Susceptibility artifacts along the transferred latissimus dorsi tendon demonstrate the new course of the tendon after transfer (*arrows*). (*B*) The sagittal T1-weighted image shows the humeral head covered by a thin layer of fibrous tissue. Susceptibility artifacts (*arrows*).

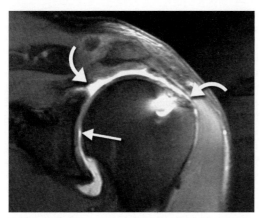

Fig. 7. Large, recurrent full-thickness tear of the supraspinatus tendon. Coronal angled proton density-weighted MR image with fat suppression shows fluid-like signal intensity (*between curved arrows*) throughout the entire tendon. Former supraspinatus substance indicates full-thickness tear. A cartilage defect is shown in the humeral head (*straight arrow*).

image did not reach the intensity of joint fluid and, therefore, was not interpreted as a retear.

MR arthrography may produce more reliable results than standard MR imaging in partial-thickness tears on the articular side. However, little has been published about the use of MR arthrography in patients with rotator cuff repair [29]. Irregularities of the tendon surfaces do not have the same relevance as in preoperative assessments because even perfect tendon repairs are associated with tendon distortion and variable diameters.

Ultrasound has been used for assessment of full-thickness retears successfully. However, the value of ultrasound for partial-thickness retears (see Fig. 4) remains debated [28].

Rotator cuff muscles

MR imaging demonstrates muscle atrophy and muscle degeneration in a quantitative and semi-quantitative fashion [30]. Cross-sectional areas of the muscles of the rotator cuff can be assessed reproducibly with parasagittal MR images obtained in a standardized fashion. For quantitative assessment, areas of the rotator cuff muscles and the area of the fossa supraspinata are measured at the most lateral angled sagittal image on which the scapular spine is imaged in continuity with the rest of the scapula. The measured value is then compared with published normal values [30].

In addition, for the qualitative diagnosis of supraspinatus muscle atrophy, the so-called "tangent sign" can be used (Fig. 8). This sign is characterized at the most lateral parasagittal image on which the scapular spine is in contact with the rest

of the scapula. A line is drawn through the superior borders of the scapular spine and the superior margin of the coracoid. The tangent sign is abnormal (positive) when the superior border of the supraspinatus muscle does not cross the tangent. The abnormal (positive) tangent sign indicates cross-sectional muscle areas are two standard deviations or more below an age-corrected normal mean [30].

CT can be used alternatively for assessment of muscle atrophy and degeneration [17].

The reliability of ultrasound in detecting rotator cuff muscle atrophy and degeneration is not clear. Based on a series of 65 patients, the authors found that ultrasound has a moderate accuracy (76% to 80%) for the diagnosis of substantial (Goutallier grade 2 to 4) supraspinatus and infraspinatus fatty muscle degeneration, with tendency to overestimate degeneration. However, MR imaging remains the standard of reference for such assessments [31].

Cartilage

Glenohumeral cartilage lesions (see Fig. 7) are found in up to one third of patients referred for MR arthrography with the clinical diagnosis of subacromial impingement syndrome [32]. Glenohumeral cartilage degeneration may become worse after rotator cuff surgery. After a mean follow-up period of 38 months, Jost et al [33] found significantly

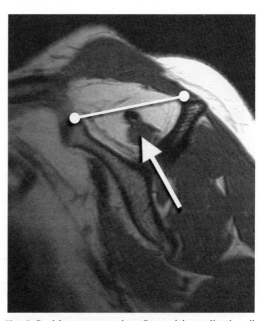

Fig. 8. Positive tangent sign. For quick qualitative diagnosis of atrophy of the supraspinatus muscle, the so-called "tangent sign" can be used. In severe atrophy, the supraspinatus muscles (*arrow*) do not cross the tangent drawn between the cranial border of the scapular spine and coracoid process.

more advanced osteoarthritis than before surgery. This evaluation was based on standard radiographs. Reliable assessment of the cartilage of the glenohumeral joint is important because articular cartilage abnormalities may simulate the symptoms of shoulder impingement syndrome [34]. Unfortunately, the performance of MR imaging in the assessment of glenohumeral cartilage appears to be inferior to that published for the knee. This may have several reasons. In contrast to the articular cartilage in the knee, which measures up to 8 mm [35], glenohumeral cartilage is much thinner (mean thickness at the humeral head, 1.24 mm; mean thickness at the glenoid fossa, 1.88 mm) [36]. Depending on the applied parameters and when chemical shift is taken into consideration, humeral cartilage may be represented by only a few pixels, which renders assessment of small lesions difficult.

MR imaging after surgery in instability

Clinical considerations

Although developmental factors may contribute to instability of the glenohumeral joint, trauma is the leading cause of subluxations and dislocations of the glenohumeral joint. The characteristic features associated with traumatic instability have been summarized by the acronym TUBS, which indicates traumatic, unidirectional, Bankart (lesion), and surgery. Atraumatic instability is less common. It is characterized by features summarized by the acronym AMBRI, which stands for atraumatic, multidirectional, bilateral, rehabilitation, and inferior capsular shift. A more sophisticated classification of instability has been described by Gerber and Nyffeler [37] describe a classification system that distinguishes between static instability, dynamic instability, and voluntary dislocation. Static instability is characterized by the absence of classic clinical symptoms of instability. Static instability may be superior, anterior, posterior, or inferior. This form of instability is associated with anatomical variants of the glenoid, rotator cuff abnormalities, and degenerative joint disease. The diagnosis is mainly radiological. Treatment may be difficult. Rotator cuff repair is commonly required. Dynamic instability becomes apparent after trauma and may be associated with capsulolabral lesions and lesions of the glenoid rim. Dynamic instability may be unidirectional or multidirectional. Hyperlaxity influences the clinical course of the disease if present but is not an integral part of this type of instability. Optimal surgical treatment in hyperlax shoulders is a subject of debate. Voluntary dislocation is a separate entity because dislocations do not occur inadvertently but are actively controlled by the patient.

More than 100 different types of operations have been described for anterior instability. Some of these techniques have been abandoned but may still be encountered on MR images performed before revision surgery.

Surgical techniques

In anterior instability, two major categories of surgical techniques are used. Direct anatomical repair of the labrum, capsular, and glenoid damage (Bankart repair) is attempted in the first group of patients. The other approach includes extraanatomical palliative procedures preventing secondary dislocation.

In the classic Bankart procedure the anterior labrum and joint capsule, including the inferior glenohumeral ligament, are readapted to the anterior glenoid rim. They are sutured in this position through three to five holes in the glenoid rim. For access to the glenoid rim, the subscapularis tendon is detached and reattached.

If the anterior capsule is insufficient, capsular reconstruction may be performed, according to Neer [38] or Matsen [39]. The capsule is cut in a T-shaped fashion and then sutured back in an overlapping fashion, resulting in three-dimensional reduction of anteroinferior capsular volume [38]. Inferior capsular shift is a more extensive variant of this technique, which is used in multidirectional instability.

Osteosynthesis and with screw fixation is performed in fractures of the glenoid rim [40]. For patients with significant glenoid bone loss, reconstruction of the glenoid with a bone graft is performed [41].

Coracoid transfer is a typical example of an extraanatomical procedure. The coracoid tip is transferred to the anterior inferior glenoid. Different variants have been described (such as the Bristow and Latarjet procedures), which vary with regard to the extent of coracoid osteotomy, the type of fixation, and the position of the transferred coracoid tip in relation to the subscapularis tendon. These procedures tighten the subscapularis tendon, change the position of the short flexors of the arm, and may have an effect on stability by correcting glenoid defects [42].

For posterior instability, rehabilitation of the shoulder muscles is the primary treatment method. If symptoms persist, the posterior capsule-labrum complex may be reconstructed [43].

SLAP lesion

Lesions at the biceps anchor from the anterior to the posterior portion of the superior labrum (SLAP lesions) occur as isolated findings or in combination with anterior instability. Repair of a SLAP lesion is usually performed arthroscopically.

Locked dislocation

Locked dislocation, such as posterior locked dislocation in patients with epilepsy, may be difficult to treat. Commonly, implantation of a prosthesis is required. Reconstruction of the humeral head may occasionally be possible.

Potential postoperative problems

Regardless of the procedure performed, the most common posttherapeutic problem is recurrence of instability. Earlier reports about arthroscopic procedures have demonstrated higher recurrence rates than those published for open procedures. More recent reports, however, have indicated that arthroscopic Bankart repair will be the preferred method in the future [44–46]. Other complications relate to staples and screws used during surgery. They may migrate and they may come into contact with articular cartilage and lead to early degeneration. Coracoid transfer procedures may fail because of nonunion of the coracoid. Overtightening and shortening of the capsules may produce subluxation in the opposite direction. Overconstraint may result in osteoarthritis of glenohumeral joint.

MR findings in successfully treated patients

Whether performed as open surgery or arthroscopically, postoperative MR images should demonstrate restoration of normal anatomy, including a normally wide joint capsule, normal capsular insertion

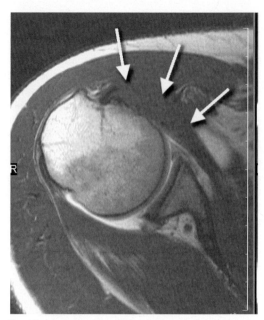

Fig. 10. After capsular shift. The subscapularis tendon (*arrows*) and the anterior capsule are thickened after capsular shift.

site, and anatomic position of the labrum [47]. Suture anchors may produce susceptibility artifacts. Suture anchors may interfere with the MR diagnosis of a recurrent tear. However, MR arthrography can be used reliably for the postoperative assessment of Bankart repair performed with sutures and

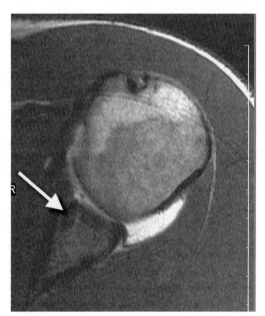

Fig. 9. Normal postoperative finding after Bankart repair. Axial T1-weighted MR arthrogram demonstrates normal transglenoid sutures leaving a channel in the glenoid (*arrow*).

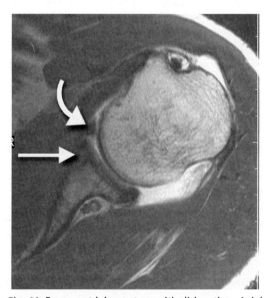

Fig. 11. Recurrent labrum tear with dislocation. Axial T1-weighted MR arthrogram demonstrates recurrent labral tear with dislocation (*curved arrow*). The postoperative channel in the glenoid (*straight arrow*) after labrum fixation is shown.

anchors [48]. Transglenoid sutures are associated with channels (Fig. 9) traversing the glenoid neck and scapula, which are seen on MR images. The subscapular tendon and the anterior joint capsule are thickened after capsular shift (Fig. 10). The labrum-like structure found after Bankart repair is typically rounded and may have inhomogeneous signal. Persons who have undergone a Bristow or Latarjet procedure have a shortened coracoid process and a changed shape of the anterior inferior glenoid.

MR findings in symptomatic patients after instability surgery

MR imaging may demonstrate a recurrent labral tear with or without dislocation (Fig. 11), a recurrent tear of the capsular insertion, a subscapularis tear, or secondary abnormalities, such as articular cartilage damage. Metallic anchors in the anterior glenoid from a previous Bankart repair may occasionally produce artifacts mimicking a recurrent anterior labral tear [47]. They also may hide recurrent labral abnormalities. In the absence of joint fluid, assessment of labrum and capsule may be difficult, however, and MR arthrography may be indicated. According to Sugimoto et al [48], MR arthrography is reliable for postoperative assessment after Bankart repair. The authors prefer oblique sagittal MR images (angled parallel to the glenoid fossa) for assessing whether the capsulolabral complex was stable or detached. MR arthrography was most reliable when performed with the shoulders in the abduction and external rotation (ABER) position.

Indirect MR arthrography (imaging 20 minutes after intravenous injection of gadopentetate) is a potentially useful alternative to direct MR arthrography. Wagner et al [47] found excellent sensitivity (100%) and specificity (100%) for indirect MR arthrography in recurrent labral tears. However, their study was characterized by small prevalences (two true positive cases, four true negative cases). In the same study, direct MR arthrography and nonenhanced MR imaging demonstrated 67% and 75% accuracy, respectively, in depicting recurrent labral tears. At least one of the false-positive diagnoses of a labral tear may not relate to the enhancement technique but rather to the chosen image sequence (susceptibility artifact).

In patients with bony reconstruction, CT arthrography may be the preferred imaging method [49,50]. The presence or absence of bony fusion and the integrity of articular cartilage can be assessed on CT arthrograms. MR imaging performed with spin-echo sequences with and without fat suppression is moderately accurate in the detection of

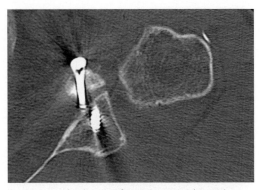

Fig. 12. Pseudarthrosis after Bristow and Latarjet procedures. The bone block is not fused with the glenoid on the axial CT.

glenohumeral cartilage lesions (see Fig. 7), even after the injection of intraarticular gadopentetate [32]. CT arthrography may replace MR imaging in joints with thin cartilage, such as the glenohumeral joint. This has been suggested in a study of the ankle joint with similarly thin cartilage. Interobserver variability and sensitivity in detecting cartilage defects was superior in CT arthrography [51]. CT also is preferred for postoperative assessment of the position and fusion of the bone block after coracoid transfer procedures (Fig. 12).

MR imaging after shoulder arthroplasty

Surgical techniques

Cemented unconstrained total shoulder arthroplasty (TSA) has been successfully used in the management of degenerative, posttraumatic, and inflammatory conditions of the shoulder. Current systems are modular on the humeral side, with varying head diameters and neck lengths [52].

Besides complete replacement of the proximal humerus, more limited prosthesis designs have been considered, including resurfacing of the humeral head. In cup arthroplasty a hemispheric surface prosthesis is cemented onto the residual humeral head. This eliminates the need to resect the humeral head and to ream the medullary canal, thus maintaining bone substance for future use [53]. Bipolar shoulder prostheses are humeral shaft prostheses with a mobile head system. Their indication is limited to patients with lesions of the rotator cuff or lesions of the glenoid surface. The inverse total shoulder prosthesis reverses the articular surface morphology of the humeral head and the glenoid. The hemispheric glenoid component serves as the center of rotation for the concave epiphyseal proximal humerus component. This implant may be used in the presence of massive rotator cuff tears [54].

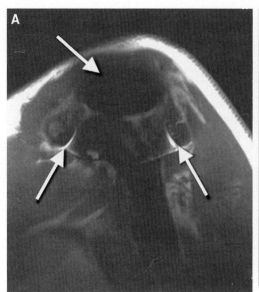 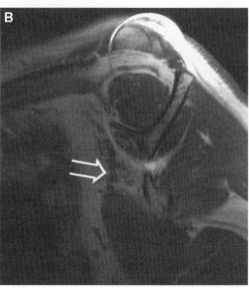

Fig. 13. Muscle quality of the rotator cuff can be analyzed in the presence shoulder of arthroplasty. Sagittal T1-weighted MR images demonstrate substantial susceptibility artifacts (*arrows*), which interfere with the evaluation of the rotator cuff tendons. (*B*) A more medially located sagittal T1-weighted MR image demonstrates that muscle assessment is possible in the presence of a prosthesis. Slight degeneration of the subscapularis muscle (*open arrow*) is visible.

Common problems after TSA

Causes of painful shoulder arthroplasty include rotator cuff tears, cartilage wear over the glenoid in hemiarthroplasty, synovitis, and infection.

Aseptic glenoid component loosening is the most frequently encountered long-term complication. Its prevalence increases with suboptimal component positioning, rotator cuff tears, and adhesive capsulitis. Minimally retracted or nonretracted rotator cuff tears that are limited to the supraspinatus tendon rarely affect outcome parameters. Conversely, fatty degeneration of the infraspinatus and, less importantly, subscapularis musculature adversely affects many of these parameters [55]. When patients are seen with persistent pain after arthroplasty, therefore, muscle quality should be analyzed (Fig. 13).

The role of shoulder prosthesis in treating acute humeral head fractures needs special consideration. A fracture prosthesis has to restore the length of the humerus, the center of rotation, and the anatomical retroversion. Positioning of the tubercula and their adequate osteosynthesis is most critical to ensure a correct healing process. Failed consolidation of the tubercula is associated with persistent symptoms.

MR findings

MR is rarely performed after shoulder arthroplasty. However, MR images may demonstrate findings not evident on standard radiographs [56,57], at least when MR sequences are optimized to the presence of a metallic implant. These findings include osteolysis at the prosthesis component-bone interface, subacromial bursitis, scarring of the joint capsule, abnormalities of the rotator cuff, and abscess formation. Subscapularis tears appear to be the most common type of rotator cuff abnormality in patients with shoulder prosthesis. A circumscribed fluid collection in a case of infection was noted as well as a focus of extruded cement in another case in close proximity to the axillary nerve.

After shoulder arthroplasty, MR imaging is competing with ultrasound, which does not suffer from susceptibility artifacts in proximity to the implant. Westhoff et al [58] found that many abnormalities, such as rotator cuff lesions, subdeltoid bursitis, changes around the long biceps tendon, and an increase in intraarticular volume resulting from effusion or synovitis, can be detected by sonography even when directly abutting the implant. Sonography may be used in combination with MR imaging, or it may replace it for the indications described above.

Glenoid loosening appears to be best addressed with CT (morphological approach) or roentgen stereophotogrammetric analysis (RSA) ("dynamic" approach relating to early migration associated with loosening) [59]. In glenoid loosening, CT arthrography demonstrates contrast between the keel and pegs of the glenoid component, though such contrast may be present between the plate of the prosthesis and bone without clinical significance.

Summary

Many types of surgical procedures are performed in the shoulder. Postoperative assessment by MR imaging is not usually indicated in most of them, including osteosynthesis of proximal humeral fractures, arthrodesis, and surgery of the clavicle and the sternoclavicular joint. In three major surgical groups, however, MR imaging is relevant, including rotator cuff surgery, surgery performed in glenohumeral joint, instability, and occasionally following total joint replacement. MR imaging is more difficult to perform after surgery than in nonoperated shoulders because of the presence of susceptibility artifacts and because the anatomy may be distorted without any clinical significance. Standard MR imaging with parameters optimized for avoiding susceptibility artifacts is most commonly performed. MR arthrography may be useful in the assessment of the labrum. MR imaging and MR arthrography are not the only available imaging methods available for the assessment of the postoperative shoulder. Standard radiographs provide accurate information on many relevant problems occurring after surgery, including recurrent glenohumeral dislocation, graft dislocation cranial migration in rotator cuff problems, and loosening of prostheses. CT is superior to MR imaging in the assessment of bone details, including integration of bone blocks or after osteosynthesis of the glenoid rim. Sonography may replace or complement MR imaging with regard to soft tissue abnormalities, especially those found close to any implant causing susceptibility artifacts.

MR imaging has advanced in many regards since 1993 when Haygood et al [1] predicted that it would be more reliable by 2003. Such advances include improved sequences and coils and a better understanding of the variability of shoulder morphology after surgery. There remains a long way to go until findings relevant for further decision making are precisely described and the role of different MR techniques has been clarified.

References

[1] Haygood TM, Oxner KG, Kneeland JB, Dalinka MK. Magnetic resonance imaging of the postoperative shoulder. Magn Reson Imaging Clin N Am 1993;1(1):143–55.

[2] Owen RS, Iannotti JP, Kneeland JB, Dalinka MK, Deren JA, Oleaga L. Shoulder after surgery: MR imaging with surgical validation. Radiology 1993;186(2):443–7.

[3] Gaenslen ES, Satterlee CC, Hinson GW. Magnetic resonance imaging for evaluation of failed repairs of the rotator cuff. J Bone Joint Surg Am 1996;78(9):1391–6.

[4] Guermazi A, Miaux Y, Zaim S, Peterfy CG, White D, Genant HK. Metallic artifacts in MR imaging: effects of main field orientation and strength. Clin Radiol 2003;58(4):322–8.

[5] Hilfiker P, Zanetti M, Debatin JF, McKinnon G, Hodler J. Fast spin-echo inversion-recovery imaging versus fast T2-weighted spin-echo imaging in bone marrow abnormalities. Invest Radiol 1995; 30(2):110–4.

[6] Hauger O, Dumont E, Chateil JF, Moinard M, Diard F. Water excitation as an alternative to fat saturation in MR imaging: preliminary results in musculoskeletal imaging. Radiology 2002; 224(3):657–63.

[7] Gartsman GM. Arthroscopic management of rotator cuff disease. J Am Acad Orthop Surg 1998;6(4): 259–66.

[8] Altchek DW, Carson EW. Arthroscopic acromioplasty: indications and technique. Instr Course Lect 1998;47:21–8.

[9] Blaine TA, Freehill MQ, Bigliani LU. Technique of open rotator cuff repair. Instr Course Lect 2001;50:43–52.

[10] Cordasco FA, Bigliani LU. The treatment of failed rotator cuff repairs. Instr Course Lect 1998;47: 77–86.

[11] Ogilvie-Harris DJ, Wiley AM, Sattarian J. Failed acromioplasty for impingement syndrome. J Bone Joint Surg Br 1990;72(6):1070–2.

[12] Warner JJ, Gerber C. Massive tears of the posterosuperior rotator cuff. In: Warner JJ, Ianotti JP, Gerber C, editors. Complex and revision surgery in shoulder surgery. Philadelphia: Lippincott-Raven; 1997. p. 177–201.

[13] Zlatkin MB. MRI of the postoperative shoulder. Skeletal Radiol 2002;31(2):63–80.

[14] Yamaguchi K, Levine WN, Marra G, Galatz LM, Klepps S, Flatow EL. Transitioning to arthroscopic rotator cuff repair: the pros and cons. Instr Course Lect 2003;52:81–92.

[15] Warner JJ. Management of massive irreparable rotator cuff tears: the role of tendon transfer. Instr Course Lect 2001;50:63–71.

[16] Goutallier D, Postel JM, Bernageau J, Lavau L, Voisin MC. Fatty muscle degeneration in cuff ruptures. Pre- and postoperative evaluation by CT scan. Clin Orthop Relat Res 1994;(304): 78–83.

[17] Fuchs B, Weishaupt D, Zanetti M, Hodler J, Gerber C. Fatty degeneration of the muscles of the rotator cuff: assessment by computed tomography versus magnetic resonance imaging. J Shoulder Elbow Surg 1999;8(6):599–605.

[18] Norwood LA, Fowler HL. Rotator cuff tears. A shoulder arthroscopy complication. Am J Sports Med 1989;17(6):837–41.

[19] Warner JJ. Overview: avoiding pitfalls and managing complications and failures of rotator cuff surgery. In: Warner JJ, Ianotti JP, Gerber C, editors. Complex and revision problems in shoulder surgery. Philadelphia: Lippincott-Raven; 1997. p. 161–3.

[20] Uri DS, Kneeland JB, Herzog R. Os acromiale: evaluation of markers for identification on sagittal and coronal oblique MR images. Skeletal Radiol 1997;26(1):31–4.

[21] Bencardino JT, Beltran J, Rosenberg ZS, Rokito A, Schmahmann S, Mota J, et al. Superior labrum anterior-posterior lesions: diagnosis with MR arthrography of the shoulder. Radiology 2000; 214(1):267–71.

[22] Zanetti M, Weishaupt D, Gerber C, Hodler J. Tendinopathy and rupture of the tendon of the long head of the biceps brachii muscle: evaluation with MR arthrography. AJR Am J Roentgenol 1998;170:1557–61.

[23] Pfirrmann CW, Zanetti M, Weishaupt D, Gerber C, Hodler J. Subscapularis tendon tears: detection and grading at MR arthrography. Radiology 1999;213(3):709–14.

[24] Weishaupt D, Zanetti M, Tanner A, Gerber C, Hodler J. MR imaging of subtle lesions of the rotator interval and the superior border of the subscapularis with or without biceps tendon subluxation (pulley lesion). [abstract]. Radiology 1997;205:237.

[25] Zanetti M, Jost B, Hodler J, Gerber C. MR imaging after rotator cuff repair: full-thickness defects and bursitis-like subacromial abnormalities in asymptomatic subjects. Skeletal Radiol 2000; 29(6):314–9.

[26] Spielmann AL, Forster BB, Kokan P, Hawkins RH, Janzen DL. Shoulder after rotator cuff repair: MR imaging findings in asymptomatic individuals—initial experience. Radiology 1999;213(3):705–8.

[27] Itoi E, Minagawa H, Sato T, Sato K, Tabata S. Isokinetic strength after tears of the supraspinatus tendon. J Bone Joint Surg Br 1997;79(1):77–82.

[28] Prickett WD, Teefey SA, Galatz LM, Calfee RP, Middleton WD, Yamaguchi K. Accuracy of ultrasound imaging of the rotator cuff in shoulders that are painful postoperatively. J Bone Joint Surg Am 2003;85(6):1084–9.

[29] Rand T, Freilinger W, Breitenseher M, Trattnig S, Garcia M, Landsiedl F, et al. Magnetic resonance arthrography (MRA) in the postoperative shoulder. Magn Reson Imaging 1999;17(6):843–50.

[30] Zanetti M, Gerber C, Hodler J. Quantitative assessment of the muscles of the rotator cuff with MR imaging. Invest Radiol 1998;33:163–70.

[31] Strobel K, Hodler J, Meyer D, Pfirrmann CW, Pirkl C, Zanetti M. Accuracy of ultrasound in diagnosis of fatty atrophy of supraspinatus and infraspinatus muscles. In: RSNA Scientific Assembly and Annual Meeting Program. Chicago; 2003. p. 398.

[32] Guntern DV, Pfirrmann CW, Schmid MR, Zanetti M, Binkert CA, Schneeberger AG, et al. Articular cartilage lesions of the glenohumeral joint: diagnostic effectiveness of MR arthrography and prevalence in patients with subacromial impingement syndrome. Radiology 2003; 226(1):165–70.

[33] Jost B, Pfirrmann CW, Gerber C, Switzerland Z. Clinical outcome after structural failure of rotator cuff repairs. J Bone Joint Surg Am 2000; 82(3):304–14.

[34] Ellman H, Harris E, Kay SP. Early degenerative joint disease simulating impingement syndrome: arthroscopic findings. Arthroscopy 1992;8(4): 482–7.

[35] Hall FM, Wyshak G. Thickness of articular cartilage in the normal knee. J Bone Joint Surg Am 1980;62(3):408–13.

[36] Yeh LR, Kwak S, Kim YS, Chou DS, Muhle C, Skaf A, et al. Evaluation of articular cartilage thickness of the humeral head and the glenoid fossa by MR arthrography: anatomic correlation in cadavers. Skeletal Radiol 1998;27(9):500–4.

[37] Gerber C, Nyffeler RW. Classification of glenohumeral joint instability. Clin Orthop 2002; (400):65–76.

[38] Neer CEI. Shoulder reconstruction. Philadelphia: W.B. Saunders; 1990.

[39] Matsen FA III, Lippitt SB, Sidles JA, Harryman DT II. Practical evaluation and management of the shoulder. Philadelphia: W.B. Saunders; 1994.

[40] Aston JW Jr, Gregory CF. Dislocation of the shoulder with significant fracture of the glenoid. J Bone Joint Surg Am 1973;55(7):1531–3.

[41] Bigliani LU, Newton PM, Steinmann SP, Connor PM, McLlveen SJ. Glenoid rim lesions associated with recurrent anterior dislocation of the shoulder. Am J Sports Med 1998;26(1):41–5.

[42] Allain J, Goutallier D, Glorion C. Long-term results of the Latarjet procedure for the treatment of anterior instability of the shoulder. J Bone Joint Surg Am 1998;80(6):841–52.

[43] Williams RJ III, Strickland S, Cohen M, Altchek DW, Warren RF. Arthroscopic repair for traumatic posterior shoulder instability. Am J Sports Med 2003;31(2):203–9.

[44] Kim SH, Ha KI. Bankart repair in traumatic anterior shoulder instability: open versus arthroscopic technique. Arthroscopy 2002;18(7):755–63.

[45] Weiss KS, Savoie FH III. Recent advances in arthroscopic repair of traumatic anterior glenohumeral instability. Clin Orthop 2002;(400):117–22.

[46] Kailes SB, Richmond JC. Arthroscopic vs. open Bankart reconstruction: a comparison using expected value decision analysis. Knee Surg Sports Traumatol Arthrosc 2001;9(6):379–85.

[47] Wagner SC, Schweitzer ME, Morrison WB, Fenlin JM Jr, Bartolozzi AR. Shoulder instability: accuracy of MR imaging performed after surgery in depicting recurrent injury—initial findings. Radiology 2002;222(1):196–203.

[48] Sugimoto H, Suzuki K, Mihara K, Kubota H, Tsutsui H. MR arthrography of shoulders after suture-anchor Bankart repair. Radiology 2002; 224(1):105–11.

[49] Kreitner KF, Runkel M, Grebe P, Just M, Schweden F, Oberbillig C, et al. MR tomography versus CT arthrography in glenohumeral

instabilities [in German]. Fortschr Geb Rontgenstr Nuklearmed 1992;157(1):37–42.

[50] Imhoff AB, Hodler J. Correlation of MR imaging, CT arthrography, and arthroscopy of the shoulder. Bull Hosp Joint Dis 1996;54(3):146–52.

[51] Schmid MR, Pfirrmann CW, Hodler J, Vienne P, Zanetti M. Cartilage lesions in the ankle joint: comparison of MR arthrography and CT arthrography. Skeletal Radiol 2003;32(5):259–65.

[52] Skirving AP. Total shoulder arthroplasty—current problems and possible solutions. J Orthop Sci 1999;4(1):42–53.

[53] Arredondo J, Worland RL. Bipolar shoulder arthroplasty in patients with osteoarthritis: short-term clinical results and evaluation of birotational head motion. J Shoulder Elbow Surg 1999;8(5):425–9.

[54] Habermeyer P, Ebert T. Current status and perspectives of shoulder replacement [in German]. Unfallchirurg 1999;102(9):668–83.

[55] Edwards TB, Boulahia A, Kempf JF, Boileau P, Nemoz C, Walch G. The influence of rotator cuff disease on the results of shoulder arthroplasty for primary osteoarthritis: results of a multicenter study. J Bone Joint Surg Am 2002;84-A(12): 2240–8.

[56] Sofka CM, Potter HG. MR imaging of joint arthroplasty. Semin Musculoskelet Radiol 2002; 6(1):79–85.

[57] Sperling JW, Potter HG, Craig EV, Flatow E, Warren RF. Magnetic resonance imaging of painful shoulder arthroplasty. J Shoulder Elbow Surg 2002;11(4):315–21.

[58] Westhoff B, Wild A, Werner A, Schneider T, Kahl V, Krauspe R. The value of ultrasound after shoulder arthroplasty. Skeletal Radiol 2002; 31(12):695–701.

[59] Nagels J, Valstar ER, Stokdijk M, Rozing PM. Patterns of loosening of the glenoid component. J Bone Joint Surg Br 2002;84(1):83–7.

RADIOLOGIC
CLINICS
OF NORTH AMERICA

Radiol Clin N Am 44 (2006) 553–567

ELSEVIER
SAUNDERS

Normal MR Imaging Anatomy of the Elbow

Keir A.B. Fowler, MD, Christine B. Chung, MD*

- Osseous and articular anatomy
- Capsular anatomy
- Ligament anatomy
- Muscle anatomy
- Nerve anatomy
- Bursal anatomy
- Summary
- References

The elbow is a compound trochoginglymoid joint formed by the articulations of three osseous structures: the humerus, the radius, and the ulna. The ulnohumeral articulation approximates a hinge (glymoid) joint, whereas the radiohumeral and radioulnar articulations allow for axial rotation, corresponding to a trochoid joint. The morphology and alignment of these structures result in a biomechanical milieu that necessitates complex motion of the articulation. This milieu is created, in part, by the mild valgus alignment of the humeroulnar articulation, referred to as the carrying angle. This alignment pattern, coupled with the complex osseous and soft tissue anatomy of the elbow, affords the elbow a wide range of motion with little inherent instability.

To better understand the complex anatomy of this joint, the following discussion is divided into sections describing the osseous, capsuloligamentous, muscular, neurovascular, and bursal components of the elbow. In some instances, these elements are discussed in the setting of functional anatomy of the articulation.

Osseous and articular anatomy

The proximal aspect of the elbow joint is formed by the humerus, which flares distally forming two central condyles that comprise the articular surfaces of the humerus, and two peripheral epicondyles that serve as attachment sites for soft tissue structures (Fig. 1). The articular surface of the distal humerus is divided into two components, the trochlea and the capitellum, which articulate with the ulna and radius respectively. The articular surfaces of the trochlea and capitellum are smooth and lined with articular cartilage. The capitellum and trochlea are oriented with 30 degrees of anterior angulation relative to the long axis of the humerus [1].

The trochlea is a pulley-like central depression of the distal humerus. The capitellum or lateral humeral condyle is nearly spherical in configuration and allows for rotation of the radial head. The capitellum approximates a sphere superiorly but narrows inferiorly with a distinct contour change where the anteriorly placed capitellum intersects the more posterior lateral epicondyle. The imaging appearance of the abrupt contour change at the posterolateral margin of the capitellum has been termed the "pseudodefect of the capitellum" (Fig. 2). The pseudodefect of the capitellum is most conspicuous on coronal images through the posterior aspect of the capitellum. In the sagittal imaging plane, the defect appears exaggerated on more

This article was previously published in *Magnetic Resonance Imaging Clinics of North America* 2004; 12:191–206.
Department of Radiology, Veterans Affairs Medical Center, University of California, 3350 La Jolla Village Drive, San Diego, CA 92161, USA
* Corresponding author.
E-mail address: cbchung@ucsd.edu (C.B. Chung).

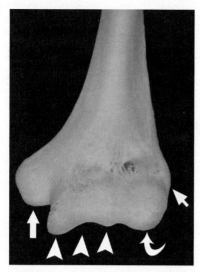

Fig. 1. Specimen photograph of the anterior aspect of the humerus shows the flared distal end of the bone. The articular surface is comprised of the trochlea (*arrowheads*) and the capitellum (*curved arrow*). The lateral epicondyle (*short arrow*) is seen to poorer advantage than the medial epicondyle (*long arrow*) because of its more posterior location.

lateral images [2]. True osteochondral lesions result in flattening and deformity of the normally smoothly convex anterior surface of the capitellum and are usually associated with subjacent marrow edema in the acute setting. However, increased marrow signal adjacent to a pseudodefect of the capitellum may be seen on MR arthrogram studies, which may relate to filling of the defect with contrast material [3].

Whereas the capitellum and trochlea have smooth surfaces lined by articular cartilage, the epicondyles are extraarticular structures with a rough, irregular contour. The prominent medial epicondyle is accentuated by the concave medial supracondylar ridge and serves as the origin of the anterior and posterior bands of the ulnar collateral ligament complex and, more superficially, the common flexor tendon. The less conspicuous lateral epicondyle is located just distal to the lateral supracondylar ridge and serves as the attachment site for portions of the lateral collateral ligament complex as well as the more superficial common extensor tendon.

Several bony fossae of the distal humerus are common sites for accumulation of intraarticular bodies in the elbow. The radial fossa is a shallow depression just proximal to the capitellum. Centrally, a deep excavation in the bone exists forming the coronoid fossa. This fossa is separated by a thin, fenestrated piece of bone from the posterior olecranon fossa. The olecranon fossa forms a solitary midline depression posteriorly for articulation with the olecranon.

The proximal ulna is formed by the confluence of the olecranon and coronoid processes and has several important anatomic landmarks (Fig. 3). The posterior olecranon process and anterior coronoid process possess articular surfaces that join to form

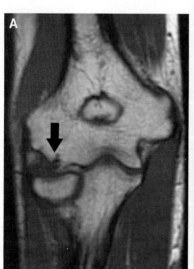
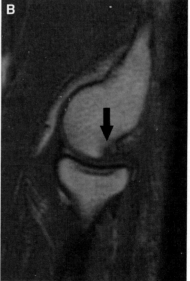

Fig. 2. (*A*) Coronal T1-weighted image shows apparent irregularity (*arrow*) at what appears to be the articular surface of the capitellum. (*B*) Cross-reference with the sagittal T1-weighted image in this patient reveal that the irregularity is the junction (*arrow*) of the anterior capitellar articular surface and the more posterior lateral epicondyle.

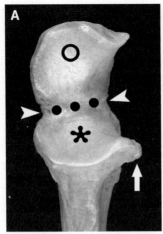
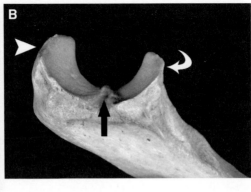

Fig. 3. (A) Specimen photograph of the frontal view of the ulna show the figure-eight configuration that results from the junction of the olecranon (O) and coronoid (*) articulating surfaces. The waist of the figure eight results in the trochlear groove (*arrowheads*), whereas the central junction results in a raised area of the articular surface devoid of cartilage, the trochlear ridge (*dots*). The medial-most portion of the coronoid process is referred to as the sublime tubercle (*arrow*) and serves as the attachment of the anterior band of the ulnar collateral ligament complex. (B) Specimen photograph of a lateral view of the ulna shows the coronoid tip (*curved arrow*), the olecranon tip (*arrowhead*), and the trochlea ridge (*arrow*).

the concave trochlear (greater sigmoid) notch. It is named for its articulation with the adjacent trochlea of the humerus. The radial (lesser sigmoid) notch is a small impression along the lateral margin of the coronoid process that articulates with the radial head. Articular hyaline cartilage covers most of the trochlear notch and the entirety of the radial notch.

Viewed en face, the trochlear notch has a figure-eight configuration with slight constriction midway between the coronoid and olecranon processes, traversed by a slight bony elevation called the trochlear ridge (Fig. 4A). The trochlear ridge lacks articular cartilage and is approximately 2 to 3 mm wide and 3 to 5 mm high [4]. Because the height corresponds to that of adjacent articular cartilage, the articular surface remains smooth and congruent. In most cases, the trochlear ridge completely traverses the trochlear notch, but occasionally can be incomplete (traversing only the medial or lateral aspect of the notch). Sagittal MR images may reveal a central elevation of the trochlear articular surface corresponding to the trochlear ridge. The ridge has been reported in 81% of MR studies of normal volunteers [5]. This anatomic structure may simulate either a central osteophyte or an olecranon stress fracture.

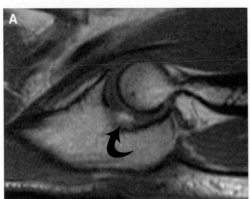
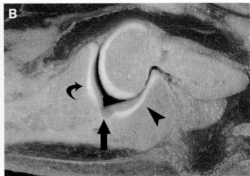

Fig. 4. (A) Sagittal T1-weighted MR image shows the appearance of the trochlear ridge, commonly mistaken for a central osteophyte (*curved arrow*). (B) Specimen photograph in the sagittal plane in the region of the waist of the figure-eight articular surface of the ulna shows the coronoid articular surface (*curved arrow*), the olecranon articular surface (*arrowhead*), and the area devoid of cartilage at their junction referred to as the trochlear groove (*straight arrow*). This can be mistaken for an osteochondral defect.

Normal cortical irregularity may be seen at the peripheral margins of the trochlear ridge, termed "the trochlear groove" (Fig. 4B). The contour change encountered at the peripheral margins of the trochlear ridge corresponds to the waist of the figure eight-shaped articular surface of the ulna. This normal variant can be distinguished from a true osteochondral lesion by recognition of its characteristic location.

The posterior surface of the olecranon process serves as the insertion of the triceps. Its marrow space is predominately fatty with sparse trabeculation, predisposing this part of the ulna to fracture [6]. The coronoid process acts as a buttress to prevent posterior translation of the ulnohumeral articulation. Fractures involving greater than 50% of the coronoid often result in elbow instability, necessitating internal fixation [7]. Although no discrete anatomic structure inserts on the tip of the coronoid process, the joint capsule inserts approximately 6 mm distal to this bony landmark [8]. The brachialis tendon inserts approximately 11 mm distal to the coronoid tip at the ulnar tuberosity.

Changes in osseous contour often correspond to the attachment of soft tissue structures. In the ulna, two important soft tissue attachment sites are noted. The sublime tubercle is a small bony eminence along the most medial aspect of the coronoid process where the anterior bundle of the ulnar collateral ligament inserts. This small tubercle may be avulsed in throwing athletes [9]. The supinator crest (crista supinatoris) is a thin linear ridge along the lateral aspect of the ulna, representing an attachment site for the lateral ulnar collateral ligament.

The proximal radius includes the discoid-shaped radial head and the tapered radial neck (Fig. 5). The radial head articular surface has a central depression that accommodates the capitellum. The outer margin of the radial head articulates with the radial notch of the ulna [10]. Hyaline cartilage of the articular surface of the radial head is contiguous with its outer margin, except for the anterolateral portion of the articular periphery, which is devoid of cartilage [6]. The anterolateral portion of the articular periphery also lacks a subchondral bone plate, predisposing to fracture [1].

In the radius, an important soft tissue attachment site is the radial tuberosity, located medially well below the joint line. The posterior aspect of the radial tuberosity serves as the insertion for the biceps brachii tendon, whereas the anterior portion of the tuberosity is covered by the bicipitoradial bursa.

In a minority of individuals a bony excrescence termed the "supracondylar process" extends anteromedially from the distal humerus approximately 7 cm proximal to the medial epicondyle (Fig. 6). The supracondylar process is considered an atavistic

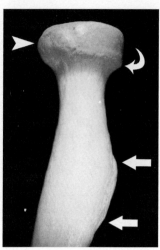

Fig. 5. Specimen photograph of the frontal view of the radius profiles the radial head (*arrowhead*), radial neck (*curved arrow*), and radial tuberosity (*arrows*).

structure typically found in amphibians, reptiles, and some mammals. This normal variant may be seen in 0.3% to 2.7% of humans and has been characterized on MR imaging [11]. The ligament of Struthers is a fibrous band extending from the tip of the supracondylar process to the medial epicondyle, creating a fibro-osseous tunnel through which passes the median nerve and brachial artery. Compression of the median nerve may occur, causing in pain and numbness of the hand with weakness of the forearm muscles.

Capsular anatomy

The joint capsule invests the three articulations of the elbow forming a single contiguous joint space. The capsule is comprised of two layers: a deep synovial lining and a more superficial fibrous layer. Three major fat pads are situated between the synovial and deep fibrous layers, making their location intraarticular but extrasynovial. Two anterior fat pads correspond to the capitellar and trochlear fossae, while a single posterior fat pad is concealed within the olecranon fossa. Therefore, in the presence of a joint effusion confined by the synovial capsule, the extrasynovial fat pads are elevated, resulting in the radiographic signs of a visible posterior fat pad and an elevated anterior fat pad, the "anterior sail" sign.

Knowledge of the capsular attachments can prove instrumental for the localization of pathology. Joint fluid that does not respect capsular boundaries implies capsular insufficiency in that location. In the case of the elbow, the capsule attaches anteriorly to the humerus at the superior margin of the coronoid and radial fossae, and to the ulna at the

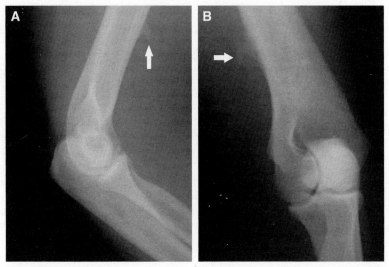

Fig. 6. Lateral (*A*) and oblique (*B*) radiographs of the distal humerus and elbow show an osseous excrescence (*arrow*) emanating from the anteromedial aspect of the humerus, the so-called "supracondylar process."

coronoid process. Posteriorly, the capsule inserts above the olecranon fossa. Medially, the capsule is attached to the medial margin of the olecranon and trochlear notch, and laterally along the lateral margin of the trochlear notch as well as the annular ligament [1].

Five principle recesses of the elbow joint are recognized, including the anterior humeral recess, the olecranon recess, the annular recess, and the recesses of the collateral ligaments (Fig. 7) [3]. The olecranon recess is the largest and is found along the posterior margin of the joint. The medial and lateral olecranon recesses are extensions of the olecranon recess along either side of the olecranon process and are best depicted on axial images. The anterior humeral recess is found along the anterior margin of the joint and is composed of the two smaller coronoid and radial fossae recesses. The collateral ligament recesses are found at the periphery of the anterior humeral recess. The peripheral margin of each collateral ligament recess is formed by the respective collateral ligament. As such, in

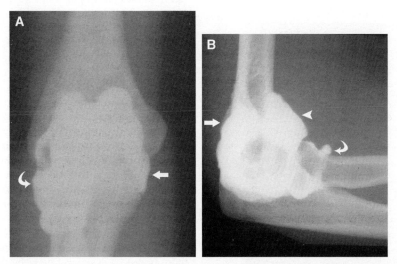

Fig. 7. (*A*) Frontal arthrogram image of the elbow shows the normal distribution of fluid within the articulation, including the recesses beneath the ulnar collateral ligament complex (*arrow*) and the radial collateral ligament complex (*curved arrow*). (*B*) Lateral arthrogram image of the elbow shows recess of the coronoid fossa (*arrowhead*), the olecranon fossa (*arrow*), and the normal extension of contrast beneath the annular ligament (*curved arrow*).

a distended joint no fluid should extend along beyond the margin of the epicondyles [3]. The periradial or annular recess may be noted anteriorly where the capsule passes in close proximity to, as well as beneath, the annular ligament. It may appear as an extension of the radial collateral ligament recess.

Several synovial folds or plica have been described throughout the elbow joint and may be confused with intraarticular bodies or normal fat pads. The lateral synovial fold or synovial fringe is one of the most frequent and is seen between the radial head and capitellum (Fig. 8). The lateral synovial fold may be associated with chondromalacia of the radial head [12]. Recent work indicates the lateral synovial fold is common, being present in 86% of cadaver elbow specimens and most commonly found along the dorsal aspect of the radiocapitellar articulation [13]. Two distinct histologic types of the lateral synovial fold have been demonstrated: (1) a true synovial fold described as a pliable structure composed of two layers of synovium and (2) a rigid triangular fibrous structure lined by synovium.

Synovial folds or plica occur elsewhere in the elbow, including a curved synovial fold at the superior margin of the lateral olecranon recess (Fig. 9) [3]. Additional small nodular or curved plica may be encountered in the medial and lateral olecranon recesses. Plica may cause mechanical symptoms of locking. Though larger synovial folds may be suspected of causing mechanical symptoms, Awaya and coworkers [14] found considerable overlap in the size of symptomatic and asymptomatic plica.

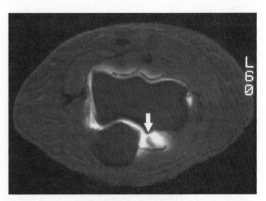

Fig. 9. Axial T1-weighted fat-suppressed fast spin-echo post arthrogram image shows a thickened piece band of synovium emanating from the posterior capsule (*arrow*), a posterior synovial plica.

Ligament anatomy

Ligamentous structures of the elbow are comprised of focal condensations of the fibrous joint capsule, thus forming a capsuloligamentous complex similar to that encountered in the shoulder. The ulnar collateral ligament (UCL) originates from the inferior aspect of the medial epicondyle slightly posterior to the center axis of elbow rotation, and is thus under greater tension with elbow flexion [15]. The humeral origin of the UCL corresponds to approximately two-thirds of the width of the inferior aspect of the medial epicondyle and has no insertion on the adjacent medial condyle [16]. The lateral collateral ligamentous complex arises from the lateral epicondyle at the central axis of rotation of the elbow joint and is thus under constant tension regardless of elbow position.

In general, the collateral ligament complexes are best demonstrated on coronal images. Axial and sagittal images are useful to confirm suspected pathology. As is the case elsewhere in the musculoskeletal system, ligaments are generally uniformly low in signal on all pulse sequences except where magic-angle effects or volume averaging may occur.

Three components of the UCL are classically described: the anterior, posterior, and transverse bundles. The largest and most important component of the UCL is the anterior bundle, a discrete focal thickening of the medial capsule arising from the inferior margin of the medial epicondyle that inserts at the sublime tubercle of the proximal ulna (Fig. 10). Timmerman and coworkers [17] have demonstrated two histologic components of the anterior bundle, a deep layer between the two fibrous layers of the capsule and a superficial layer external to medial capsule. The superficial or extracapsular layer may represent deep fibers of the ulnohumeral head of the flexor digitorum superficialis [18].

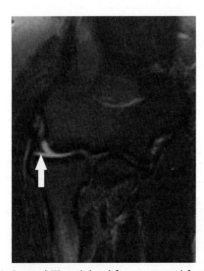

Fig. 8. Coronal T2-weighted fat-suppressed fast spin-echo image through the elbow shows a tongue of synovial tissue extending from the lateral capsule (*arrow*), the synovial fringe.

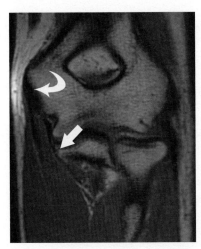

Fig. 10. Coronal T1-weighted image shows the attachment of the anterior band of the ulnar collateral ligament (*arrow*) to the sublime tubercle of the coronoid process. The common flexor tendon (*curved arrow*) is located just superficial to the ligament.

Whereas the ulnar insertion of the anterior bundle is classically described as being flush with the articular margin of the medial coronoid, there may be some variability of the ulnar insertion at the sublime tubercle. Timmerman has reported the ulnar insertion of the anterior bundle is in close proximity (1 mm) of the joint line [19]. In contradistinction, Munshi et al [18] found the anterior bundle may insert either at the articular margin or approximately 3 mm distally. The more distal insertion may create a small recess on arthrograms, simulating a partial undersurface tear of the anterior bundle. Therefore, differentiating partial undersurface tears of the UCL from a normal distal insertion of the anterior bundle may be clinically important.

On coronal images the anterior bundle of the UCL is seen as a uniformly low signal structure. The proximal fibers of the anterior bundle may appear indistinct and lax [6]. Typically the anterior bundle insertion at the sublime tubercle is flush with the articular margin. In a distended joint, fluid undercutting the ulnar insertion of the anterior bundle may represent an undersurface tear, the so-called "T sign." However, as previously mentioned, caution is warranted as variations in attachment may occur in this region.

The posterior bundle is a focal thickening of the medial capsule, which, unlike the anterior bundle, lacks a distinct superficial component. The posterior bundle originates from the inferior aspect of the medial epicondyle and inserts at the posteromedial margin of the trochlear notch, forming the floor of the cubital tunnel. On coronal MR images, the humeral origin of the posterior bundle is seen posterior to a plane bisecting the epicondyles and extends to the posteromedial aspect of the olecranon. MR imaging identification of the posterior band is most facile in the axial plane when localizing the floor of the cubital tunnel at the joint line. The transverse bundle, also termed the "Ligament of Cooper," extends between the ulnar insertions of the anterior and posterior bundles and plays little if any functional role. It is not readily visualized on routine MR imaging.

Variants of the UCL complex have been described and include a strong oblique pattern in which the transverse bundle flares in a fanlike configuration as it inserts on the anterior bundle and coronoid [20]. In nearly a quarter of specimens, Beckett and coworkers [20] identified a fourth component of the ulnar collateral ligament termed the "accessory" or "extra bundle." The accessory bundle originates from the posteromedial aspect of the capsule and inserts on the transverse bundle. There is little or no variation of the anterior or posterior bundles of the UCL.

The lateral collateral ligament complex consists of the radial collateral ligament (RCL), lateral ulnar collateral ligament (LUCL), and the annular (orbicular) ligament (Fig. 11). A fourth component, the accessory lateral collateral ligament, is variably present, extending from the annular ligament to the supinator crest. The LUCL and RCL may appear contiguous at their origin on the lateral epicondyle. On gross inspection the RCL and LUCL are difficult to visually distinguish from one another at the humeral origin [21]. The RCL inserts broadly on the annular ligament, whereas the LUCL passes along the posterolateral margin of the radial head where it blends with fibers of the annular ligament and continues medially to insert on the supinator crest of the ulna. The course of the LUCL is such that the radial head is "cradled" by the ligament, which may explain its important role in posterolateral instability. The annular ligament originates from the anterior and posterior margins of the radial notch, encircling the radial head and acting as the primary stabilizer of the proximal radioulnar joint. Less important ligamentous structures include the quadrate ligament (ligament of Denuce) and oblique cord; the former may play a role in stabilization of the proximal radioulnar joint [1].

Compared with the medial ligamentous complex, the lateral ligamentous complex is not as well demonstrated on MR imaging because of the smaller size of the individual ligamentous structures. Joint distension with saline or gadolinium solution may improve overall visualization and better demonstrate undersurface tears. The radial collateral ligament forms the lateral capsular margin on coronal images and the extensor carpi radialis brevis is seen closely applied to its outer margin. In a distended

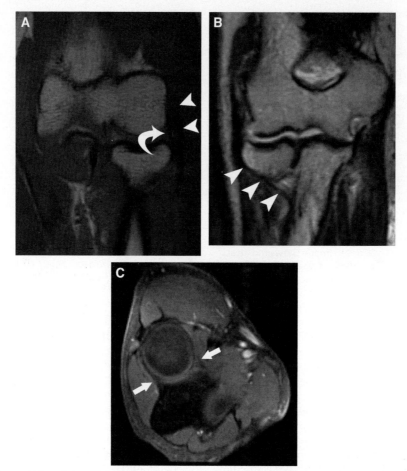

Fig. 11. (*A*) Coronal T1-weighted image shows the radial collateral ligament (*curved arrow*) extending from the undersurface of the lateral epicondyle to the region of its distal annular ligament attachment. The common extensor tendon (*arrowheads*) is located just superficial to the ligament. (*B*) Coronal T1-weighted image at the posterior aspect of the joint show the fibers of the lateral ulnar collateral ligament (*arrowheads*) extending around the posterior aspect of the radial head to attach to the supinator crest of the ulna. (*C*) Axial proton density-weighted fat-suppressed image shows the anterior and posterior attachments (*arrows*) of the annular ligament, which encircles the radial head neck junction, to the ulna.

joint, fluid may slightly separate the radial collateral ligament and the radial head as the ligament inserts on the annular ligament. The lateral ulnar collateral ligament can be difficult to visualize completely because of its oblique course, but its midportion can be demonstrated on coronal images along the posterior margin of the radial head and neck. Identification of the ulnar insertion of the lateral ulnar collateral ligament at the supinator crest can be facilitated by noting a triangular focus of fatty tissue separating the distal LUCL from the annular ligament [22].

Given the oblique course of the collateral ligaments, specialized imaging planes may provide better demonstration of the radial collateral ligament and anterior bundle of the ulnar collateral ligament without partial-volume effects [22]. Imaging of the elbow in mild flexion (20 to 30 degrees) with the coronal plane aligned along the humeral axis was found to produce optimal ligamentous visualization.

Muscle anatomy

Organization of the complex muscular anatomy about the elbow lends itself to division into anterior, posterior, medial, and lateral groups. Though this method allows delineation of the specific muscles and their respective tendons about the elbow, it is important to emphasize that the common flexor and common extensor tendons are involved in the vast majority of musculotendinous pathology about the elbow, thus obviating the need for localizing pathology to a single muscle (**Fig. 12**). To this

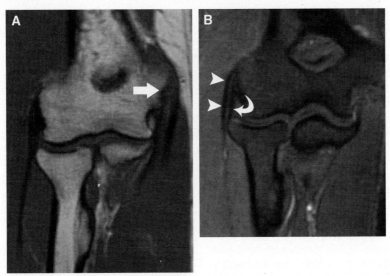

Fig. 12. (*A*) Coronal T1-weighted image shows the attachment of the common flexor tendon (*arrow*) to the medial epicondyle. (*B*) Coronal T2-weighted fat-suppressed fast spin-echo image shows the intimate relationship of the radial collateral ligament (*curved arrow*) to the overlying common extensor tendon arising from the lateral epicondyle (*arrowheads*).

end, the coronal imaging plane provides optimal visualization of the common flexor and common extensor tendons, underscoring the importance of obtaining high signal-to-noise ratio fluid-sensitive images in the coronal plane.

The lateral muscle group can be thought of consisting of three components—a superficial group, the common extensors, and the supinator. The superficial group includes the brachioradialis and extensor carpi radialis longus (ECRL). Together with the extensor carpi radialis brevis, the superficial group forms a bulky muscular mass termed "the mobile wad," which surrounds much of the anterolateral aspect of the elbow [1]. The brachioradialis forms the most anterior portion of the lateral muscle group, arises from the supracondylar ridge of the humerus, and inserts near the radial styloid process. The extensor carpi radialis longus originates from the supracondylar ridge just distal to the brachioradialis and inserts distally at the base of the second metacarpal.

The common extensor group is composed of four muscles: the extensor carpi radialis brevis (ECRB), extensor digitorum (ED), extensor digiti minimi (EDM), and extensor carpi ulnaris (ECU). The common extensors originate from the lateral epicondyle by way of the common extensor tendon and are found along the posterolateral aspect of the elbow, blending with the more substantial superficial muscle group. The most lateral component of the common flexor tendon is the extensor carpi radialis brevis, which lies immediately deep to the ECRL. The radiohumeral bursa is an adventitial bursa deep

to the ECRB, which may distend in cases of epicondylitis, thereby separating the LCL and ECRB [23].

The common extensor tendon is seen as a hypointense band arising from the lateral epicondyle on MR imaging. The extensor carpi radialis brevis and lateral collateral ligamentous complex are closely applied to each other and may not be resolved as discrete structures. The tendinous origins of the extensor carpi radialis longus and brevis can be distinguished from one another, with the ECRL slightly superficial to the ECRB with intervening intermediate signal between the two tendons. The extensor carpi radialis brevis is the initial site of signal abnormalities in cases of tennis elbow [23]. Given the close proximity of the ECRB and LUCL, it is not surprising that severe lateral epicondylitis is associated with secondary abnormalities of the LUCL on MR imaging [24].

The supinator, the deepest of the lateral muscle group, arises from the lateral epicondyle and the supinator crest of the ulna, inserting distally on the radial shaft, enveloping much of the proximal radius along its course. The muscle typically has thin superficial and bulky deep components. The posterior interosseous nerve innervates the supinator and travels between the deep and superficial portions of the muscle.

The medial muscle group includes the pronator teres and four superficial flexors—the flexor carpi radialis (FCR), palmaris longus (PL), flexor carpi ulnaris (FCU), and flexor digitorum superficialis (FDS). The pronator teres forms most of the anteromedial muscle mass at the level of the elbow. The bulk of the pronator teres arises from a large humeral head proximal to the medial epicondyle. A smaller ulnar head of pronator teres arises from the medial aspect of coronoid process. The pronator teres proceeds distally to insert on the lateral aspect of the radial shaft.

The common flexor tendon arises from the medial epicondyle and includes the FCR, PL, FCU, FDS (humeroulnar head), and a portion of the pronator teres. The common flexor muscles at the level of the elbow form a confluent muscular mass at the posteromedial aspect of the joint. On coronal MR images, the common flexor tendon appears as a hypointense band that gradually blends with proximal fibers of the ulnar collateral ligament arising from the undersurface of the medial epicondyle. The palmaris longus, which blends with the posteromedial border of pronator teres, may be absent in up to 13% of cases [6]. The FDS arises from two heads, a humeroulnar head arising from the common flexor tendon and a radial head arising from the anterior radius. A fibrous arch is formed where the two heads of the FDS coalesce, beneath which passes the anterior interosseous branch of the median nerve. The FCU also arises from two heads near the cubital tunnel. The first head is the most medial portion of the common flexor tendon, and the second head arises from the medial aspect of the olecranon. A fibrous arch between the two heads forms the roof of the cubital tunnel has been variously termed "the arcuate ligament," "Osborne's band," and "the cubital tunnel retinaculum."

The deep flexors include the flexor digitorum profundus (FDP) and flexor pollicis longus (FPL). This group originates from the proximal ulna, just distal to the cubital tunnel, thus forming a small muscular mass as the posteromedial aspect of the ulna. Gantzer's muscle, an accessory slip of the flexor pollicis longus, may be encountered in 45% of individuals [25] and may rarely cause impingement of the median nerve [26].

The anterior muscle group includes the two primary flexors of the elbow, the biceps brachii and brachialis. The brachialis arises from the distal humerus and inserts at the ulnar tuberosity. The biceps brachii muscle arises from long and short heads and terminates in a single insertion at the radial tuberosity (Fig. 13). The short head arises from the coracoid process and the long head from the supraglenoid tubercle of the scapula. The distal biceps tendon is formed from the two muscle bellies, which unite approximately 7 cm proximal to the elbow joint. Like the Achilles tendon, the distal biceps tendon has no tendon sheath. The distal portion of the biceps tendon may be at risk for attritional changes and tearing in a fashion similar to the supraspinatus tendon of the shoulder in cases of impingement [27]. A relative hypovascular zone has been described in the distal tendon subject to mechanical impingement between the radial tuberosity and ulna [28]. The bicipital aponeurosis, or lacertus fibrosis, arises from the distal biceps tendon and passes medially to blend with the fascia covering the flexor-pronator mass of the medial aspect of the elbow. This fibrous band may prevent proximal retraction of the complete biceps rupture, thereby masking the typical clinical findings of a balled-up muscular mass.

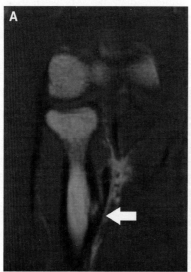
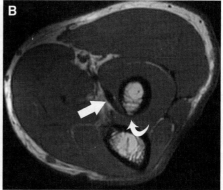

Fig. 13. (*A*) Coronal T1-weighted image shows the biceps tendon attaching to the radial tuberosity (*arrow*). (*B*) Axial T1-weighted image shows the biceps tendon (*arrow*) moving to its attachment at the radial tuberosity (*curved arrow*).

Axial images generally provide the best visualization of the biceps tendon as it inserts on the radial tuberosity. Sagittal images of biceps may help confirm suspect pathology. Fluid distension of the bicipitoradial bursa can be easily seen all three standard imaging planes, although axial images best illustrate the close relation of the bursa and biceps tendon.

The anconeus and triceps form the posterior muscle group (Fig. 14). The triceps arises from three heads, the lateral head from the posterolateral proximal humerus, the long head from the infraglenoid tubercle of the scapula, and the medial head from the posterior distal humerus. These form a common tendon that inserts at the olecranon, which normally may have a striated appearance [5]. Rarely, a portion of the medial triceps may insert on the medial epicondyle and compress the ulnar nerve [29]. The medial head of the triceps may subluxate, causing a snapping sensation similar to that of ulnar nerve subluxation [30]. The anconeus arises from the posterior margin of the lateral epicondyle and courses medially to insert on the lateral margin of the olecranon. The role of the anconeus is somewhat controversial, although it is thought to help stabilize the elbow joint [1]. The triceps insertion is clearly seen on sagittal and axial MR images. The anconeus is easily seen on axial images, serving as a useful landmark for the lateral aspect of the elbow.

The anconeus epitrochlearis is an anomalous muscle found to occur in 11% of anatomic specimens that may cause cubital tunnel syndrome [31]. The anconeus epitrochlearis arises from the medial humeral condyle, passes superficial to the ulnar nerve, and inserts on the olecranon.

Nerve anatomy

The three primary nerves about the elbow demonstrate signal characteristics similar to peripheral nerves elsewhere in the body. Nerves are normally intermediate in signal intensity on T1-weighted images, similar to that of adjacent muscle, and may be slightly brighter on T2-weighted images. Nerves are made more conspicuous by surrounding perineural fat, and this effect is most pronounced with the ulnar nerve as it passes through the cubital tunnel.

The cubital tunnel is a fibro-osseous conduit along the posterior aspect of the medial epicondyle (Fig. 15). The posterior bundle of the ulnar collateral ligament forms the floor of the cubital tunnel and the arcuate ligament the roof. The arcuate ligament may be absent in up to 23% of subjects [31]. Fatty tissue usually surrounds the ulnar nerve and posterior recurrent ulnar artery as they pass through the cubital tunnel. The ulnar nerve continues distally traversing the flexor carpi ulnaris muscle and deep flexor pronator aponeurosis. The nerve may be identified in the proximal forearm along the medial aspect of the ulna within a small triangular focus of fat just lateral to the flexor digitorum superficialis.

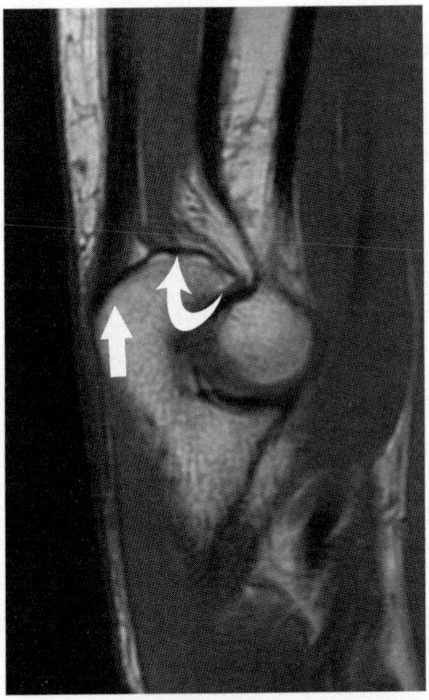

Fig. 14. Sagittal T1-weighted image demonstrates the tendinous (*arrow*) and muscular (*curved arrow*) attachments of the triceps to the olecranon process.

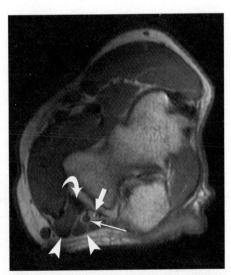

Fig. 15. Axial T1-weighted image portrays the spatial relationships of the cubital tunnel. The floor is comprised of the posterior band of the ulnar collateral ligament (*thick arrow*) complex. The two heads of the flexor carpi ulnaris (*arrowheads*) arise from the common flexor tendon (*curved arrow*) and surround the ulnar nerve (*thin arrow*).

The cubital tunnel is best demonstrated on axial images. Predominantly fat signal is present throughout the cubital tunnel surrounding the ulnar nerve, which demonstrates intermediate signal intensity. A few small, dotlike structures adjacent to the nerve represent posterior recurrent ulnar vessels, which are hypointense on T1-weighted images and of variable signal intensity on T2-weighted images depending on the degree of blood flow. The arcuate ligament, forming the roof of the tunnel, is seen as a slender hypointense band.

Cubital tunnel syndrome results from narrowing of the cubital tunnel or repetitive stress and traction on the ulnar nerve. The pathoanatomy of cubital tunnel syndrome is predicated on diminished canal volume, increased intraneural pressure, and ulnar nerve elongation and excursion [32]. In normal subjects, the arcuate ligament becomes taut and more closely apposed to the floor of the cubital tunnel with flexion of the elbow. The cross-sectional area of the tunnel decreases with subsequent elevation of intraneural pressure [33]. This fact likely accounts for the occurrence of the syndrome in certain occupations prone to repetitive elbow flexion, such as carpentry, painting, sewing, and playing a musical instrument. Anomalous anatomic structures, such as the anconeus epitrochlearis, may cause cubital tunnel syndrome. The ligament of Struthers, normally associated with median nerve compression, rarely involves the ulnar nerve [34].

Excessive mobility of the ulnar nerve may result in traction neuritis. The nerve may subluxate to the posteromedial margin of the cubital tunnel or frankly dislocate and be found anteromedial to medial epicondyle. Because the ulnar nerve may sublux in 10% to 16% of healthy subjects [32], clinical correlation regarding the presence of ulnar nerve symptoms is necessary.

The radial nerve extends distally along the spiral groove of the humerus and then passes along the anterolateral aspect of the elbow between the brachioradialis and brachialis muscles (Fig. 16) [25]. At the proximal margin of the supinator muscle, just superficial to the radiohumeral joint, the nerve divides into the superficial and deep branches. The deep motor branch, commonly referred to as the posterior interosseous nerve, passes between the superficial and deep portions of the supinator muscle. The superficial branch of the radial nerve continues distally deep to the brachioradialis. The radial nerve is classically described as innervating the triceps, anconeus, brachioradialis, ECRL, and ECRB. The posterior interosseous nerve usually innervates the supinator and extensors of the hand, although there is significant variability regarding innervation patterns of the extensor muscles by the radial and posterior interosseous nerves [35].

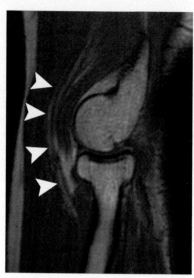

Fig. 16. Sagittal T1-weighted image shows the radial nerve (*arrowheads*) running between the deep brachialis and superficial brachioradialis muscles.

The posterior interosseous nerve courses distally through a fibromuscular tunnel termed the radial tunnel. The radial tunnel commences at the level of the capitellum near the proximal border of the supinator and extends to the distal margin of the supinator muscle [26,35]. The supinator tunnel refers to the distal portion of the radial tunnel and corresponds to the fatty space between the superficial and deep portions of the supinator muscle through which the posterior interosseous nerve passes. The roof of the radial tunnel is formed by fibrous bands of adjacent muscles, the Leash of Henry (recurrent radial artery vessels) and the Arcade of Frohse. The Arcade of Frohse is the fibrous arch formed by the proximal border of the superficial portion of the supinator and demarcates the proximal portion of the supinator tunnel. The radial tunnel is prone to compression at four primary sites: fibrous bands forming the proximal roof of the tunnel, the Leash of Henry, the Arcade of Frohse, and the ECRB muscle [35]. Various terms have been used to describe impingement of posterior interosseous nerve within the radial tunnel, including radial tunnel syndrome, supinator syndrome, posterior interosseous nerve syndrome, and resistant tennis elbow syndrome [36].

The radial nerve is best shown on axial images, and is most consistently seen at the proximal margin of the elbow joint within a strip of fat between brachioradialis and brachialis muscles [26]. In many cases the superficial and posterior interosseous branches can be demonstrated where the radial nerve bifurcates at the level of the radiocapitellar joint. The posterior interosseous nerve is identified within the supinator tunnel between the superficial and deep portions of the supinator muscle.

At the level of the elbow the median nerve lies deep to the lacertus fibrosis along the medial aspect of the brachialis muscle. The median nerve is slightly medial to the brachial artery and biceps tendon at the level of the elbow joint. The brachial artery bifurcates at the level of the radial head into radial and ulnar arteries, which continue distally with the superficial branch of the radial nerve and ulnar nerve, respectively. The median nerve passes superficial to the ulnar head of the pronator teres, thus separated from the ulnar artery, and then passes deep to the fibrous arch formed by the two heads of the flexor digitorum superficialis. Muscular branches of the median nerve at the level of the elbow joint provide motor innervation to the pronator teres and flexor muscles. Visualization of the median nerve can be difficult, particularly if there is little surrounding perineural fat. The nerve often can be seen between the pronator teres and brachialis muscles on axial MR images at the proximal margin of the elbow joint.

Impingement of the median nerve, or pronator syndrome, usually occurs as it passes between the ulnar and humeral heads of the pronator teres. Less commonly the median nerve may be entrapped by a thickened lacertus fibrosis or fibrous arch of the flexor digitorum superficialis. In patients with a supracondylar process, the nerve may be impinged as it passes through the fibro-osseous tunnel created by the ligament of Struthers.

The anterior interosseous nerve is the major branch of the median nerve in the forearm, arising 5 to 8 cm distal from the elbow joint at the inferior margin of the pronator teres. The nerve courses distally along the interosseous membrane, deep to the flexor digitorum profundus and flexor pollicis longus, which receive motor supply from the nerve. Impingement of the anterior interosseous nerve, termed "Kiloh Nevin syndrome," may mimic pronator syndrome clinically.

Routine axial images with the elbow in full extension and the wrist supinated allow consistent identification of all major nerves [37]. Occasionally, specialized axial views with the elbow in flexion may be useful for further characterization of the ulnar nerve and cubital tunnel. Images obtained during elbow flexion reveal narrowing of the cubital tunnel, attenuation of the perineural fat, bulging of the medial head of the triceps, and flattened morphology of the ulnar nerve. Specialized axial views with pronation of the forearm may be helpful for better characterization of the median and radial nerves [37].

Bursal anatomy

Several bursa may occur about the elbow, the most important of which are the cubital and olecranon bursae. The cubital bursae include the bicipitoradial bursa and the interosseous bursa [38]. The bicipitoradial bursa covers the anterior aspect of the radial tuberosity and is intimately associated with the insertion of the biceps brachii. With pronation of the forearm, the radial tuberosity impinges the bicipitoradial bursa and biceps tendon between the radius and ulna. The bicipitoradial bursa may become distended with repetitive mechanical trauma, infection, or an inflammatory arthropathy. The interosseous bursa is stated to occur in approximately 20% of individuals and is located along the medial aspect of the antecubital fossa adjacent to the biceps tendon and along the brachialis muscle [1].

Three bursae occur posteriorly, the best known being the superficial olecranon bursa that is found in the subcutaneous tissue dorsal to the olecranon. This bursa is reported to develop at the age of 7 years and may become inflamed following direct acute trauma, chronic repetitive stress, infection, and various inflammatory disorders, such as gout and rheumatoid arthritis. The deep intratendinous bursa occurs within the substance of the triceps near its insertion on the olecranon, and the deep subtendinous bursa is found deep to the triceps tendon near the tip of the olecranon. Less common bursa include subcutaneous medial and lateral epicondylar bursae, ulnar nerve bursa, and the subanconeus bursa [1].

Summary

The elbow is a complex joint consisting of three separate but intimate articulations, which in simplest terms, is classified as a hinge joint. Stability of the elbow is provided by the biomechanical axis of the osseous infrastructure and superimposed soft tissue supporting structures, most notably the ligamentous complexes. The anterior bundle of the ulnar collateral ligament, the lateral ulnar collateral ligament, and the ulnohumeral articulation play the most important role in maintaining joint stability. The numerous muscles surrounding the elbow provide supplemental dynamic stabilization of the joint and can be classified according to their position relative to the joint. Three major nerves pass about the elbow and are predisposed to impingement as they traverse soft tissue and fibro-osseous tunnels.

The superior soft tissue contrast resolution of MR imaging affords excellent demonstration of the joint and supporting structures and is thus an important tool for patients with suspected elbow or neuromuscular derangement. Knowledge of normal imaging anatomy is imperative for diagnosis of elbow pathology, and normal anatomic variants must be recognized to prevent misdiagnosis.

References

[1] Morrey BF. The elbow and its disorders. Philadelphia: W.B. Saunders; 2000.

[2] Rosenberg ZS, Beltran J, Cheung YY. Pseudodefect of the capitellum: potential MR imaging pitfall. Radiology 1994;191:821–3.

[3] Cotten A, Jacobson J, Brossmann J, et al. MR arthrography of the elbow: normal anatomy and diagnostic pitfalls. J Comput Assist Tomogr 1997;21:516–22.

[4] Rosenberg ZS, Beltran J, Cheung Y, Broker M. MR imaging of the elbow: normal variant and potential diagnostic pitfalls of the trochlear groove and cubital tunnel. AJR Am J Roentgenol 1995; 164:415–8.

[5] Rosenberg ZS, Bencardino J, Beltran J. MR imaging of normal variants and interpretation pitfalls of the elbow. Magn Reson Imaging Clin N Am 1997;5:481–99.

[6] Mallisee TA, Boynton MD, Erickson SJ, Daniels DL. Normal MR imaging anatomy of the elbow. Magn Reson Imaging Clin N Am 1997;5:451–79.

[7] Closkey RF, Goode JR, Kirschenbaum D, Cody RP. The role of the coronoid process in elbow stability. A biomechanical analysis of axial loading. J Bone Joint Surg [Am] 2000;82:1749–53.

[8] Cage DJ, Abrams RA, Callahan JJ, Botte MJ. Soft tissue attachments of the ulnar coronoid process. An anatomic study with radiographic correlation. Clin Orthop 1995;320:154–8.

[9] Glajchen N, Schwartz ML, Andrews JR, Gladstone J. Avulsion fracture of the sublime tubercle of the ulna: a newly recognized injury in the throwing athlete. AJR Am J Roentgenol 1998;170:627–8.

[10] Gray H, Williams PL, Bannister LH. Gray's anatomy: the anatomical basis of medicine and surgery. New York: Churchill Livingstone; 1995.

[11] Pecina M, Boric I, Anticevic D. Intraoperatively proven anomalous Struthers' ligament diagnosed by MRI. Skeletal Radiol 2002;31:532–5.

[12] Clarke RP. Symptomatic, lateral synovial fringe (plica) of the elbow joint. Arthroscopy 1988; 4:112–6.

[13] Duparc F, Putz R, Michot C, et al. The synovial fold of the humeroradial joint: anatomical and histological features, and clinical relevance in lateral epicondylalgia of the elbow. Surg Radiol Anat 2002;24:302–7.

[14] Awaya H, Schweitzer ME, Feng SA, et al. Elbow synovial fold syndrome: MR imaging findings. AJR Am J Roentgenol 2001;177:1377–81.

[15] Morrey BF, An KN. Functional anatomy of the ligaments of the elbow. Clin Orthop 1985; 201:84–90.

[16] O'Driscoll SW, Jaloszynski R, Morrey BF, An KN. Origin of the medial ulnar collateral ligament. J Hand Surg [Am] 1992;17:164–8.

[17] Timmerman LA, Andrews JR. Histology and arthroscopic anatomy of the ulnar collateral ligament of the elbow. Am J Sports Med 1994; 22:667–73.

[18] Munshi M, Pretterklieber M, Chung C, et al. Anterior bundle of the ulnar collateral ligament: evaluation of anatomic relationships using MR imaging, MR arthrography and gross anatomic and histologic analysis. RSNA 2002 Scientific Program. Radiology 2003;225(Suppl):1627.

[19] Timmerman LA, Andrews JR. Undersurface tear of the ulnar collateral ligament in baseball players. A newly recognized lesion. Am J Sports Med 1994;22:33–6.

[20] Beckett KS, McConnell P, Lagopoulos M, Newman RJ. Variations in the normal anatomy of the collateral ligaments of the human elbow joint. J Anat 2000;197(Pt 3):507–11.

[21] Dunning CE, Zarzour ZD, Patterson SD, et al. Ligamentous stabilizers against posterolateral rotatory instability of the elbow. J Bone Joint Surg [Am] 2001;83:1823–8.

[22] Cotten A, Jacobson J, Brossmann J, et al. Collateral ligaments of the elbow: conventional MR imaging and MR arthrography with coronal oblique plane and elbow flexion. Radiology 1997; 204:806–12.

[23] Potter HG, Hannafin JA, Morwessel RM, et al. Lateral epicondylitis: correlation of MR imaging, surgical, and histopathologic findings. Radiology 1995;196:43–6.

[24] Bredella MA, Tirman PF, Fritz RC, et al. MR imaging findings of lateral ulnar collateral ligament abnormalities in patients with lateral epicondylitis. AJR Am J Roentgenol 1999;173:1379–82.

[25] Boles CA, Kannam S, Cardwell AB. The forearm: anatomy of muscle compartments and nerves. AJR Am J Roentgenol 2000;174:151–9.

[26] Rosenberg ZS, Bencardino J, Beltran J. MR features of nerve disorders at the elbow. Magn Reson Imaging Clin N Am 1997;5:545–65.

[27] Williams BD, Schweitzer ME, Weishaupt D, et al. Partial tears of the distal biceps tendon: MR appearance and associated clinical findings. Skeletal Radiol 2001;30:560–4.

[28] Seiler JG III, Parker LM, Chamberland PD, et al. The distal biceps tendon. Two potential mechanisms involved in its rupture: arterial supply and mechanical impingement. J Shoulder Elbow Surg 1995;4:149–56.

[29] Matsuura S, Kojima T, Kinoshita Y. Cubital tunnel syndrome caused by abnormal insertion of triceps brachii muscle. J Hand Surg [Br] 1994;19:38–9.

[30] Spinner RJ, Hayden FR Jr, Hipps CT, Goldner RD. Imaging the snapping triceps. AJR Am J Roentgenol 1996;167:1550–1.

[31] Dellon AL. Musculotendinous variations about the medial humeral epicondyle. J Hand Surg [Br] 1986;11:175–81.

[32] Bozentka DJ. Cubital tunnel syndrome pathophysiology. Clin Orthop 1998;351:90–4.

[33] Gelberman RH, Yamaguchi K, Hollstien SB, et al. Changes in interstitial pressure and cross-sectional area of the cubital tunnel and of the ulnar nerve with flexion of the elbow. An experimental study in human cadavera. J Bone Joint Surg [Am] 1998;80:492–501.

[34] O'Hara JJ, Stone JH. Ulnar nerve compression at the elbow caused by a prominent medial head of the triceps and an anconeus epitrochlearis muscle. J Hand Surg [Br] 1996;21:133–5.

[35] Mazurek MT, Shin AY. Upper extremity peripheral nerve anatomy: current concepts and applications. Clin Orthop 2001;383:7–20.

[36] Resnick D, Kang HS. Internal derangements of joints: emphasis on MR imaging. Philadelphia: W.B. Saunders; 1997.

[37] Kim YS, Yeh LR, Trudell D, Resnick D. MR imaging of the major nerves about the elbow: cadaveric study examining the effect of flexion and extension of the elbow and pronation and supination of the forearm. Skeletal Radiol 1998; 27:419–26.

[38] Skaf AY, Boutin RD, Dantas RW, et al. Bicipitoradial bursitis: MR imaging findings in eight patients and anatomic data from contrast material opacification of bursae followed by routine radiography and MR imaging in cadavers. Radiology 1999;212:111–6.

ELSEVIER
SAUNDERS

RADIOLOGIC
CLINICS
OF NORTH AMERICA

Radiol Clin N Am 44 (2006) 569–581

Normal MR Imaging Anatomy of the Wrist and Hand

Joseph S. Yu, MD*, Paula A. Habib, BA

- Technical considerations
- Wrist anatomy
  - *Distal radioulnar joint*
  - *Triangular fibrocartilage complex*
  - *Ligaments*
  - *Tendons*
  - *Carpal tunnel*

- *Guyon's canal*
- Hand anatomy
  - *Ligaments*
  - *Tendons*
- Summary
- References

MR imaging is widely used in the evaluation of internal derangement of joints. In the past, the use of hand and wrist MR imaging lagged behind imaging of larger joints, largely because of technical limitations of spatial resolution and signal-to-noise (SNR) ratio when imaging the small anatomic structures [1]. However, with recent technical advances in extremity coil design, MR imaging has provided us with new insights into the difficult anatomy of the wrist by allowing improved visualization of the relationship of the muscles, ligaments, tendons, and bone [2,3]. Although the limits of spatial resolution afforded by specialized surface coils and signal processing methods may not have yet been completely realized at 1.5 Tesla, the potential for significant improvements in hand and wrist imaging is likely to rest with the advent of higher strength magnets [4–6].

Technical considerations

To visualize the small structures of the hand and wrist, spatial resolution and image quality must be optimized. At 1.5 Tesla, MR image quality is enhanced with the application of dedicated extremity coils, a small field of view (8–12 cm), and thin-slice thickness, on the order of 1 to 2 mm [7–10]. Recently, microscopy coils have been shown to elicit higher resolution images than standard production coils, but these coils require meticulous positioning and are limited by less than optimal depiction of deeper structures [2]. Higher field strength magnets have the ability to produce images that are high in both SNR and contrast-to-noise (CNR) ratios and, thus, have the capability of generating images with higher spatial resolution. Recent investigations of the wrist at 3.0 Tesla have shown that the effect of the field strength alone increases the CNR ratio by a magnitude of 2.0 to 2.9 times compared with 1.5 Tesla, if all other parameters are kept constant [11]. Efficient high resolution imaging at 3.0 Tesla can also be achieved, allowing the prescription of thinner slices than are possible at 1.5 Tesla while preserving the image quality [12]. Super high-field magnets hold the promise of surpassing current limitations in spatial resolution. Early images acquired at 8.0

This article was previously published in *Magnetic Resonance Imaging Clinics of North America* 2004;12: 207–219.
Department of Radiology, Ohio State University Medical Center, 633 Means Hall, 1654 Upham Drive, Columbus, OH 43210, USA
* Corresponding author.
E-mail address: yu-1@medctr.osu.edu (J.S. Yu).

doi:10.1016/j.rcl.2006.04.008

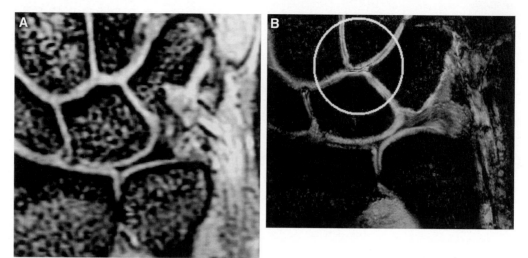

Fig. 1. Effect of magnet strength on spatial resolution. (*A*) Coronal three-dimensional gradient recalled echo (3D GRE) images on 1.5 Tesla (T) magnet acquired with a dedicated wrist coil. (*B*) Coronal two-dimensional (2D) GRE images on an 8 T system with a prototype radio-frequency (RF) coil. Note that the spatial resolution is exquisite, allowing unparalleled imaging of the cartilage layers between the carpal bones (*circle*).

Tesla have been shown to have an in-plane resolution of 100 to 140 μm (**Fig. 1**) [4,13–16].

Numerous pulse sequences are currently available from which to choose: spin-echo, two- and three-dimensional Fourier transformation sequences, and fat-suppression techniques all have been used in the assessment of the wrist [9]. More sophisticated software has introduced newer techniques, including thin-slice spin-echo techniques. The use of volumetric gradient-recalled echo (GRE) sequences provides thin sections at a higher SNR ratio than routine two-dimensional Fourier transform imaging [17]. T1-weighted sequences and short tau inversion recovery are useful for depiction of marrow pathology. The outstanding contrast afforded by these MR imaging techniques provides excellent depiction of the anatomy of the hand and wrist, including the intrinsic and extrinsic ligaments and components of the triangular fibrocartilage complex (TFCC) of the wrist, the components of the carpal tunnel, and the tendons, ligaments, and interstitial soft tissues of the hand and fingers.

Wrist anatomy

The wrist is a complex and unusual joint because normal function depends on the integrated action

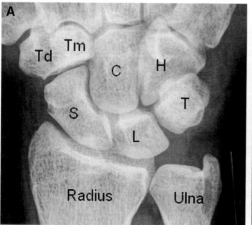
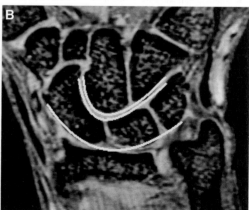

Fig. 2. Carpal anatomy. (*A*) Frontal view of the wrist shows the osseous structures. The pisiform (not labeled) lies adjacent to the triquetrum (T). C, capitate; H, hamate; L, lunate; S, scaphoid; Td, trapezoid; Tm, trapezium. (*B*) The carpal arcs (*white lines*) delineate normal carpal alignment. Any break in the arcs indicates a shift in the position of a carpal bone from instability or trauma.

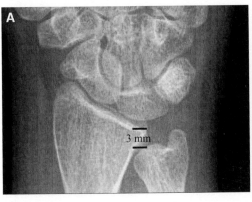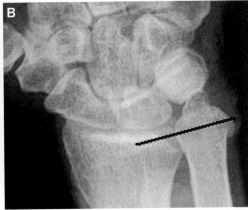

Fig. 3. Ulnar variance. (*A*) Negative ulnar variance. There is an association with Keinbock's disease (avascular necrosis of the lunate) when the length discrepancy exceeds 3 mm. (*B*) Positive ulnar variance. This condition increases the risk of abutment syndrome and triangular fibrocartilage (TFC) tears.

of a number of tissue structures including the carpal and forearm bones, the intrinsic and extrinsic ligaments, tendons, and the components of the TFCC. The wrist is composed of eight carpal bones that are aligned in two groups of four, comprising the proximal and distal carpal rows (Fig. 2). The proximal carpal row consists of the scaphoid, lunate, triquetrum, and pisiform bones, and the distal row consists of the trapezium, trapezoid, capitate, and hamate bones. The carpus is concave on its palmar surface, and it forms the roof of the carpal tunnel, which confines the flexor tendons and adjacent median nerve [18]. The distal radius articulates with the scaphoid and lunate, as well as with the ulna through the radiocarpal and distal radioulnar joints (DRUJs), respectively.

The wrist, as seen arthrographically, is actually composed of a series of articulations that are separated into several major compartments including the DRUJs, radiocarpal, pisiform-triquetral, midcarpal, common carpometacarpal, first carpometacarpal, and intermetacarpal compartments.

The ulnar variance denotes the relative length of the ulna with respect to the articular margin of the radius (Fig. 3). A negative ulnar variance indicates that the ulna is shorter than the radius, and a positive ulnar variance indicates a relatively longer ulna. Neutral variance occurs when both bones are equal in length.

Distal radioulnar joint

The distal radius has a quadrilateral appearance, and its articular surface has two concave depressions that articulate with the scaphoid and lunate bones. The articular surface tilts ulnarly and volarly. A medial depression, the sigmoid notch, receives

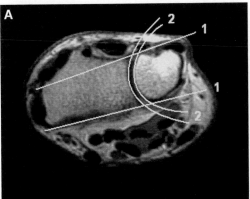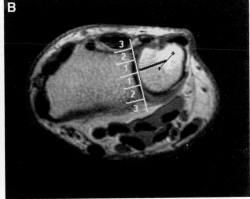

Fig. 4. Assessing DRUJ stability. (*A*) In the Mino method (*1*), the head of the ulna lies between the dorsal and volar marginal lines of the radius. In the congruency method (*2*), the arcs formed by the articular surfaces of the sigmoid notch of the radius and the head of the ulna are virtually parallel. (*B*) In the epicenter method, a perpendicular line (*thick black line*) drawn to the midpoint of a line between the epicenter of the ulnar styloid and the head of the ulna aligns with the middle of the sigmoid notch (zone *1*).

the rounded head of the distal ulna, forming the DRUJ. Cross-sectional imaging techniques such as CT and MR imaging are useful for assessment of the DRUJ because they allow direct inspection of the articulation. Assessment of instability should be performed with full pronation and supination. Between full pronation and supination, the distal radius can rotate approximately 150° around the ulnar head. Maximum contact between the ulnar head and radius occurs when the forearm is in mid-rotation. In the neutral position, the distal ulna articulates with the radius in the sigmoid notch. During pronation, the ulna moves dorsally, and during supination the ulnar head moves volarly. There are three different techniques (the Mino, congruency, and epicenter methods) for evaluating the integrity of the DRUJ on CT or MR imaging (Fig. 4) [19,20].

Triangular fibrocartilage complex

The TFCC is the primary stabilizer of the DRUJ. It also cushions the ulnar head and lunate during axial loading of the wrist. It is composed of the articular disk, the triangular ligament, the meniscal homolog, the volar and dorsal radioulnar ligaments, the volar ulnolunate and ulnotriquetral ligament, and the sheath of the extensor carpi ulnaris (ECU) tendon [2,21–23].

Four osseous structures border the TFCC. The head of the ulna and the sigmoid notch of the radius form the proximal border of the TFCC. The articular disk, which is composed of fibrocartilage, is triangular in shape and situated on a horizontal, crescent-shaped articular surface of the ulnar head. It inserts on the radius at the prominence of the sigmoid notch distally (Fig. 5). The ulnar portion of the disk is broader, inserting at the

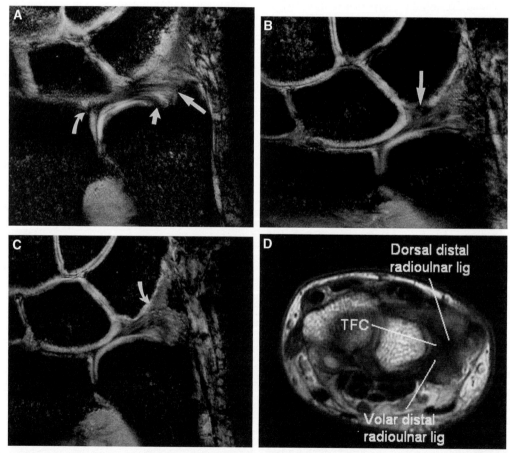

Fig. 5. Triangular fibrocartilage complex. (*A*) Coronal 2D GRE 8 T image shows the insertions of the TFC on the prominence of the sigmoid notch (*curved arrow*), the styloid process (*long arrow*), and the ulnar fovea (*short arrow*). (*B*) Coronal 2D GRE 8 T image shows the triquetral (*arrow*) insertion of the TFC. (*C*) The meniscal homolog insertion is shown on the ulnar border of the triquetrum (*curved arrow*). (*D*) Axial spin-echo T1-weighted image show the thickened margins of the TFC, which are referred to as the *dorsal* and *volar radioulnar ligaments.*

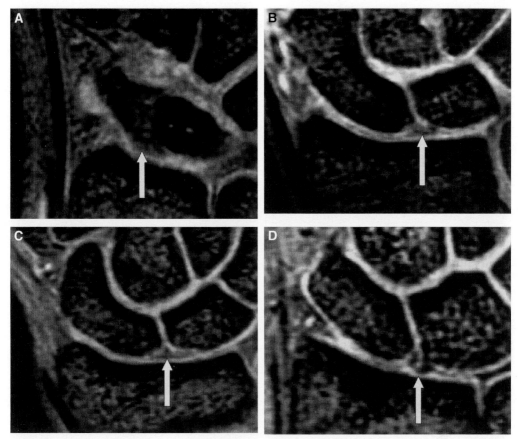

Fig. 6. Scapholunate ligament. (*A–D*) Coronal 3D GRE images show the variability of appearances of the scapholunate ligament (*arrows*) depending on the level and anatomic variation in thickness.

base of the ulnar styloid process and the adjacent ulnar fovea through the upper and lower lamina of the triangular ligament [22]. The volar and dorsal margins of the articular disk are thickened, referred to as the *radioulnar ligaments*, and the center of the disk is thin. The disk is usually two to three times thicker ulnarly than radially and is vascularized by branches of the ulnar and posterior interosseous arteries. The central and radial aspects of the disc are relatively avascular [24]. The meniscal homolog is a structure that resides between the ulna and triquetrum, having a common origin with the triangular ligament, and inserting on the ulnar border of the triquetrum.

The volar ulnolunate and ulnotriquetral ligament arise from the volar aspect of the middle third of the articular disk and insert on the volar aspect of the lunate and triquetrum, forming the anterior band of the triquetral sling [25]. The dorsal radiotriquetral ligament forms the posterior band of the triquetral sling and is oriented obliquely from the posteromedial aspect of the distal radius to the dorsal proximal surface of the triquetrum. The sheath of the ECU tendon merges with the dorsal triangular ligament to form the posteromedial margin of the TFCC.

Ligaments

The intrinsic carpal ligaments originate and insert onto the carpal bones and act to restrict motion between the carpal bones [26]. The two most important interosseous ligaments are the scapholunate (Fig. 6) and lunotriquetral (Fig. 7) ligaments, which connect the bones in the proximal row thus preventing communication between the radiocarpal and midcarpal compartments [27–31]. These ligaments tend to be C-shaped and are thicker dorsally and ventrally. The central portion is membranous. The radial collateral ligament is a thickening in the radiocarpal joint that extends from the tip of the radial styloid process to the radial side of the scaphoid and trapezium. The ulnar collateral ligament is a connective tissue cord that extends from the ulnar styloid process and below the base of the pisiform to the adjacent medial part of the flexor retinaculum (Fig. 8).

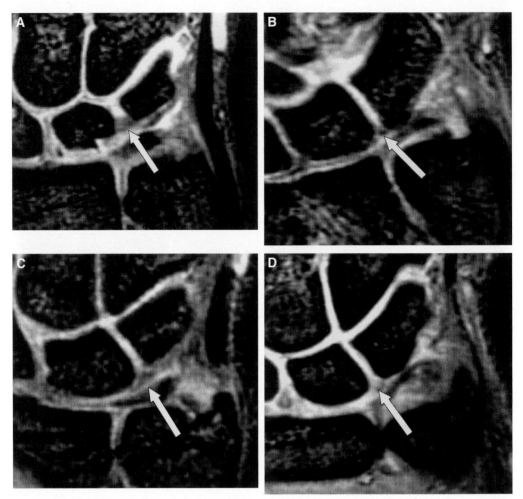

Fig. 7. Lunotriquetral ligament. (*A–D*) Coronal 3D GRE images show the variability of appearances of the lunotriquetral ligament (*arrows*), which is similar to the scapholunate ligament depending on the level and anatomic variation in thickness.

The extrinsic carpal ligaments limit motion and stabilize the proximal carpal row [32]. The extrinsic ligaments originate in the forearm, insert onto the carpal bones, and are classified by their locations as either volar or dorsal. The volar radiocarpal ligaments (Fig. 9) are stronger and thicker than the dorsal ligaments (Fig. 10). The most important of these ligaments are the radioscaphocapitate, short and long radiolunate, volar deltoid, and dorsal radiotriquetral ligaments [28,31,33].

The integrity of the intrinsic and extrinsic ligaments is critical for the maintenance of carpal stability [32]. The arcs define the normal relationship between carpal bones and are composed of three parallel arcs along the proximal articular margins of the proximal carpal row, the distal articular margins of the proximal carpal row, and the proximal articular margins of the distal carpal row. Disruption of the carpal arcs can be an indication of a ruptured ligament, which can destabilize the central column. The central column of the wrist is composed of the lunate and capitate. In normal anatomy, a continuous line can be drawn through the long axis of the radius, lunate, capitate, and third metacarpal bone. A normal lunocapitate angle is less than 20°. An intersecting line drawn through the long axis of the scaphoid creates an angle (scapholunate angle) of 30° to 60° degrees. Intercalary segmental instability denotes disruption of the scapholunate angle, lunocapitate angle, or both, and can occur in either the dorsal or volar direction.

Tendons

The tendons of the wrist are grouped into flexor and extensor compartments. The extensor tendons are divided into six compartments on the dorsal aspect of the wrist and are sequentially numbered from the radial to the ulnar side (Fig. 11A). These tendons

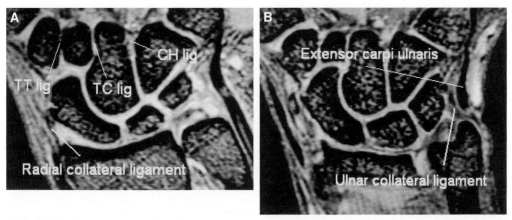

Fig. 8. Collateral ligaments of the wrist. (*A*) Coronal 3D GRE image shows the relationship of the radial collateral ligament to the radial styloid and the distal aspect of the scaphoid. CH, capitohamate; TC, trapeziocapitate; TT, trapeziotrapezoid. (*B*) The ulnar collateral ligament is part of the triangular fibrocartilage complex.

lie superficial to the carpal bones and interosseous ligaments. The first compartment is located lateral to the distal radius and contains the abductor pollicis longus and extensor pollicis brevis tendons. The second compartment is located lateral to Lister's tubercle, an osseous protuberance on the dorsal distal radius, and contains the extensor carpi radialis brevis and longus tendons. The tendons of the first and second compartments are frequently traumatized during injuries in which the hand is outstretched. The third compartment is located medial to Lister's tubercle and contains the extensor pollicis longus tendon. The fourth extensor compartment contains the extensor indicis proprius and extensor digitorum communis tendons, and the fifth compartment contains the extensor digiti minimi

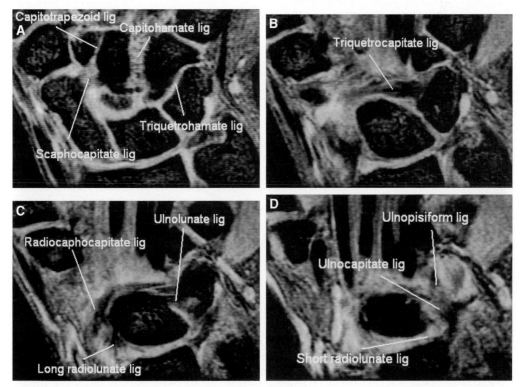

Fig. 9. Volar extrinsic ligaments of the wrist. (*A–D*) Coronal 3D GRE images at different levels show the dominant volar carpal ligaments.

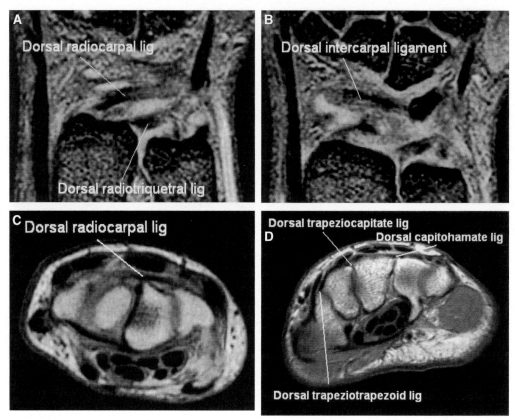

Fig. 10. Dorsal extrinsic ligaments of the wrist. (*A, B*) Coronal 3D GRE images at different levels show the dominant dorsal carpal ligaments. (*C, D*) Axial spin-echo T1-weighted images show the dorsal radiocarpal ligaments and the dorsal intercarpal ligaments.

tendon. The sixth compartment, located medial to the ulnar styloid, contains the ECU tendon and also is frequently injured during wrist trauma.

The flexor tendons, which begin in the distal forearm, are located on the volar aspect of the wrist and reside either within or adjacent to the carpal tunnel (see Fig. 11B). The flexor pollicis longus is dorsal and lateral to the median nerve. It inserts on the distal phalanx of the thumb and is enveloped by the radial bursa [34]. The flexor digitorum superficialis and

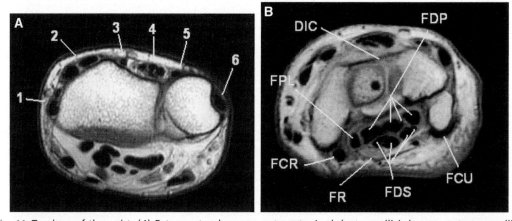

Fig. 11. Tendons of the wrist. (*A*) Extensor tendon compartments: 1, abductor pollicis longus, extensor pollicis brevis; 2, extensor carpi radialis longus, extensor carpi radialis brevis; 3, extensor pollicis longus; 4, extensor digitorum and indicis; 5, extensor digiti minimi; 6, extensor carpi ulnaris. (*B*) Flexor tendons: DIC, dorsal intercarpal ligament; FCR, flexor carpi radialis; FCU, flexor carpi ulnaris; FDP, flexor digitorum profundus; FDS, flexor digitorum superficialis; FPL, flexor pollicis longus; FR, flexor retinaculum.

profundus tendons reside medial to the median nerve, enveloped by the ulnar bursa. The flexor carpi radialis tendon is located outside the carpal tunnel, coursing just lateral to the tunnel, and inserts on the base of the second metacarpal bone. The flexor carpi ulnaris tendon is located medial to the ulnar nerve and inserts principally on the pisiform but with fibers extending to the hamulus and the base of the fourth and fifth metacarpal bones [35].

Carpal tunnel

The normal carpal tunnel anatomy is accurately delineated on MR imaging (**Fig. 12**) [36–38]. The anterior boundary of the carpal tunnel is the flexor retinaculum, also known as the *transverse carpal ligament*, which appears as a broad low-signal intensity structure that extends from the hamate hamulus to the scaphoid and trapezial tuberosities. The posterior boundary is formed by the deep palmar carpal ligaments and the carpal bones. Because of the rigidity of the boundaries of the carpal tunnel, any process that either increases the volume of the contents of the tunnel or decreases the size of the tunnel can result in symptoms. The median nerve is located in the superficial radial portion of the canal, immediately deep to the flexor

retinaculum. Morphologically, it typically is round or flat, and on MR imaging it appears intermediate in signal intensity. It is constant in caliber throughout the carpal canal, but its location or position varies with wrist flexion or extension; flexion can produce anatomic crowding in the canal [39,40]. The axial plane is the most optimal imaging plane for evaluating the contents of the carpal tunnel.

Guyon's canal

On the anteromedial aspect of the wrist, there is a fibro-osseous tunnel approximately 4 cm long containing the ulnar nerve and accompanying ulnar artery and vein. This space is called *Guyon's canal* (see **Fig. 12**). The conspicuity of the ulnar nerve is enhanced by the adipose tissue surrounding the nerve. This anatomic region is well depicted with MR imaging and is clinically relevant because the ulnar nerve may become entrapped in this location by masses, other space-occupying processes, and post-traumatic osseous deformities [39,41–44].

Hand anatomy

The metacarpophalangeal and interphalangeal joints are structurally similar. They are both condyloid in morphology, with a rounded head

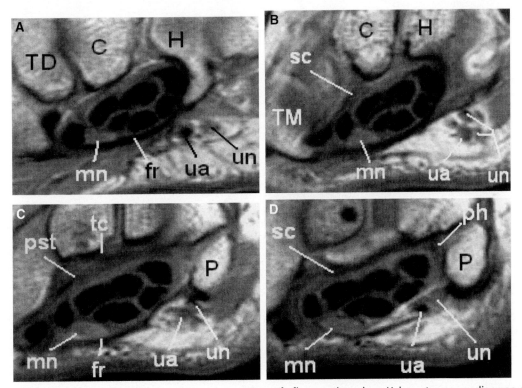

Fig. 12. (*A–D*) Carpal tunnel and Guyon's canal: C, capitate; fr, flexor retinaculum; H, hamate; mn, median nerve; P, pisiform; ph, pisohamate ligament; pst, palmar scaphotriquetral ligament; sc, scaphocapitate ligament; tc, triquetrocapitate ligament; TD, trapezoid; TM, trapezium; ua, ulnar artery; un, ulnar nerve.

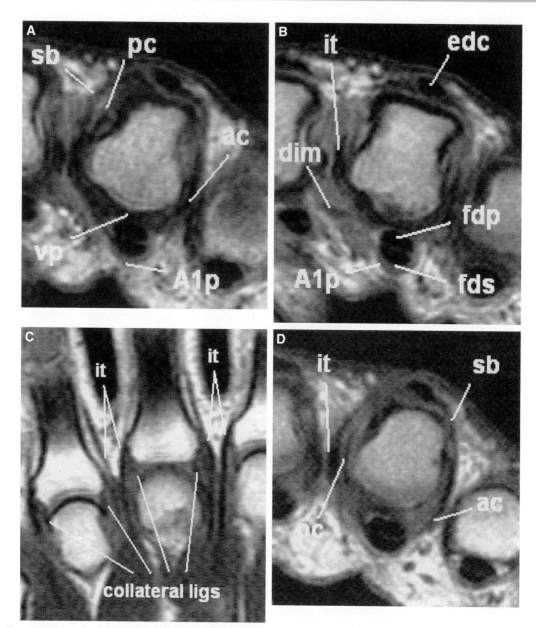

Fig. 13. Anatomy of the metacarpophalangeal joint. (A–C) Axial spin-echo T1-weighted images show the ligaments, muscles, tendons, and osseous structures of the metacarpophalangeal joint: A1p, A1 pulley; ac, accessory collateral ligament; dim, deep intermetatarsal ligament; edc, extensor digitorum communis tendon; fdp, flexor digitorum profundus; fds, flexor digitorum superficialis; it, interosseous tendon; pc, proper collateral ligament; sb, sagittal band; vp, volar plate. (D) Coronal T1-weighted image shows the relationship of the interosseous tendons to the collateral ligaments.

proximally articulating with a concave distal articular surface. The shape of the articular surface, which allows a greater degree of flexion than extension, dictates the range of motion of these hinge-type joints.

Ligaments

The ligamentous anatomy of the metacarpophalangeal and interphalangeal joints is similar [45]. The collateral and palmar ligaments form a bridge that binds the bones together (Fig. 13). The palmar ligament (also referred to as the *volar plate*) is a dense band of fibrocartilaginous tissue adhering firmly to the proximal edge of the phalanges and spreading at the sides to merge with the collateral ligament fibers. The collateral ligaments are strong cords that attach proximally to depressions on the condylar

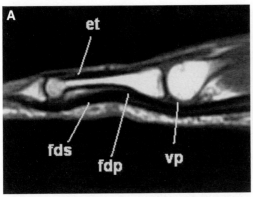
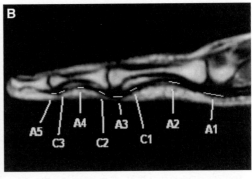

Fig. 14. Anatomy of the pulley system of the finger. (*A*) Sagittal spin-echo T1-weighted image shows the flexor tendons and a portion of the extensor tendon complex: et, extensor tendon communis; fdp, flexor digitorum profundus; fds, flexor digitorum superficialis; vp, volar plate. (*B*) Sagittal spin-echo T1-weighted image shows the locations of the retinacular sheaths that act as the pulleys of the flexor tendons. There are five annular (A1–A5) and three C-shaped (C1–C3) pulleys that prevent "bow-stringing" during flexion. (*Adapted from* Berquist TH. Anatomy. In: Berquist TH, editor. MRI of the hand and wrist. Philadelphia: Lippincott Williams & Wilkins; 2003. p. 1–32; with permission).

heads and spread distally to the palmar aspect of the base of the phalanges.

Tendons

The flexor tendons of the hand are held in place in the digits by fibrous sheaths that attach along the borders of the proximal and middle phalanges, to the interphalangeal joint capsules, and to the surface of the distal phalanx [46]. The attachments of these sheaths form semicylindrical tunnels that allow the passage of tendons (Fig. 14). Transversely oriented across the shafts of the proximal and middle phalanges are thickened connective tissue bands that create the pulley system of the fingers.

The extensor tendons of the hand arise from a common compartment in the dorsum of the wrist, occupying a space beneath the extensor retinaculum [47]. Over the dorsum of the proximal interphalangeal joint, the extensor tendon divides into three slips. The central slip is broad and inserts on the dorsal lip of the middle phalanx. The two lateral slips merge with fibers of the tendons of the lumbrical muscles on the radial side and the interosseous tendons on both sides; they then converge into a common band that inserts on the dorsal lip of the distal phalanx.

Summary

MR imaging of the wrist has been used in the evaluation of a wide spectrum of diseases. Its multiplanar and exquisite soft tissue contrast capabilities allow for depiction of subtle osseous and soft tissue pathology. Although the anatomy is complex, the reader has gained a thorough understanding of the indications for MR imaging of the wrist, as well as the clinically relevant anatomy and pathology.

References

[1] Yu JS. Magnetic resonance imaging of the wrist. Orthopedics 1994;17:1041–8.

[2] Yoshioka H, Ueno T, Tanaka T, Shindo M, Itai Y. High-resolution MR imaging of the triangular fibrocartilage complex (TFCC): comparison of microscopy coils and a conventional small surface coil. Skeletal Radiol 2003;32:575–81.

[3] Robittaille PML, Abduljalil AM, Kangarlu A. Ultra high resolution imaging of the human head at 8 Tesla: 2K × 2K for Y2K. J Comput Assist Tomogr 2000;24:2–8.

[4] Farooki S, Ashman CJ, Yu JS, Abduljalil A, Chakeres D. In-vivo high resolution MR imaging of the carpal tunnel at 8.0 Tesla. Skeletal Radiol 2002;31:451–6.

[5] Ashman CJ, Farooki S, Abduljalil AM, Chakeres DW. In vivo high-resolution coronal MRI of the wrist at 8.0 T. J Comput Assist Tomogr 2002;26:387–91.

[6] Constable RT, Henkelman RM. Contrast, resolution, and detectability in MR imaging. J Comput Assist Tomogr 1991;15:297–303.

[7] Totterman SMS, Miller RJ. Triangular fibrocartilage complex: normal appearance on coronal three-dimensional gradient-recalled-echo MR images. Radiology 1995;195:521–7.

[8] Zlatkin MB, Chao PC, Osterman AL, Schnall MD, Dalinka MK, Kressel HY. Chronic wrist pain: evaluation with high-resolution MR imaging. Radiology 1989;173:723–9.

[9] Yu JS, Brahme SK, Resnick D. MR imaging of the wrist. RSNA Categorical Course in Musculoskeletal Radiology Syllabus 1993;87–96.

[10] Weiss KL, Beltran J, Shamam OM, Stilla RF, Levey M. High-field MR surface-coil imaging of the hand and wrist. I. Normal anatomy. Radiology 1986;160:143–6.

[11] Saupe N. Pruessmann KP, Luechinger R, Boesiger P, Marincek B, Weishaupt D. MR imaging of the wrist at 3T: comparison between 1.5T and 3T [abstract 1374]. Presented at the Annual Meeting of the Radiological Society of North America. November 30–December 5, 2003. p. 656.

[12] Gold GE, Han E, Stainsby J, Wright GA, Brittain JH, Beaulieu CF. Relaxation times and contrast in musculoskeletal MR imaging at 3. 0 Tesla [abstract 1372]. Presented at the Annual Meeting of the Radiological Society of North America. November 30–December 5, 2003. p. 655.

[13] Robittaille PML, Abduljalil AM, Kangarlu A. Ultra high resolution imaging of the human head at 8 Tesla: 2K × 2K for Y2K. J Comput Assist Tomogr 2000;24:2–8.

[14] Robittaille P-ML, Abduljalil AM, Kangarlu A, Zhang X, Yu Y, Burgess R, et al. Human magnetic resonance imaging at 8 T. NMR Biomed 1998; 11:263–5.

[15] Abuljalil AM, Kangarlu A, Zhang X, Burgess RE, Robitaille P-ML. Acquisition of human multi-slice MR images at 8 Tesla. J Comput Assist Tomogr 1999;23:335–40.

[16] Kangarlu A, Abduljalil AM, Robitaille P-ML. T1- and T2-weighted imaging at 8 Tesla. J Comput Assist Tomogr 1999;23:875–8.

[17] Totterman SM, Miller R, Wasserman B, Blebea JS, Rubens DJ. Intrinsic and extrinsic carpal ligaments: evaluation by three-dimensional Fourier transform MR imaging. AJR Am J Roentgenol 1993;160:117–23.

[18] Mesgarzadeh M, Schneck CD, Bonakdarpour A. Carpal tunnel: MR imaging. I. Normal anatomy. Radiology 1989;171:743–8.

[19] Wechsler RJ, Wehbe MA, Rifkin MD, Edeiken J, Branch HM. Computed tomography diagnosis of distal radioulnar subluxation. Skeletal Radiol 1987;16:1–5.

[20] Mino DE, Palmer AK, Levinsohn EM. The role of radiography and computed tomography in the diagnosis of subluxation and dislocation of the distal radioulnar joint. J Hand Surg [Am] 1983; 8:23–31.

[21] Golimbu CN, Firooznia H, Melone CP Jr, Rafii M, Weinreb J, Leber C. Tears of the triangular fibrocartilage of the wrist: MR imaging. Radiology 1989;173:731–3.

[22] Nakamura T, Makita A. The proximal ligamentous component of the triangular fibrocartilage complex. Functional anatomy and three-dimensional changes in length of the radioulnar ligament during pronation and supination. J Hand Surg [Br] 2000;25:479–86.

[23] Tubiana R, Thomine JM, Mackin E. Functional anatomy. In: Examination of the hand and wrist. 2nd ed. London: Mosby; 1996. p. 1–39.

[24] Berquist TH. Anatomy. In: Berquist TH, editor. MRI of the hand and wrist. Philadelphia: Lippincott Williams & Wilkins; 2003. p. 1–32.

[25] Smith DK. Volar carpal ligaments of the wrist: normal appearance on multiplanar reconstructions of three-dimensional Fourier transform MR imaging. AJR Am J Roentgenol 1993; 161:353–7.

[26] Taleisnik J. The ligaments of the wrist. J Hand Surg [Am] 1976;1(2):110–8.

[27] Smith DK, Snearly WN. Lunotriquetral interosseous ligament of the wrist: MR appearances in asymptomatic volunteers and arthrographically normal wrists. Radiology 1994; 191:199–202.

[28] Totterman SMS, Miller RJ. Scapholunate ligament: normal MR appearance on three-dimensional gradient-recalled-echo images. Radiology 1996;200:237–41.

[29] Brown RR, Fliszar E, Cotten A, Trudell D, Resnick D. Extrinsic and intrinsic ligaments of the wrist: normal and pathologic anatomy at MR arthrography with three-compartment enhancement. Radiographics 1998;18:667–74.

[30] Rominger MB, Bernreuter WK, Kenney PJ, Lee DH. MR imaging of anatomy and tears of wrist ligaments. Radiographics 1993;13:1233–46.

[31] Smith DK. Scapholunate interosseous ligament of the wrist: MR appearances in asymptomatic volunteers and arthrographically normal wrists. Radiology 1994;192:217–21.

[32] Yeager B, Dalinka M. Radiology of trauma to the wrist: dislocations, fracture dislocations, and instability patterns. Skeletal Radiol 1985; 13:120–30.

[33] Smith DK. Dorsal carpal ligaments of the wrist: normal appearance on multiplanar reconstructions of three-dimensional Fourier transform MR imaging. AJR Am J Roentgenol 1993; 161:119–25.

[34] Ham SJ, Konings JG, Wolf RFE, Mooyaart EL. Functional anatomy of the soft tissues of the hand and wrist. In vivo excursion measurement of the flexor pollicis longus tendon using MRI. Magn Reson Imaging 1993;11:163–7.

[35] Anderson MW, Kaplan PA, Dussault RG, Degnan GG. Magnetic resonance imaging of the wrist. Curr Probl Diagn Radiol 1998;27:187–229.

[36] Zeiss J, Skie M, Ebraheim N, Jackson WT. Anatomic relations between the median nerve and flexor tendons in the carpal tunnel: MR evaluation in normal volunteers. AJR Am J Roentgenol 1989;153:533–6.

[37] Maurer J, Bleschkowski A, Tempka A, Felix R. High resolution MR imaging of the carpal tunnel and the wrist. Acta Radiol 2000;41:78–83.

[38] Middleton WD, Kneeland JB, Kellman GM, Cates JD, Sanger JR, Jesmanowicz A, et al. MR imaging of the carpal tunnel: Normal anatomy and preliminary findings in the carpal tunnel syndrome. AJR Am J Roentgenol 1987;148: 307–16.

[39] Zeiss J, Jakab E, Khimji T, Imbriglia J. The ulnar tunnel at the wrist (Guyon's canal): normal MR anatomy and variants. AJR Am J Roentgenol 1992;158:1081–5.

[40] Mesgarzadeh M, Schneck CD, Bonakdarpour A. Carpal tunnel: MR imaging. Normal anatomy. Radiology 1989;171:743–8.

[41] Ruocco MJ, Walsh JJ, Jackson JP. MR imaging of ulnar nerve entrapment secondary to an anomalous wrist muscle. Skeletal Radiol 1998; 27:218–21.

[42] Subin GD, Mallon WJ, Urbaniak JR. Diagnosis of ganglion in Guyon's canal by magnetic resonance imaging. J Hand Surg [Am] 1989; 14A:640–3.

[43] Dodds GA III, Hale D, Jackson WT. Incidence of anatomic variants in Guyon's canal. J Hand Surg [Am] 1990;15A:352–5.

[44] Netscher D, Cohen V. Ulnar nerve compression at the wrist secondary to anomalous muscles: a patient with a variant of abductor digiti minimi. Ann Plast Surg 1997;39(6):647–51.

[45] Theumann NH, Pfirrmann CWA, Drape JL, Trudell DJ, Resnick D. MR imaging of the metacarpophalangeal joint of the fingers. Conventional MR imaging and MR arthrographic findings in cadavers. Radiology 2002;222:431–45.

[46] Hauger O, Chung CB, Lektrakul N, Botte MJ, Trudell D, Boutin RD, et al. Pulley system in the fingers: normal anatomy and simulated lesions in cadavers at MR imaging, CT and US with and without contrast material distension of the tendon sheath. Radiology 2000;217:201–12.

[47] Kaplan PA. Anatomy, injuries, and treatment of the extensor apparatus of the hand and fingers. Clin Orthop 1959;13:24–41.

ELSEVIER
SAUNDERS

RADIOLOGIC
CLINICS
OF NORTH AMERICA

Radiol Clin N Am 44 (2006) 583–594

MR Imaging of Ligament Injuries to the Elbow

Liat J. Kaplan, MD, Hollis G. Potter, MD*

- Imaging technique
  Coil selection
  Patient positioning
  Pulse sequences
- Ligamentous pathology
  Anatomy

- Medial (ulnar) collateral ligament complex
  Lateral collateral ligament complex
  Elbow dislocation
- Summary
- References

The elbow joint has many features that render it particularly amenable to evaluation using MR imaging. Its inherent obliquity makes it difficult to image with conventional radiographs and CT. The multiplanar capabilities of MR imaging enable the joint to be imaged in true sagittal and coronal planes, facilitating more accurate diagnosis of ligamentous injuries. In addition, stability of the elbow joint is imparted by osseous as well as soft tissue constraints, and injuries often involve several of these structures. The superior soft tissue contrast of MR imaging provides simultaneous evaluation of bone and soft tissue, allowing for assessment of all the static and dynamic stabilizers, making accurate diagnoses possible using a single examination. Recent advances have improved visualization of the physes in children, which, combined with a lack of ionizing radiation, is of considerable utility in imaging the pediatric elbow. As clinical and conventional imaging techniques are often limited in the assessment of elbow instability, direct visualization of the anatomy is helpful in guiding clinical management.

Imaging technique

Coil selection

The use of surface coils is essential if adequate images of the ligamentous structures in the elbow are to be obtained. Circumferential and phased-array coils improve signal to noise and are therefore preferable. Shoulder or dedicated elbow coils confer optimal signal to noise; anterior loop coils may also be used but visualization of posterior structures may be limited by poor signal to noise.

Patient positioning

As with all musculoskeletal imaging, proper patient positioning is of paramount importance. Care should be taken to position the patient as comfortably as possible to minimize motion. Imaging is best performed with the patient supine, with the arm at his or her side, the elbow fully extended, and the forearm in supination. Positioning the patient prone with the arm over the head and the elbow in an extremity coil should be avoided as this position places traction on the brachial plexus. In addition, it often is a difficult position for symptomatic

This article was previously published in *Magnetic Resonance Imaging Clinics of North America* 2004;12: 221–232.
Department of Radiology and Imaging, Division of Magnetic Resonance Imaging, Hospital for Special Surgery, 535 East 70th Street, New York, NY 10021, USA
* Corresponding author.
E-mail address: potterh@hss.edu (H.G. Potter).

doi:10.1016/j.rcl.2006.04.007

patients to maintain and image quality may therefore be compromised by patient motion [1].

Pulse sequences

Imaging in the axial, sagittal, and coronal planes should be performed for comprehensive evaluation of ligamentous structures in the elbow. Technique should impart adequate slice and spatial resolution, afforded by a combination of thin slices and high-imaging matrix, respectively, to adequately demonstrate the ligaments. High-resolution gradient-echo sequences are especially useful in evaluating the low-intensity ligaments and tendons. In patients who cannot maintain full extension, such as those with intraarticular bodies, posterolateral impingement, or posterolateral rotatory instability, coronal thin slice (slice thickness 1.5 to 2 mm) gradient recalled-echo images can be useful. If necessary, three-dimensional acquisitions may be obtained and can be easily reformatted into a true coronal plane, which is helpful for evaluating the oblique fibers of some of the ligaments [2]. Cartilage-sensitive pulse sequences are also necessary, particularly in the evaluation of the throwing athlete [3]. Fat suppression techniques also are useful to discern subtle areas of traumatic bone marrow edema and fluid collections. Because of the diminished uniformity of the static field at the peripheral margins of the bore, fast-inversion recovery sequences are recommended over frequency-selective techniques.

In postoperative patients, the utility of gradient-echo sequences is significantly diminished as a result of the artifact caused by paramagnetic hardware. In this population, therefore, fast-spin echo techniques are the most useful, and gradient-echo images may be eliminated [3].

The use of intraarticular gadolinium or saline has been advocated as previous studies reported increased sensitivity, particularly for partial-thickness ligament tears, with MR arthrography as compared with conventional MR imaging [4–6]. However, proper imaging techniques obviate the need for intraarticular contrast. One of the advantages of MR imaging is its noninvasive nature; arthrography compromises this and makes the examination more time-consuming and costly. In addition, the administration of intraarticular contrast prevents the capsule and ligaments from being visualized in their "native" state, leading to the loss of potentially useful information. A sample protocol is described in Box 1 [3].

Ligamentous pathology

Anatomy

The elbow is a hinge joint stabilized by osseous and soft tissue structures. The most important bony

---

Box 1:   Sample protocol

Series 1: Coronal inversion recovery (fat saturation): TR/TE (milliseconds) 4900/15 (Ef); TI 150; matrix 256 × 192; two excitations; FOV 11 to 12 cm; slice thickness 3 mm.

Series 2: Axial fast spin echo: TR/TE (milliseconds) 3000 to 4000/34 (Ef); echo train length, 6 to 8; matrix 512 × 256; two excitations; FOV 11 to 12 cm; slice thickness 3.5 to 4 mm with no interslice gap.

Series 3: Coronal multiplanar gradient recalled: TR/TE (milliseconds) 400 to 450/20; flip angle 45 degrees; matrix 256 × 256; two excitations; slice thickness 1.6 to 1.8 mm with no interslice gap.

Series 4: Sagittal fast spin echo: TR/TE (milliseconds) 3500 to 4000/34 (Ef) ; echo train length 6 to 8; matrix 512 × 256 to 320; 2 excitations; FOV 12 to 13 cm; slice thickness 3.5 mm with no interslice gap.

Series 5: Coronal fast spin echo: TR/TE (milliseconds) 3500 to 4000/34; echo train length 6 to 8; matrix 512 × 384; two excitations; FOV 11 to 12 cm; slice thickness 3.5 mm with no interslice gap.

Abbreviations: Ef, effective; FOV, field of view; TI, time to inversion; TE, time to echo; TR, time to repetition.

---

stabilizer is the articulation between the trochlea and olecranon; this is particularly significant when the elbow is in extension [7]. Soft tissue stabilizers include ligaments, muscles, and the joint capsule [8]. Two ligamentous structures are primarily responsible for maintaining joint stability. These are the anterior bundle of the medial collateral ligament (A-MCL) and the ulnar band of the lateral collateral ligament (also known as the lateral ulnar collateral ligament) [8].

Medial (ulnar) collateral ligament complex

The medial or ulnar collateral ligament complex consists of the anterior and posterior bundles of the medial collateral ligament (MCL), which arise from the medial humeral epicondyle and insert on the medial aspect of the coronoid process of the ulna and posteromedial olecranon respectively, and the transverse bundle [9]. The anterior bundle (A-MCL) runs deep to the origin of the flexor-pronator tendon. It is the strongest ligament in the elbow and comprises the largest component of the medial collateral ligament complex [7,10]. The horizontally oriented transverse bundle connects the distal portions of the anterior and posterior bands along the medial olecranon, is usually thin, and has a negligible role in joint stability [11,12]. It is not present in all patients; in addition, its clinical significance is minor and it is therefore not routinely evaluated on MR examinations of the elbow [13].

The anterior bundle, composed of anterior and posterior bands, is the most biomechanically important portion of the medial collateral ligament, being the primary stabilizer against valgus instability [8,10,14]. It can be readily distinguished as a discrete structure separate from the joint capsule, as opposed to the posterior bundle that has a more fan-shaped configuration and is essentially a thickening of the posterior capsule [7,11]. The anterior bundle, on average, is 21.1 mm long and 7.6 mm wide, and the average dimensions of the posterior bundle are 16.5 mm in length by 8.8 mm wide [7]. It is taut in extension and is therefore best visualized on the coronal sequences outlined in Box 1 [7]. Like all ligaments, the MCL is composed primarily of type I collagen and is therefore normally homogeneously low in signal (Fig. 1A). It has a broad-based origin from the humerus, but once it tapers, it should be uniform in thickness to its attachment on the ulna. A potential pitfall in the evaluation of the A-MCL is the focus of high signal intensity caused by a synovial invagination just deep to the humeral attachment of the ligament; this is normal and should not be confused with pathology [9].

A "reciprocating relationship" between the anterior and posterior bundles has been described by Regan et al [7]. In extension, the anterior bundle is taut, and as the elbow moves into flexion, the anterior bundle becomes lax, while the posterior bundle tightens [7]. This relationship is important to understand for proper patient positioning during the MR imaging examination. Though injury to the posterior bundle is uncommon, if it is clinically suspected, imaging should be performed with the elbow in flexion so that the ligament is taut and more readily evaluated [9].

Patients presenting with medial elbow pain often have a confusing clinical picture, and it may be difficult even for the most astute clinician to distinguish between pathology involving the medial collateral ligament, medial tendons, and cartilage [9]. MR imaging with thin slices (1.5 to 2 mm) can be of considerable clinical utility in the evaluation of medial elbow pain, as high spatial resolution and tissue contrast enable ligamentous and tendinous structures to be readily distinguished.

Injury to the A-MCL usually is caused by a valgus stress. On MR imaging, acute injury is manifest as signal hyperintensity, discontinuity of some or all of the fibers, and in cases of complete rupture, total discontinuity with or without retraction (Figs. 2 and 3). The authors' experience dictates that proximal tears are more common; however, careful scrutiny of the entire ligament is necessary, particularly for acute superimposed on chronic injuries. An avulsion fracture of the medial epicondyle may or may not be present.

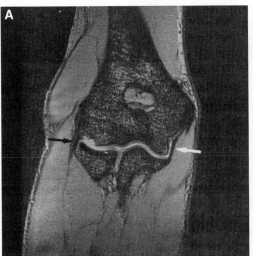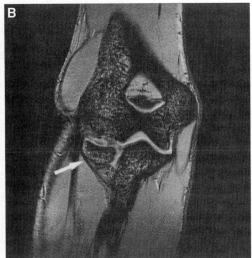

Fig. 1. Normal medial and radial collateral ligaments and lateral ulnar collateral ligament. Coronal gradient echo images demonstrate the normal homogeneously low signal intensity of the collateral ligaments. (*A*) The anterior bundle of the medial collateral ligament (*white arrow*) is taut in extension and courses from the medial humeral epicondyle to the coronoid process of the ulna, deep to the origin of the flexor-pronator tendon. The radial collateral ligament (*black arrow*) extends from the lateral humeral epicondyle to the proximal radius. (*B*) The lateral ulnar collateral ligament (*white arrow*) originates on the lateral humeral epicondyle and courses posteriorly around the radial neck to insert on the supinator crest of the ulna. As it is obliquely oriented, it may not be seen in its entirety on a single coronal image.

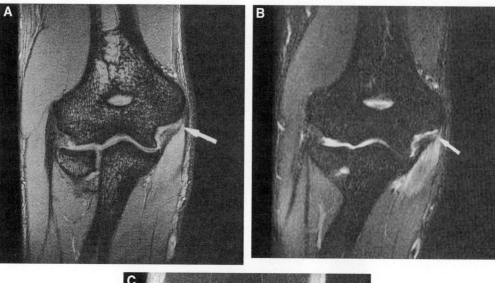

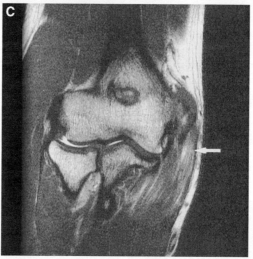

Fig. 2. Medial collateral ligament injury with flexor-pronator contusion. Coronal gradient-echo (*A*) and fat-saturated (*B*) images demonstrate hyperintensity of the medial collateral ligament with focal thinning (*arrows in A and B*), reflecting a focal complete tear of the anterior band, with only a few fibers remaining in continuity. In addition, hyperintensity in the surrounding muscle of the flexor-pronator mass (*white arrow in C*) represents concomitant muscle/tendon junction injury, seen on the coronal fat-saturated (*B*) and fast spin-echo (*C*) images.

In a 1992 study, Mirowitz and London [12] demonstrated a high correlation between abnormalities of the MCL seen on MR imaging and pathologic findings. High signal on T1 and T2-weighted images was found to correspond to hemorrhage and edema, and morphologic changes such as increased laxity and attenuation of the MCL also were confirmed pathologically. Nakanishi et al [4] performed MR saline arthrography in symptomatic throwing athletes and obtained histologic correlation; they concluded that increased T2 signal surrounding the ligament represented scar formation. They also found that extracapsular leakage of saline indicated the presence of a complete MCL tear or an avulsion fracture [4].

It is important to distinguish between complete and partial-thickness tears. Whereas complete tears usually produce signs of valgus instability on clinical examination, partial-thickness tears are more variable in presentation, and the clinical signs of instability may not be present. MR imaging can be useful in determining the precise location of partial-thickness tears, aiding in clinical management and potential surgical planning [9]. In particular, a characteristic lesion—a partial-thickness under-surface tear of the A-MCL—has been described [5,6,15] in which the deep fibers of the ligament avulse off of the ulnar rather than the humeral attachment. The typical MR appearance of this lesion has been described as a "T sign." It was initially

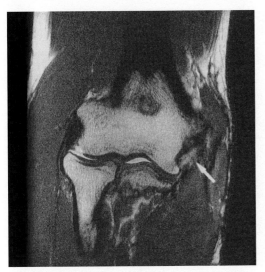

Fig. 3. Tear of medial collateral ligament reconstruction in a professional pitcher. Coronal fast spin-echo image demonstrates complete disruption (*arrow*) of a palmaris tendon graft used for reconstruction of the medial collateral ligament.

described on CT arthrography as leakage of contrast around the detached portion of the MCL and within the intact superficial fibers of the MCL and capsule, but has since been seen on MR arthrography as well [6,15]. Timmerman et al [15], in a prospective study, performed CT arthrography and MR imaging on 25 baseball players with medial elbow pain. They found that the sensitivity of CT arthrography was 100% for full-thickness tears and 71% for partial-thickness tears, with a specificity of 91%, using surgical inspection as a standard. In the same study, MR imaging was 100% sensitive for full-thickness tears but only 14% sensitive for partial-thickness tears. Specificity was 100%. The discrepancy in the sensitivity of MR imaging for full-thickness and partial-thickness tears may be related to technical factors; this is difficult to judge because specific parameters for the MR images were not provided [15]. Schwartz et al [6] found that when intraarticular gadolinium was administered, sensitivity for partial-thickness tears increased to 86%, with 100% specificity. This led them to conclude that MR arthrography is necessary for the diagnosis of partial-thickness tears; however, if proper MR imaging technique is used, partial-thickness tears can be accurately diagnosed without arthrography. Careful evaluation of the anterior bundle is of paramount importance, particularly because it is often not well seen arthroscopically, and MR imaging is often the only way in which it can be fully evaluated [5,16].

In addition to causing injury to the MCL, valgus load may lead to other injuries, and a comprehensive evaluation of the elbow must include these structures. Cartilage injury may be seen, particularly involving the radiocapitellar joint in the case of an acute valgus overload, and in the posterior margin of the trochlea with valgus extension overload. Cartilage-sensitive fast spin-echo images should be scrutinized to exclude the presence of such lesions, and a careful search for intraarticular bodies should be performed. Muscle strains and contusions to the medial flexors may be seen as areas of signal hyperintensity (see Fig. 2). Valgus load also can lead to tears of the posteromedial capsule, as well as ulnar neuropathy; all of these are well evaluated on the fast spin-echo sequences outlined in Box 1 [3].

Chronic A-MCL pathology is prevalent in throwing athletes, who sustain tremendous repetitive valgus stresses at the elbow [17]. Imaging findings in chronic injury include plastic deformation, manifest as a diffuse increase in signal intensity, thickening of the ligament, "microtears," and remodeling, manifest as thickening and increased signal intensity [1,3,9]. An acute on chronic pattern also may be seen, in which a remodeled ligament demonstrates focally increased signal intensity with adjacent soft tissue edema [1]. Associated findings in patients with chronic A-MCL injury include hypertrophic spurring at the coronoid attachment [3], capsular scarring, and loose bodies. With eventual ligament failure, the MCL is reconstructed with a soft tissue (typically tendon) graft, and MR imaging may be used to assess for tears of the construct (see Fig. 3).

Chronic A-MCL injury often is associated with valgus extension overload or posteromedial impingement, a clinical syndrome common in throwing athletes and other patients who experience repetitive valgus stresses. In this syndrome, extreme repetitive valgus stresses (such as those incurred during the early acceleration phase of pitching) create high contact pressures at the posterior medial margin of the humeral ulnar joint and cause osteophytes to form off the medial olecranon. During elbow extension, these osteophytes impinge on the olecranon fossa, causing reduced range of motion as well as pain, and they may become detached and form intraarticular loose bodies [18]. These posteromedial osteophytes are often difficult to visualize on conventional radiographic views, although a lateral view obtained in maximum flexion may be helpful. Other findings associated with MCL injury include capsular scarring, or cartilage loss over the posterior trochlea or medial olecranon [9,18]. If a patient is unable to achieve full extension during MR imaging (best appreciated on sagittal images), posteromedial impingement should be a consideration, particularly if osteophytes are seen on the medial olecranon or if there is associated MCL pathology (Fig. 4).

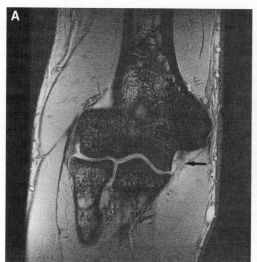
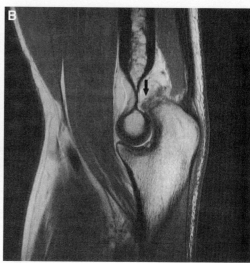

Fig. 4. Medial collateral ligament tear with posteromedial impingement. Coronal gradient-echo image (*A*) demonstrates a high-grade partial tear (*arrow*) of the medial collateral ligament. Sagittal fast spin-echo image (*B*) demonstrates a fracture through a posteromedial olecranon osteophyte (*arrow*), the presence of which indicates posteromedial impingement syndrome. Intermediate signal intensity surrounding the osteophyte reflects scarring of the adjacent capsule.

In children with medial elbow pain, MR imaging can be helpful in evaluating the physes and apophyses, as well as soft tissue constraints. Before fusion of the medial epicondylar apophysis, the A-MCL appears as a low signal linear structure that blends distally with the periosteum of the ulna [19]. The periosteum at this point is not completely apposed to the underlying bone and a high-signal zone of demarcation may be noted at the interface [19]. As the apophysis fuses, the zone of demarcation between the periosteum and ulnar cortex disappears and the A-MCL appears to insert directly onto the cortex [19]. A notable difference between the normal appearance of the A-MCL in children and in adults is that in children (before and after apophyseal fusion), the proximal insertion of the A-MCL typically exhibits high signal on fluid-sensitive sequences. This is thought to be the result of the higher elastin content as compared with type I collagen, which makes up most of the substance of the ligament in adults, and care should be taken not to confuse this with pathology [19].

Before apophyseal fusion, valgus stresses are imparted to the physis rather than to the MCL, causing physeal widening, often with surrounding soft tissue edema, or fragmentation and resorption of the ossification center of the medial epicondyle (Figs. 5 and 6) [3,19]. This Salter fracture through the medial epicondylar physis reflects "Little League elbow." This is best evaluated on a physeal-sensitive pulse sequence such as a coronal fat-suppressed gradient echo sequence [3]. If untreated, the fracture through the growth plate may lead to deformity

(Fig. 7) or even eventual nonunion (Fig. 8) of the epicondyle. As the apophysis begins to fuse, valgus stress preferentially affects the MCL and apophyseal pathology is less prevalent [19]. With proper imaging techniques, the physis and the MCL are well evaluated on MR imaging, making it a useful modality in distinguishing between ligamentous and physeal injury in the pediatric population.

Lateral collateral ligament complex

The lateral collateral ligament complex consists of the radial collateral ligament, the annular ligament, and the lateral ulnar collateral ligament. In general, the lateral collateral ligament complex is a less robust and less well-defined structure than its medial counterpart, and unlike the MCL, its appearance can vary considerably among individuals [11]. On average, it measures approximately 19.9 mm in length by 9.7 mm wide [7]. The radial collateral ligament proper runs deep to the common extensor tendon, extending from the lateral humeral epicondyle to the proximal radius, and blends with the annular ligament anteriorly (see Fig. 1A) [20]. The annular ligament surrounds the radial head, acts primarily to stabilize the proximal radioulnar joint, and contributes minimally to elbow joint stability [21]. The lateral ulnar collateral ligament (LUCL) is a posterior structure extending from the lateral humeral epicondyle, where it is closely apposed to the common extensor tendon, to course around the radial neck posteriorly and insert on the supinator crest of the ulna (see Fig. 1B) [22,23].

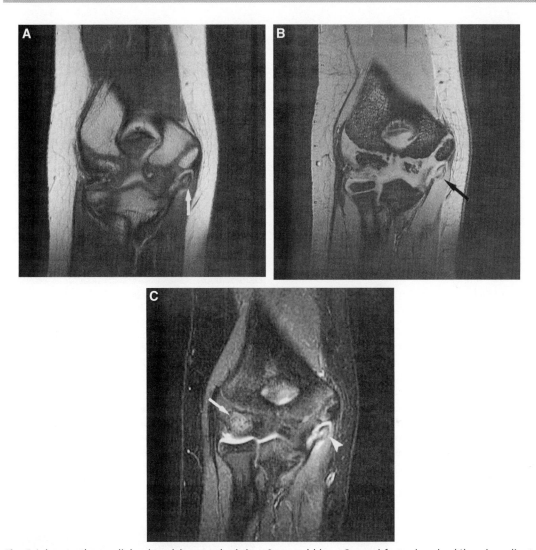

Fig. 5. Injury to the medial epicondylar apophysis in a 9-year-old boy. Coronal fast spin-echo (*A*) and gradient-echo (*B*) images demonstrate avulsion of the inferior portion of the medial epicondylar apophysis (*arrows*), to which the anterior bundle of the medial collateral ligament is attached. Coronal fat-saturated image (*C*) demonstrates hyperintensity in the soft tissues surrounding the avulsion (*arrowhead in C*). In addition, there is a bone marrow edema pattern (*arrow in C*) in the capitellum, indicative of early osteochondritis dissecans.

There has been some controversy over the relative importance of the various components of the lateral collateral ligament complex. Olsen et al [24] found that the radial collateral ligament was primarily responsible for stability. Dunning et al [21] found that though the LUCL was an important stabilizer, it was not solely responsible for protecting against posterolateral rotatory instability. However, the majority of studies have shown the LUCL to be one of the most important ligamentous stabilizers in the lateral elbow, and it should be carefully evaluated on every MR imaging examination (see references [2,7,14,22,23]).

The LUCL, like the A-MCL, is taut in extension and is best evaluated on coronal images, ideally obtained with a slice thickness of 2 mm or less. As it is an obliquely oriented structure, it is usually not seen on a single coronal image but can be followed from posterior to anterior on sequential images. The normal ligament is homogeneously low in signal intensity (Fig. 1B). MR imaging findings in acute LUCL injury resemble those described for the MCL: hyperintensity, discontinuity, and surrounding soft tissue edema (Figs. 8C and 9A). Tears more commonly occur at the proximal humeral attachment [2]. The appearance of a chronically torn and remodeled LUCL is similar to that described for the MCL, with findings including thickening, abnormally increased signal, and discontinuity.

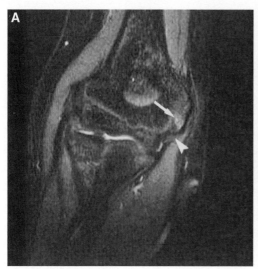
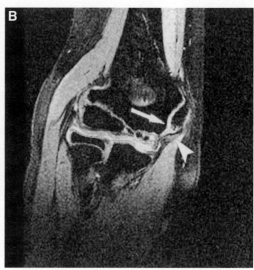

Fig. 6. Little League elbow in a 12-year-old boy. The patient sustained a valgus stress which caused injury to the medial epicondylar apophysis, manifest on a coronal fat-saturated image (*A*) as a bone marrow edema pattern and irregularity in the apophysis (*white arrow*) and on a physeal-sensitive coronal gradient-echo sequence (*B*) as physeal widening (*white arrow*). The valgus stress also caused injury to the medial collateral ligament (*arrowheads*), which is hyperintense on both pulse sequences. Although both structures are affected, most of the stress was imparted to the physis rather than the ligament, as is typical before apophyseal fusion.

Patients who have sustained an injury to the LUCL may have associated findings including cartilage loss, particularly over the medial humeral-ulnar joint, and intraarticular bodies [3]. LUCL pathology also has been shown to be associated with lateral epicondylitis, particularly if the latter is severe. In one study, Bredella et al demonstrated abnormalities of the LUCL in 63% of 35 patients with lateral epicondylitis, and if the epicondylitis was severe, the association was 100% [25]. Additionally, the LUCL is at risk for injury during open surgery for lateral epicondylitis and special care should be taken to evaluate the ligament in these cases [3].

Injury to the lateral ulnar collateral ligament has been implicated in posterolateral rotatory instability (PLRI), a clinical syndrome within the spectrum of elbow dislocation. PLRI usually is caused by a fall onto an outstretched hand with the forearm supinated, with a resultant axial and valgus load causing injury to the LUCL. This results in rotatory subluxation of the ulnohumeral joint, allowing posterolateral subluxation of the radial head with respect to the capitellum when the elbow is extended and the forearm supinated [23]. Symptoms may include lateral elbow pain, clicking, locking, and apprehension as the elbow approaches full extension, instability, and dislocation [23].

O'Driscoll et al [23] have shown the "lateral pivot shift test" to be useful in the diagnosis of PLRI. The test is performed with the patient's arm overhead;

the elbow is slowly flexed while axial compression and valgus and supination forces are applied. In a positive test, as elbow flexion approaches 40 degrees, the humeral-ulnar joint subluxates, and the forearm hinges on the biceps and brachialis tendons and on the medial soft tissues, allowing the radius to shift posterolaterally with respect to the

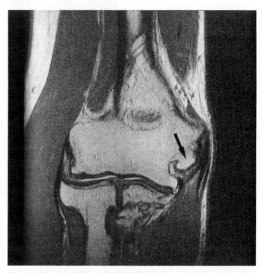

Fig. 7. Coronal fast spin-echo image demonstrating deformity of the medial epicondyle (*arrow*) in a 43-year-old man due to an apophyseal injury sustained before physeal closure, which led to bony overgrowth and deformity.

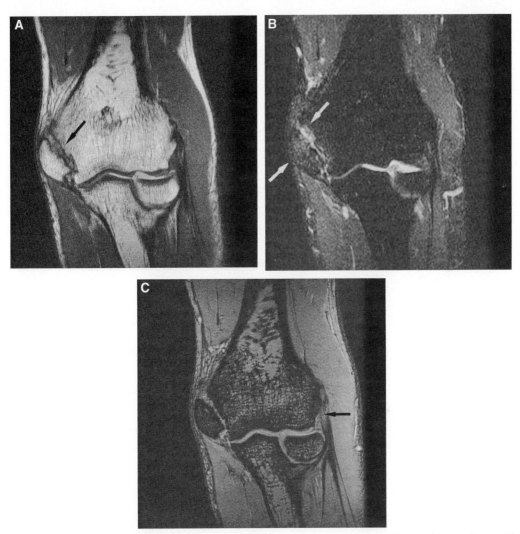

Fig. 8. Nonunion of Salter fracture through the medial epicondylar apophysis in a 25-year-old man. Coronal fast spin-echo image (*A*) demonstrates widening and irregularity of the physis (*arrow*), with intermediate signal in the fracture site representing fibrous union. Coronal fat-saturated image (*B*) demonstrates stress reaction in the surrounding bone, manifest as a bone marrow edema pattern (*arrows*). The patient had also sustained an elbow subluxation, causing injury to the lateral ulnar collateral ligament (LUCL). On a coronal gradient-echo image (*C*), partial disruption of the proximal LUCL is demonstrated (*arrow*).

humerus. As the elbow is flexed further, the radius snaps back into place, resulting in a palpable "clunk" [2]. Diagnosis often is difficult, as the clinical exam can be misleading unless performed under anesthesia; MR imaging can therefore be extremely useful in evaluating for tears of the ulnar collateral ligament in patients presenting with lateral elbow pain or instability [23]. Potter et al [2] have shown that MR imaging is a highly sensitive and specific for LUCL pathology in these patients. In addition to the findings in the ligament described above, secondary findings may be present on MR imaging that can suggest the presence of PLRI. For example, because patients often

demonstrate apprehension as the joint approaches full extension, inability to maintain full extension during the examination, as well as posterior subluxation of the radial head, may be seen on sagittal images in patients with PLRI (Fig. 9) [2,3].

Elbow dislocation

Elbow dislocations can result from complete disruption of the two primary ligamentous stabilizers of the elbow: the MCL and LUCL; however, clinical signs of dislocation and instability also may occur in the absence of a complete ligamentous disruption [14]. The mechanism of elbow dislocation usually involves external rotation of the forearm with

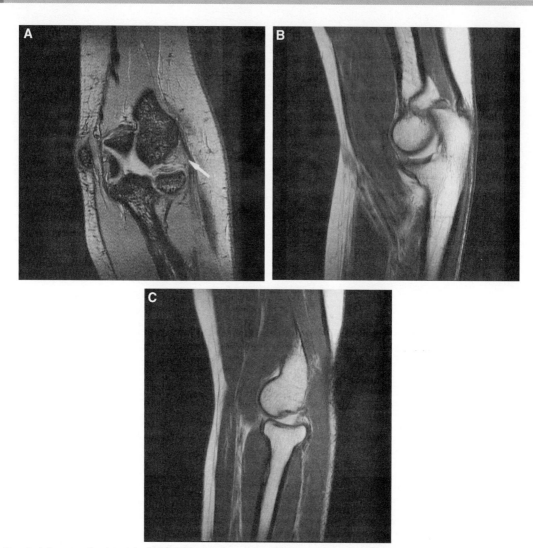

Fig. 9. Injury to the lateral ulnar collateral ligament (LUCL), resulting in posterolateral rotatory instability. Coronal gradient-echo (A) image demonstrates complete disruption of the proximal LUCL (arrow). Sagittal fast spin-echo images (B, C) demonstrate the sequelae of posterolateral rotatory instability: inability to maintain full extension (B) and posterior subluxation of the radial head with respect to the capitellum (C).

a valgus moment and a compressive load at the elbow, such as is experienced when a patient falls onto an outstretched arm [14]. O'Driscoll et al [14] described elbow dislocation as a spectrum consisting of three stages, with the site of injury progressing in a "circular" fashion from the lateral to the medial elbow. In stage 1 instability, there is injury to the LUCL, with or without injury to the RCL and posterolateral capsule. This manifests clinically as posterolateral rotatory instability. Stage 2 instability results from a more severe stress and involves the lateral collateral ligament complex as well as the anterior and posterior capsule. These patients will have a "perched" dislocation, in which the coronoid process is perched on the trochlea.

Stage 3a instability is characterized by additional involvement of the P-MCL, allowing the coronoid to travel more posteriorly behind the trochlea. Proper identification of stage 2 and 3a instability is important. Because the A-MCL is intact in these patients, they will maintain valgus stability after reduction. This is in contrast to patients who sustain greater loads to the elbow and develop stage 3b instability, in which the A-MCL is injured and the only remaining stabilizers are the muscles and osseous structures [14].

In chronic or severe dislocations, "telescoping" of the humerus into the ulna may be seen on sagittal MR images as a result of inferior migration and lack of support of the humerus. Concomitant osseous or chondral injury to the coronoid may also be seen in these patients. Feldman et al [26] described an osseous impaction injury to the radial head and capitellum. This may be seen on MR imaging as abnormal signal in the radial head and nonarticular posterior surface of the capitellum, or a frank defect may be seen.

Summary

MR imaging is a highly valuable tool in the evaluation of ligamentous injuries to the elbow. Its multiplanar capabilities and superior tissue contrast afford detailed evaluation of complex anatomy. Proper coil selection, pulse sequence parameters, and patient positioning enhance the ability of MR imaging to demonstrate subtle injuries to the ligaments and the regional osseous and soft tissue structures, including those not easily visualized at surgery. The primary ligamentous stabilizers of the elbow are the A-MCL and LUCL. Pathology of the MCL, encompassing acute and chronic injury, as well as the associated findings of posteromedial impingement, is often a difficult clinical diagnosis to establish, and MR imaging can be helpful in distinguishing ligamentous from tendinous or cartilaginous injury. Similarly, the LUCL is well evaluated on MR imaging and in the presence of pathology, the diagnosis of posterolateral rotatory instability can also be made. MR imaging is useful in the evaluation of children with elbow pain, as it can demonstrate physeal as well as ligamentous and osseous injury. With further advances in imaging technique and software, the ability to detect ligamentous injuries will continue to improve, allowing for more expeditious and accurate diagnoses.

References

[1] Potter HG, Sofka CM. Imaging. In: Altchek DW, Andrews JR, editors. The athlete's elbow. New York: Lippincott, Williams & Wilkins; 2001. p. 59–80.

[2] Potter HG, Weiland AJ, Schatz JA, Paletta GA, Hotchkiss RN. Posterolateral rotatory instability of the elbow: usefulness of MR imaging in diagnosis. Radiology 1997;204(1):185–9.

[3] Potter HG. Imaging of posttraumatic and soft tissue dysfunction of the elbow. Clin Orthop 2000; 370:9–18.

[4] Nakanishi K, Masatomi T, Ochi T, Ishida T, Hori S, Ikezoe J, et al. MR arthrography of elbow: evaluation of the ulnar collateral ligament of elbow. Skeletal Radiol 1996;25(7):629–34.

[5] Timmerman LA, Andrews JR. Undersurface tear of the ulnar collateral ligament in baseball players: a newly recognized lesion. Am J Sports Med 1994;22(1):33–6.

[6] Schwartz ML, Al-Zahrani S, Morwessel RM, Andrews JR. Ulnar collateral ligament injury in the throwing athlete: evaluation with saline-enhanced MR arthrography. Radiology 1995; 197(1):297–9.

[7] Regan WD, Korinek SL, Morrey BF, An K. Biomechanical study of ligaments around the elbow joint. Clin Orthop 1991;271:170–9.

[8] Morrey BF, An K. Articular and ligamentous contributions to the stability of the elbow joint. Am J Sports Med 1983;11(5):315–9.

[9] Gaary EA, Potter HG, Altchek DW. Medial elbow pain in the throwing athlete: MR imaging evaluation. Am J Roentgenol 1997;168(3):795–800.

[10] Hotchkiss RN, Weiland AJ. Valgus stability of the elbow. J Orthop Res 1987;5(3):372–7.

[11] Morrey BF, An K. Functional anatomy of the ligaments of the elbow. Clin Orthop 1985; 201:84–90.

[12] Mirowitz SA, London SL. Ulnar collateral ligament injury in baseball pitchers: MR imaging evaluation. Radiology 1992;185(2):573–6.

[13] Callaway GH, Field LD, Deng X, Torzilli PA, O'Brien SJ, Altchek DW, et al. Biomechanical evaluation of the medial collateral ligament of the elbow. J Bone and Joint Surg [Am] 1997; 79(8):1223–31.

[14] O'Driscoll SW, Morrey BF, Korinek S, An K. Elbow subluxation and dislocation: a spectrum of instability. Clin Orthop 1992;280:186–97.

[15] Timmerman LA, Schwartz ML, Andrews JR. Preoperative evaluation of the ulnar collateral ligament by magnetic resonance imaging and computed tomography arthrography: evaluation in 25 baseball players with surgical confirmation. Am J Sports Med 1994;22(1):26–31.

[16] Field LD, Callaway GH, O'Brien SJ, Altchek DW. Arthroscopic assessment of the medial collateral ligament complex of the elbow. Am J Sports Med 1995;32(4):396–400.

[17] Fleisig GS, Andrews JR, Dillman CJ, Escamilla RF. Kinetics of baseball pitching with implications about injury mechanisms. Am J Sports Med 1995;23(2):233–9.

[18] Wilson FD, Andrews JR, Blackburn TA, McCluskey G. Valgus extension overload in the pitching elbow. Am J Sports Med 1983;11(2):83–7.

[19] Sugimoto H, Ohsawa T. Ulnar collateral ligament in the growing elbow: MR imaging of normal development and throwing injuries. Radiology 1994;192(2):417–22.

[20] Murphy BJ. MR imaging of the elbow. Radiology 1992;184(2):525–9.

[21] Dunning CE, Zarzour ZDS, Patterson SD, Johnson JA, King GJW. Ligamentous stabilizers against posterolateral rotatory instability of the elbow. J Bone Joint Surg [Am] 2001;83(12): 1823–8.

[22] O'Driscoll SW, Horii E, Morrey BF, Carmichael SW. Anatomy of the ulnar part of

the lateral collateral ligament of the elbow. Clin Anat 1992;5:296–303.

[23] O'Driscoll SW, Bell DF, Morrey BF. Posterolateral rotatory instability of the elbow. J Bone Joint Surg [Am] 1991;73(3):440–6.

[24] Olsen BS, Søjbjerg JO, Dalstra M, Sneppen O. Kinematics of the lateral ligamentous constraints of the elbow joint. J Shoulder Elbow Surg 1996;5(5):333–41.

[25] Bredella MA, Tirman PFJ, Fritz RC, Feller JF, Wischer TK, Genant HK. MR imaging findings of lateral ulnar collateral ligament abnormalities in patients with lateral epicondylitis. Am J Roentgenol 1999;173(5):1379–82.

[26] Feldman DR, Schabel SI, Friedman RJ, Young JW. Translational injuries in posterior elbow dislocation. Skeletal Radiol 1997;26(2):134–6.

ELSEVIER
SAUNDERS

RADIOLOGIC
CLINICS
OF NORTH AMERICA

Radiol Clin N Am 44 (2006) 595–623

MR Imaging of Ligaments and Triangular Fibrocartilage Complex of the Wrist

Michael B. Zlatkin, MD*, Joel Rosner, MD

Imaging of the wrist with MR imaging can be difficult because of the small size of this joint, its complex anatomy, and its sometimes poorly understood pathologic lesions. A recent study by Hobby and co-workers [1] of 98 patients revealed that MR imaging of the wrist influences clinicians' diagnoses and management plans in most patients. This article summarizes the current diagnostic criteria that can be useful in interpreting abnormalities of the wrist ligaments and triangular fibrocartilage complex (TFCC) of the wrist in this difficult topic in joint MR imaging.

Anatomy

Ligamentous anatomy

The carpal ligaments may be classified as either extrinsic or intrinsic. The extrinsic ligaments link the carpal bones to the radius and ulna. The intrinsic or intercarpal ligaments connect the individual carpal bones.

Volar ligaments

The most functionally significant of the extrinsic ligaments are the volar radiocarpal ligaments [2]. There is considerable variation in the anatomic description of these ligaments [2–6]. These ligaments are the most important stabilizers of wrist motion. They originate from the volar aspect of the styloid process of the radius. Specifically, the radioscaphocapitate ligament (RSC; radiocapitate) connects the radius to the distal carpal row and plays an important role in preventing rotary subluxation of the scaphoid. The second and strongest, the radiolunatotriquetral

This article was previously published in *Magnetic Resonance Imaging Clinics of North America* 2004;12:301–331.
National Musculoskeletal Imaging, 13798 Northwest 4th Street, Sunrise, FL 33325, USA
* Corresponding author.
E-mail address: MBZlat@aol.com (M.B. Zlatkin).

doi:10.1016/j.rcl.2006.04.010

(RLT; radiotriquetral) ligament, connects the radius to the proximal carpal row (Fig. 1).

The volar extrinsic ligaments display low signal on MR images (see Fig. 1), although on three-dimensional (3D) images may have a striated appearance [7,8]. On coronal sequences, the volar radiocarpal ligaments are low signal intensity bands traversing obliquely from the radius to the carpal bones [9,10]. They can also be seen on sagittal images, and this is the preferred plain of review of these ligaments by some [7,8]. The radioscaphocapitate ligament is the most radial of the major volar ligaments. It originates at the radial styloid, crosses the waist of the scaphoid, and attaches to the head of the capitate. Some fibers of the radioscaphoidcapitate ligament may extend to the triquetrum. The radiolunatotriquetral ligament arises on the radial styloid process adjacent to the radioscaphocapitate ligament [9,11–13]. It courses distally and ulnarward to attach to the volar aspect of the triquetrum. It may be visualized in two portions, the radiolunate portion and the lunotriquetral portion. As such it has also been referred to as separate long radiolunate and volar lunotriquetral ligaments. This ligament serves as a volar sling for the lunate.

Of the small ligaments that attach to the palmar aspect of the scaphoid, lunate, and scapholunate interosseous ligament, that which attaches to the scapholunate is most often identified, and it originates more dorsal and medial. It is best seen on coronal images. It has a higher signal intensity than the other extrinsic ligaments. It is best described as the radioscapholunate ligament. It arises from the volar aspect of the distal portion of the radius and inserts into the proximal and volar surfaces of the scapholunate interval [5,14–16]. Some experts believe that this structure may not be a ligament but rather a neurovascular bundle, with components derived from the anterior interosseous and radial arteries and the anterior interosseous nerve [16].

The volar ulnocarpal ligaments [2,17] arise from the ulnar styloid process and the anterior margin of the TFCC (see Fig. 1). The ulnocarpal ligaments can best be seen on coronal sequences, but may also be identified on sagittal sequences [7,8]. They extend distally and laterally to the lunate and triquetral bones respectively. That which inserts on the lunate is the ulnolunate ligament. The band that inserts on the triquetrum is the ulnotriquetral ligament. There is also a distal portion of the ulnotriquetral ligament that extends on to the volar aspect of the capitate and lunate.

The deltoid ligament has a V shape (Fig. 2) and is an intrinsic ligament with a capitotriquetral (ulnar) and a capitoscaphoid (radial) arm. Disruption of the ulnar arm of the deltoid ligament may lead to dynamic midcarpal instability. The space of Pourier is an area of normal weakness in the volar aspect of the capsule, just proximal to the deltoid ligament. It is through this site of weakness where volar dislocation of the lunate occurs [18]. The deltoid ligament may be difficult to observe on conventional spin-echo images; however, Totterman [13] describes good visualization on thin section 3D fourier transform (FT) images. MR imaging arthrography also may aid in its visualization [12,19–21].

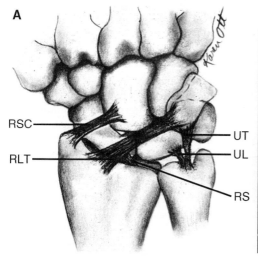
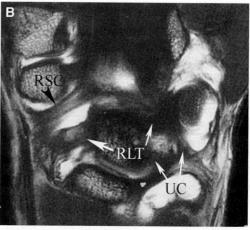

Fig. 1. Anatomy of the volar ligaments. (*A*) Diagram illustrating the volar radiocarpal and ulnocarpal ligaments. (*B*) Correlative coronal MR arthrogram image. RLT, radiolunatotriquetral ligament; RSC, radioscaphocapitate ligament; RS, radioscaphoid (radioscapholunate) ligament; UC, ulnocarpal ligaments; UL, ulnolunate ligament; UT, ulnotriquetral ligament.

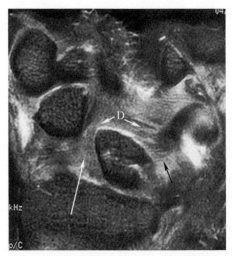

Fig. 2. Coronal MR image. The V-shaped deltoid ligament is shown (D). The volar aspects of the scapholunate (*long white arrow*) and lunate triquetral (*shorter dark arrow*) ligaments also are shown.

Dorsal ligaments

The dorsal radiocarpal ligament extends from the dorsal aspect of the radial styloid to terminate on the triquetrum [22–24]. In its course it traverses the lunate to which it is also attached (Fig. 3) [17,30]. It actually represents a thickening of the joint capsule. This structure may be viewed as a single structure or as several separate structures with a multitude of different names. The most consistent of these structures appears to be the radiotriquetral ligament. These ligaments generally are regarded as

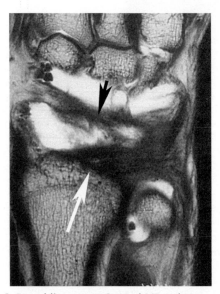

Fig. 3. Dorsal ligaments. Coronal MR arthrogram image. The dorsal radiocarpal ligament (*white arrow*) is seen. More distally the dorsal intercarpal ligament is identified (*black arrow*).

functionally less important than the volar radiocarpal ligaments.

Of the other dorsal carpal ligaments the most prominent is the dorsal intercarpal ligament (see Fig. 3). This is an intrinsic ligament that may have a common proximal origin from the triquetrum, with a proximal limb to the scaphoid (triquetroscaphoid) and a distal limb to the trapezium (triquetrotrapezium) [24].

The dorsal ligaments provide stability to wrist motion and are frequently injured in a fall on the outstretched hand, producing a "dorsal wrist sprain." The dorsal ligaments can be seen on sagittal images but are best depicted on dorsal coronal images (see Fig. 3) (see references [7,22,23,25]). Smith [7,22] has described consistent visualization of these ligaments with 3DFT imaging with multiplanar reconstruction. High-resolution MR arthrography may also depict these structures, better than which they can be visualized with conventional MR imaging [20,21].

Collateral ligaments

The collateral ligaments are thickenings of the fibrous capsule and are functionally less important than collateral ligaments in other joints, such as the knee. The ulnar collateral ligament is a poorly developed capsular thickening that arises from the ulnar styloid and inserts into the triquetrum. It has an extension more proximally to the TFCC. The radial collateral ligament is more volar than lateral and runs from the radial styloid process to the tuberosity of the scaphoid and the flexor carpi radialis tendon. The radial and ulnar collateral ligaments are seen as low signal bands on coronal sections [26].

Interosseous ligaments

The interosseous (intercarpal) ligaments are intrinsic ligaments that connect the adjacent carpal bones and separate the intercarpal compartments. The most important of these ligaments from a clinical and imaging point of view are the proximal interosseous ligaments, the scapholunate (SL) and lunatotriquetral (LT) ligaments (Fig. 4). These ligaments bridge the dorsal, proximal, and volar (palmar) aspects of their respective joints, leaving the distal aspect of each joint open to communicate with the midcarpal joint. Both of these ligaments have histologic characteristics, which justify division into dorsal, proximal, and volar (palmar) regions [27]. Both ligaments are deep in the joint, separated from and covered palmarly and dorsally by the joint capsule. These ligaments have volar and dorsal portions with thinner membranous portions in between [5,21,28]. They separate the radiocarpal from the midcarpal compartments and provide the flexible linkage for the proximal carpal row to function

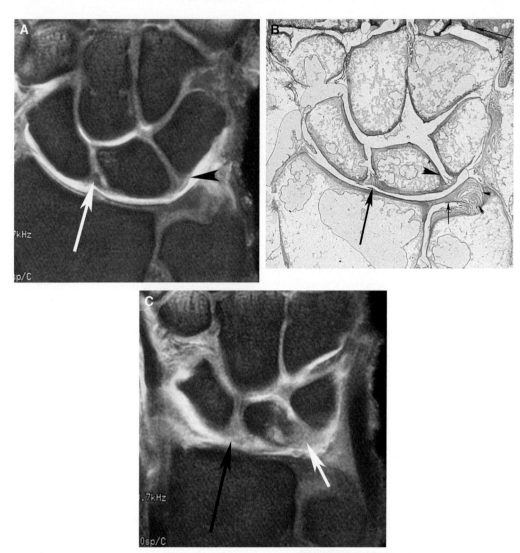

Fig. 4. Normal intercarpal ligaments. (*A, B*) Central portion. The central portion of the intercarpal ligaments are thinner. They course along the more inferior aspect of the corresponding carpal bones as seen on the coronal MR image in A, and corresponding thin coronal histologic section in B. Note the scapholunate ligament (*white arrow in A, black arrow in B*) and the lunate triquetral (*arrowhead*). The scapholunate ligament may appear triangular in this central region. Also note on the histologic section the differing characteristics of the Triangular fibrocartilage complex (TFCC), with the more fibrocartilage-like articular disc (*small black arrow*) and the more ligamentous-like peripheral ulnar attaching portion (*smaller arrowheads in B*). (*C*) Dorsal portion of the ligaments. The ligaments in this portion thicken and extend more vertically, especially the scapholunate ligament. Scapholunate ligament (*black arrow*); lunate triquetral ligament (*white arrow*).

properly. The lunatotriquetral ligament is more taut than the scapholunate ligament, thus there is a more solid relationship between these bones than that between the scaphoid and lunate. The distal carpal row has three intercarpal ligaments that unite the trapezium with the trapezoid, the trapezoid with the capitate, and the capitate with the hamate. The ligament between the capitate and hamate is the strongest. These distal interosseous ligaments do not extend from the volar to the

dorsal portions of the wrist capsule, explaining the communication of the midcarpal and common carpometacarpal compartments of the wrist [29].

The scapholunate and lunatotriquetral interosseous ligaments are identified on MR images as low signal bands traversing the inferior aspect of these bones (see Fig. 4). The scapholunate ligament is described as having either a linear or triangular configuration [30]. The triangular configuration is the most common. Most ligaments have a homogeneous low signal, but central or linear vertical intermediate signal may be seen within the scapholunate ligament [30]. Hyaline cartilage signal may be present at the interface of this ligament with the scaphoid, lunate, or both, but primarily at the central weakest portion. The lunatotriquetral ligament is more difficult to visualize because of its smaller size. It may have a linear, delta shape or amorphous configuration, though the delta shape is most common [31]. Though most LT ligaments also have homogeneously low signal, there may also be linear intermediate signal within the ligament and at its interface with the lunate, triquetrum, or both. This intermediate signal, seen in the SL and LT ligaments and at their bone interfaces, should not be mistaken for tears unless fluid signal is seen traversing the ligament or its interface. Because of the convex adjacent surfaces of the scaphoid and lunate bones, the scapholunate interosseous interval may appear wider along the far volar and dorsal aspects of the wrist [32]. This should not be mistaken for pathologic widening [32].

The appearance of the intercarpal ligaments varies from the volar to dorsal aspect, and this can be observed on MR imaging (Figs. 2, 4, and 5) [5,21,28]. The volar region of the lunotriquetral ligament is a true ligament and is the thickest region of the ligament. It is composed of transversely oriented collagen fascicles (see Fig. 2). Volarly on MR imaging exam the LT ligament may appear to attach to, and be difficult to separate from, fibers of the TFCC. The volar aspect of the scapholunate ligament is thinner than the dorsal aspect and oriented obliquely from palmar to dorsal progressing from the scaphoid to the lunate (see Fig. 2) [27]. It can appear thicker inferiorly and more

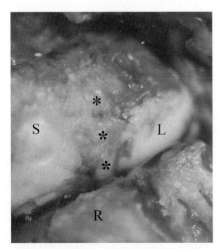

Fig. 5. Normal scapholunate ligament (*). Intraoperative photograph, viewed from below. Note the volar to dorsal extent of the ligament. L, lunate; R, radius; S, scaphoid.

posteriorly, just anterior to the central portion where the radioscapholunate ligament attaches. Both ligaments have a more linear midportion, which on MR imaging may appear slinglike, attaching at the inferior margin of the carpal bones (see Fig. 4). This central portion of the ligament may be fibrocartilaginous histologically [27]. Both ligaments thicken again dorsally and have a broader proximal to distal attachment than at the midportion, although the SL ligament is said to be thicker in the proximal to distal dimension than the LT ligament (see Fig. 4) [13,33]. The dorsal region of the scapholunate interosseous ligament is its thickest region, and is also a true ligament composed of transversely oriented collagen fascicles. The dorsal portion of the SL ligament is thought to be the most important portion for wrist stability. The appearance of these ligaments from volar to dorsal can also be characterized as hammock-like. The volar and dorsal portions extend not only linearly from medial to lateral as in the thinner central portion, but also have a more vertical course from superior to inferior along the more volar (see Fig. 2), and especially along the more dorsal (see Fig. 4), aspects of the ligaments.

Triangular fibrocartilage complex

Which structures make up the TFCC are not universally agreed upon. In most descriptions, however, the TFCC is composed of the triangular fibrocartilage (TFC), the meniscus homolog, the ulnar collateral ligament, the dorsal and volar radioulnar ligaments, and the sheath of the extensor carpi ulnaris tendon (Fig. 6) [34]. The ulnolunate and ulnotriqetral ligaments may also be considered as part of the TFCC [35]. These structures are a complex unit that function as a stabilizing element in the pivot movement of the radius and ulna and limit the lateral deviation of the carpus. The distal radioulnar joint is primarily stabilized by the TFCC. The TFC functions as a cushion between the ulnar head and carpal bones [3]. Many of the structures that make up the complex are connected by fibrous bands. Proximally, the TFCC arises from the ulnar aspect of the lunate fossa of the radius, courses toward the ulna, and inserts in the fovea at the base of the ulnar styloid process. Benjamin [36], in a histologic study, describes two ulnar attachments, a proximal one attaching to the base of the ulnar styloid and a distal one extending beyond the ulna and blending with the fibrous connective tissue of the extensor carpi ulnaris tendon sheath. The insertion of the disc may occasionally extend up the entire length of the styloid process [37] to its distal tip. Totterman [38,39] describes two ulnar styloid attachments, one at the ulnar base and one at the

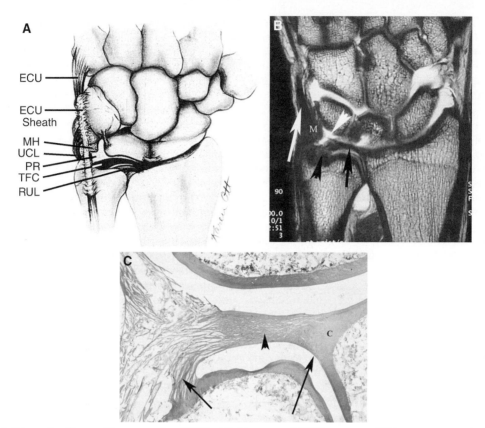

Fig. 6. Triangular fibrocartilage complex (TFCC). (*A*) Diagram of TFCC anatomy. ECU, extensor carpi ulnaris tendon; MH, meniscus homolog; PR, prestyloid recess; RUL, radioulnar ligament; TFC, triangular fibrocartilage (articular disc); UCL, ulnar collateral ligament. (*B*) Correlative coronal MR arthrogram image provides a detailed view of the TFCC anatomy. The TFC (articular disc) reveals homogeneous low signal (*black arrow*); the ulnar portion is more intermediate in character, as it attaches to the ulnar styloid (*arrowhead*). Note the contrast outlining the region of the prestyloid recess (*white arrowhead*). ECU tendon (*white arrow*). M, meniscus homolog. (*C*) Normal histologic specimen of the triangular fibrocartilage. Radial attachment (*long arrow*), central portion (*arrowhead*), ulnar foveal attachment (*short arrow*). Note how the radial-sided TFC fibers attach to the articular cartilage (c), and the striated pattern of the ulnar attachment.

distal tip. Palmer also describes an insertion along the ulnar head [40]. Distally, the TFCC inserts onto the hamate, triquetrum, and base of the fifth metacarpal [40]. As it extends distally, it is joined by fibers of the ulnar collateral ligament. The TFCC is firmly attached volarly to the triquetrum (ulnotriquetral ligament) and the lunatotriquetral interosseous ligament, and less strongly to the lunate (ulnolunate ligament). It is strongly attached dorsally where it incorporates the sheath of the extensor carpi ulnaris tendon [40].

Just distal to the ulnar styloid is the prestyloid recess, which is a site of communication between the TFCC and the radiocarpal joint. The prestyoid recess is fluid-filled space located between the TFC and the meniscus homolog. It protrudes inferiorly to the apex of the TFC and variably interfaces with the ulnar styloid process. The TFC separates the radiocarpal compartment from the distal radioulnar joint and acts as a cushion on the ulnar aspect of these joints. It is the most typical site of injury. It is fibrocartilaginous and thicker at its margins than at its center. It may be fenestrated centrally, especially in older individuals. The thickness of the TFC is inversely proportional to ulnar length, thus a thinner TFC in patients with ulnar positive variant may predispose to TFC tears [41,42]. The thick and strong marginal portions of the TFC, which are composed of lamellar collagen, are often referred to as the dorsal and volar radioulnar ligaments. These are stabilizers of the DRUJ in radioulnar rotation. These ligaments have superficial and deep portions. The attachments of the TFC to these ligaments is by folds on the proximal aspects of these ligaments [38,39]. Some authors regard the dorsal and volar radioulnar ligaments as simply prominent dorsal and volar portions of the TFC.

The meniscus homolog is a complex fibrous structure on the volar side of the wrist. It has a common origin with the dorsal radioulnar ligament on the dorsoulnar corner of the radius [3]. It inserts directly into the triquetrum and partially or completely separates the pisotriquetral joint from the radiocarpal joint.

The extensor carpi ulnaris tendon is located within a dorsal notch in the distal ulna (Figs. 6 and 7). The ECU tendon lies within its own synovial sheath, which in turn is surrounded by the investing fascia of the wrist. The ECU sheath makes a significant contribution to stabilization of the dorsal aspect of the TFCC as some of its fibers fuse with the TFCC [37].

The blood supply of the TFCC originates from the ulnar artery through its radiocarpal branches and the dorsal and palmar branches of the anterior interosseous artery. These vessels penetrate only the peripheral 10% to 40% of the TFCC, and the central section is avascular [43].

The TFCC, composed of fibrocartilage and ligaments, appears as low signal intensity on MR images (see Fig. 6). The TFC specifically is triangular on coronal sections with its apex attaching to the articular cartilage of the radius. Its ulnar attachment may appear bifurcated, with two bands of lower signal intensity separated by a region of higher signal intensity. Totterman [38,39] describes the low signal fibrocartilaginous portion (articular disc, TFC) ending before the ulnar attachments. The ulnar attachments thus have a more striated appearance and are less homogeneously low in signal, thus appearing more ligamentous in character (see Fig. 6).

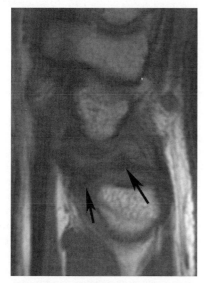

Fig. 7. Sagittal T1-weighted MR image. Note the thicker appearance of the volar and dorsal portions on sagittal section (*arrows*).

The authors have observed similar findings [21]. Increased signal may also be seen between the two ulnar attachments. The TFCC has a triangular appearance on axial images and is discoid on sagittal scans [32]. On sagittal scans it appears thicker on the volar and dorsal aspects (see Fig. 7). In older patients some signal may be seen within the low signal TFC I on short TR/TE and proton density-weighted sequences, thought to be due to mucoid degenerative changes [44]. Morphologic changes may also be evident [45]. On short TR/TE sequences, high signal intensity is normally seen in the region of the prestyloid recess as well as in the region of the ulnar attachment of the TFC, thought to represent fibrofatty tissue in this area [26,46]. Joint fluid may collect in the prestyloid recess between the TFC and meniscus homolog and appear as high signal intensity on long TR/TE images. Contrast may accumulate in this region normally at MR arthrography (see Fig. 6).

Subjacent to the radial attachment of the TFC is the mildly increased signal of hyaline articular cartilage of the distal radius (see Fig. 6). These areas of increased signal mentioned above should not be mistaken for detachments or tears. These sites of increased signal at the ulnar attachments and at the hyaline cartilage interface can be distinguished from tears by their lack of increased signal on images with T2-type contrast.

The meniscus homolog also has low signal on MR images (see Fig. 6). The course of the meniscus homolog around and just distal to the styloid process can be seen at the level where it borders the prestyloid recess. The more distal and volar portion of the meniscus homolog may be more difficult to appreciate on MR images [38,39,47].

The dorsal and volar radioulnar ligaments (Fig. 8) have a striated appearance on MR images that follows the course of the collagen fascicles that constitute these portions of the TFCC. Because of their oblique course they cannot be followed for their entire extent on any one coronal image. Their ulnar attachment may not be clearly visualized on MR images. These ligaments may also be identified on axial images (see Fig. 8).

The size of the ulnolunate and ulnotriquetral ligaments may vary considerably. Because of this variability, they may at times be difficult to appreciate on MR images. In most wrists they may be difficult to see as separate structures and may be visible on coronal images as a single inhomogeneous structure.

Distal radioulnar joint

The distal radioulnar joint (DRUJ) is composed of the sigmoid notch of the distal radius, the head of the ulna, and the TFCC [48,49]. In neutral position, the radius is centered on the ulnar head.

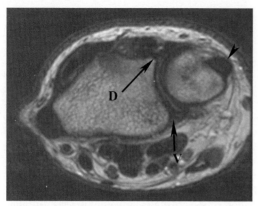

Fig. 8. Distal radioulnar joint (DRUJ). Axial FSE T2-weighted MR image. Note the distal ulna within the sigmoid notch of the radius. The volar (V) and dorsal (D) radioulnar ligaments are seen. Also note the ECU tendon within a notch in the distal ulna (*arrowhead*).

The principle motion of the DRUJ is rotation. With rotation of the radius about the ulnar head, there is some associated translational motion, such that in supination the ulna is somewhat palmar, whereas in pronation the ulna is more dorsal relative to the radius.

As discussed previously, the articular disc portion of the TFCC functions as a cushion for the ulnar head and ulnar-sided carpal bones and as the load-bearing component of the TFCC. Thus tears of the TFC may not of themselves result in DRUJ instability but require disruption of the volar and dorsal radioulnar ligaments, which are the structures primarily responsible for the stabilization of the DRUJ.

Axial MR images depict the distal ulna articulating with the distal radius (see Fig. 8). The volar and dorsal radioulnar ligaments are also delineated as low signal intensity structures on MR images. Normal congruence of the DRUJ is present when the ulnar head is articulated within the sigmoid notch of the radius, and it does not project above a line drawn through the dorsal ulnar and radial borders of the radius or below a line drawn through the volar ulnar and radial borders of the radius [26,50].

Variations of the length of the ulna relative to the radius are referred to as ulnar variance (see references [41,42,51,52]). This can significantly alter the forces borne by the distal radius and ulna. Ulnar variance is measured from the center of the distal articular surfaces of the radius and ulna. It should be measured without any pronation or supination of the forearm, which can change the relative lengths of the distal radius and ulna. If the radius and ulna are of equal length then this is considered neutral, most of the axial loading forces are then transmitted from the ulna to the radius. If the ulna is long relative to the radius, this is considered positive (or plus), and if the ulna is short relative to the radius, this is considered ulna negative (or minus) (Fig. 9).

As will be discussed in the section on pathology, ulnar minus leads to a relative decreased load on the distal portion of the ulna and is seen in association with Kienbock's disease. With such variance the TFCC is thicker (see Fig. 9) and abnormalities of the TFCC are said to be less common [41]. With an ulnar-positive situation there is an increase in the force borne by the distal portion of the ulna. The TFC portion is also thinner in such cases. This is seen in association with the ulnocarpal impaction/abutment syndrome. Ulnocarpal impaction syndrome may be associated with tears of the TFC and of the lunate triquetral interosseous ligament (see references [35,51,53–56]).

Triangular fibrocartilage complex tears

General features

Lesions of the TFCC may be variable in their extent of involvement. They may be confined to the horizontal or flat portion of the TFCC, referred to as the TFC or articular disc, or involve one or more components of the TFCC. Such injuries also can involve instability of the DRUJ. Tears of the TFC should be suspected in patients with ulnar-sided wrist pain and tenderness, although some degenerative tears or defects may not be symptomatic. A palpable or audible click or pain may be present with rotation of the forearm. Degenerative and traumatic tears of the TFC may occur.

Degenerative perforations tend to occur in the central region of the disc where it is thinnest [40]. The incidence of central degenerative tears is age related. According to Mikic [45], degeneration begins in the third decade and progressively increases in frequency and severity in subsequent decades. The changes comprise reduced cellularity, loss of elastic fibers, mucoid degeneration of the ground substance, exposure of collagen fibers, fibrillation, erosion, ulceration, abnormal thinning, and, ultimately, disc perforation. The changes are more frequent and more intense on the ulnar surface, and they are always situated in the central part of the disc. In their caveric study of 180 wrists, there were no perforations in the first two decades of life; in the third there were 7.6%, in the fourth 18.1%, in the fifth 40.0%, in the sixth 42.8%, and in specimens over 60 years of age the incidence was 53.1%. There was an associated pattern of degenerative changes in the wrist joint as a whole. The structures adjacent to the articular disc (discal surface of

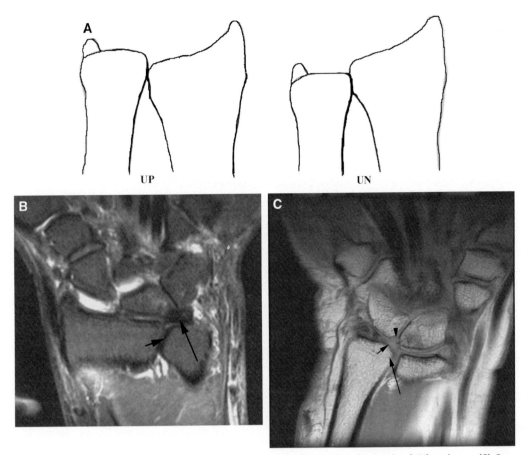

Fig. 9. Ulnar variance. (*A*) Diagrammatic representation of positive (UP) and negative (UN) variance. (*B*) Coronal T2 FSE image. There is negative ulnar variance (*short arrow*). Note the thickened TFC (*longer arrow*). (*C*) Coronal PD FSE image. There is positive ulnar variance (*long arrow*). There is a large central defect of the TFC (*short arrow*). The lunate triquetral ligament is also disrupted (*arrowhead*).

the ulnar head, discal part of the lunate) were much more often involved, and the changes were much more advanced, than on nondiscal surfaces. Because degenerative perforations may be so common in older patients, who may be asymptomatic, Gilula and Palmer [57] have objected to the use of the term "tear" or "perforation" for these lesions and prefer the term "defect."

Longer ulnae are associated with perforations of the TFCC. Positive ulnar variance may lead to increased ulnar carpal loading with resultant ulnolunate impaction syndrome (see references [40,51,53,55,58–60]). This chronic abutment leads to erosive changes in the cartilage of the ulnar head and lunate, degenerative perforation of the disc, and attrition and eventually a tear of the lunatotriquetral ligament. These associated abnormalities of the lunate triquetral interosseous ligament have been described in up to 70% of patients with degenerative perforation of the TFC [40]. Despite the stated association of ulnar-positive variance to

TFC tears and ulnocarpal abutment, Manaster [61], in a study using plain films and arthrography, was unable to find a significant correlation between ulnar-positive variance and TFC tears. This may have been because of the young age of the patients in the study, as most were under 35 years of age [61]. Tomaino [59] also has indicated that although the ulnar impaction syndrome occurs most commonly in the ulnar-positive wrist, it can also occur in wrists with either ulnar negative or neutral variance.

In patients with negative ulnar variance, TFC tears may more likely be traumatic. Many posttraumatic tears of the TFC occur closer to the radial insertion (within 2 to 3 mm) than the central degenerative tears, where the thick collagen bundles connect the avascular portion of the TFC to the radius [62]. Traumatic tears may also be more common in younger patients. Avulsions of the TFC may also occur from the ulnar attachments. This is typically a less common lesion, although in a study by Golimbu [56,63–65] most of the tears that were observed were believed to occur closer to the ulnar insertion site. Ulnar detachments may be associated with an ulnar styloid fracture [66,67]. This may be associated with instability of the distal radioulnar joint Palmer type 1B [68]. Ulnar styloid fracture associated with an avulsion of the ulnar attachment of the TFC can result in a nonunion (type 2) [67]. The ununited fracture can cause chondromalacia along the undersurface of the triquetrum [51]. Studies of the microvascular anatomy of the TFC indicate that tears that occur on the ulnar side of the TFC have the ability to heal, whereas those that are centrally or radially located do not [43,62].

The Palmer classification of TFCC tears divides TFCC tears into traumatic (classes 1A–D) and degenerative types (2A–D). Palmer indicated that the traumatic types (class 1) were uncommon. The traumatic types include central perforation, ulnar avulsion with and without distal ulnar fracture, distal avulsion, and radial avulsion with and without sigmoid notch fracture. Class 1A, the central perforation, represents a tear or perforation of the horizontal portion of the TFCC, usually occurring as a 1- to 2-mm slit, and located 2 to 3 mm medial to the radial attachment of the TFCC. The ulnar avulsion, or class 1B, represented a traumatic avulsion of the TFCC from its insertion site into the distal portion of the ulna, sometimes with an associated fracture of the base of the styloid process of the ulna. This lesion is considered to be an unstable lesion. Class 1C represents distal avulsion of the TFCC at its site of attachment to the lunate or triquetrum, reflective of a tear of the ulnolunate or ulnotriquetral ligaments. A class 1D lesion represented avulsion of the TFCC from its attachment to the radius at the distal aspect of the sigmoid notch, which may be associated with an avulsion fracture of this region [69].

The degenerative type is reflected by progressive stages of ulnocarpal impaction. Five types of degenerative lesions were detailed. Class 2A is TFC wear from the undersurface, occurring in the central horizontal portion, without perforation. Class 2B is TFC wear with ulnolunate malacia. The cartilage changes occur on the inferomedial aspect of the lunate or on the more radial portion of the head of the ulna. Stage C is TFC perforation with ulnolunate malacia. The perforation is in the central, horizontal portion of the TFCC and occurs in a more ulnar location than that seen with the traumatic injury that occurs in this region (class 1A). Stage D is a TFC perforation in the central horizontal portion, associated with ulnolunate malacia as denoted in 2C, and lunatotriquetral ligament perforation. Stage E is all of the above with ulnolunate/ulnocarpal arthritis, and there may be

degenerative arthritis about the distal radioulnar joint as well.

Imaging findings

Degenerative defects are more common than traumatic defects. The imaging characteristics, however, may be similar, and location, age, and clinical history may often be needed to differentiate their origin. Either type of lesion may result in full-thickness defects of the TFCC, and these can be visualized on MR imaging exam or at MR imaging arthrography.

Radial tears of the TFC appear as a linear band of increased signal intensity on short TR/TE and proton density-weighted spin echo (SE) or gradient echo (GRE) images [26,46]. With complete tears the signal extends to proximal and distal articular surfaces. In partial tears, believed to be less important from a clinical perspective, the signal will extend only to one articular surface, usually the proximal surface (DRUJ), as the proximal surface tends to be subject to more stresses, particularly in situations of positive ulnar variance. The signal will increase on long TR/TE images SE images, or T2*-weighted GRE images or T2-weighted FSE sequences with fat suppression (Fig. 10), consistent with synovial fluid trapped in the defect. Fluid collecting in the DRUJ is an important secondary sign [70], but the presence of fluid signal alone is not indicative of a tear of the triangular fibrocartilage. MR arthrography with either a radiocarpal or distal radioulnar joint injection will reveal contrast extending through and outlining the TFC defect (see Fig. 10).

There are no specific differentiating features on MR imaging exam separating a traumatically induced tear of the TFC from one caused by degeneration. The appearance of these lesions may also be similar in symptomatic and asymptomatic individuals; therefore, determining the clinical relevance of these lesions and their correlation with patients' symptoms (ie, radial or ulnar-sided wrist pain) may be difficult [71]. As noted previously, the age of the patient, the site of the tear, and associated lesions may help in this regard.

Ulnar-sided tears should be differentiated from central ones because of the different therapeutic strategies. Peripheral tears have a good vascular supply and are thus repaired, whereas central lesions are avascular and are treated with debridement. Ulnar-sided tears and avulsions can, however, be more difficult to diagnose [46,72]. This is especially true if there is a large amount of fluid that preferentially collects on the ulnar aspect of the wrist. Differentiating this joint fluid from focal synovitis related to a peripheral TFCC injury, either acute or chronic, is often a challenge. Oneson et al [73] in their large

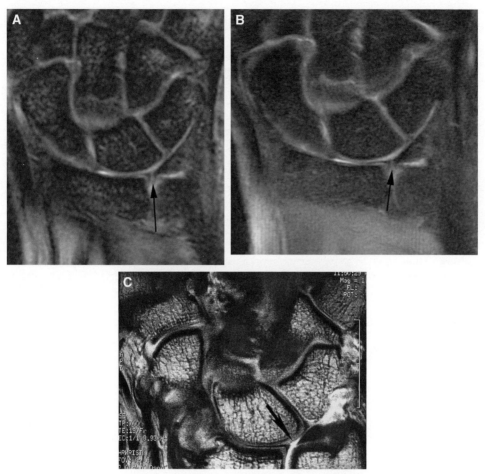

Fig. 10. Triangular fibrocartilage tears. Radial-sided tears coronal 2D T2* gradient-echo image (*A*) and T2 FSE image with fat saturation (*B*) demonstrate fluid signal intensity in the radial aspect of the TFC (*arrow*), which extends to the radiocarpal and distal radioulnar joint (DRUJ) articular surfaces. Fluid is seen in the DRUJ. (*C*) Coronal "hi-res" T1 FSE image after intraarticular contrast injection into the radiocarpal joint in another patient illustrates high signal contrast extending through a TFC defect into the DRUJ (*black arrow*).

study of TFCC tears found only a small number of ulnar tears of the TFCC. They had a poor sensitivity to these lesions. The poor sensitivity was attributed to the presence of the striated fascicles at the periphery of the TFCC, which were believed to be difficult to evaluate by MR imaging [73].

Findings that correlate with these types of tears include altered morphology of the ulnar attachments of the TFC, excessive fluid localizing to this region (especially if it extends below the expected location of the prestyloid recess), and linear fluid signal in the ulnar TFC itself extending to its surface (Fig. 11). High signal intensity at the ulnar insertion of the triangular fibrocartilage complex as the only marker for a tear of the ulnar TFC may be insensitive, as was found by Haims and coworkers [72]. Their study revealed a sensitivity of only 42%, a specificity of 63%, and an accuracy of 55%. Use

of axial and sagittal imaging may be helpful in assessing these patients. Greater attention to the findings of focal synovitis may also prove to improve sensitivity [72]. Additionally, unenhanced and enhanced MR imaging may be helpful in differentiating joint fluid from focal synovitis [72]. MR arthrography may also help outline such tears by revealing contrast extending directly into the defect. The results of indirect MR arthrography in this regard are still under investigation, and further study is needed to determine its efficacy [74,75]. Not uncommonly, fluid signal and thickening may be present along the ulnar aspect of the TFCC (Fig. 12). This appearance may be due to degenerative or inflammatory change or the result of an old healed peripheral TFC injury with scarring and chronic synovitis. This may be difficult to differentiate from an acute peripheral TFC injury. Correlation with

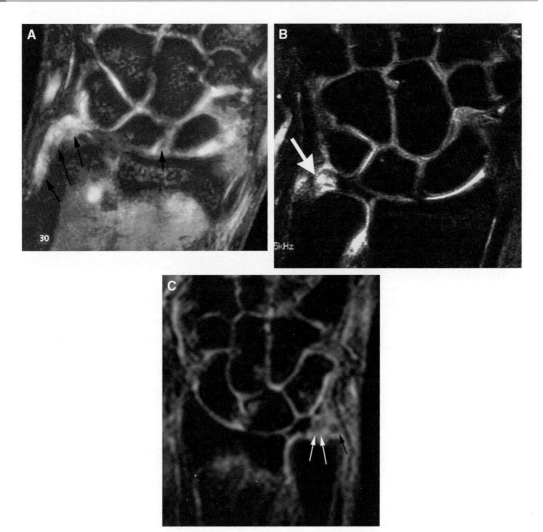

Fig. 11. Triangular fibrocartilage tears. Ulnar-sided tears. (*A*) Coronal 2D T2* gradient-echo image. A large amount of fluid signal is seen replacing the ulnar attachment of the TFC, extending beyond the ulnar capsule, along the ECU tendon sheath more proximally (*arrows*). A tear of the SL ligament is also present (*short arrow*). (*B*) Coronal T2 FSE image with fat saturation reveals fluid signal and altered morphology indicating disruption of the ulnar attachment (*arrow*) of the TFC. (*C*) Coronal STIR image. The ulnar aspect of the TFC is torn and detached (*white arrows*). There is a fracture of the ulnar styloid tip (*black arrow*).

the patient's clinical history is helpful in this regard. Such findings often are associated with significant ulnar-sided wrist pain.

Ulnocarpal impaction (abutment)

Ulnocarpal impaction syndrome (Figs. 9, 13, and 14) is considered a degenerative condition and is characterized by ulnar-sided wrist pain, swelling, and limitation of motion related to excessive load bearing across the ulnar aspect of the wrist [51,53,55]. There is typically a pattern of ulna-positive variance or a distal ulna prominent enough to allow transfer of excessive compressive force from the ulna and triquetrum and lunate by way of the TFCC. It is distinguished from ulnar impingement, which

consists of a short ulna impinging on the distal portion of the radius and causing a disabling painful pseudoarthrosis. Ulnocarpal abutment can also occur in a secondary manner, by way of an acquired ulna-positive anatomy, after malunited distal radius fractures [58].

In patients with ulnocarpal abutment (impaction), foci of low signal intensity may be seen within the articular cartilage of the ulnar head and or lunate, reflective of the presence of chondromalacia [44]. There may be thinning of the articular cartilage surface. This may be best seen on T2 FSE sequences with fat saturation or on MR arthrography, if performed. The perforations in these lesions are more centrally located. Degenerative changes in

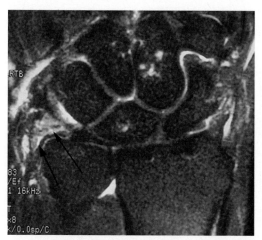

Fig. 12. Chronic peripheral triangular fibrocartilage complex (TFCC) synovitis. Coronal T2-weighted MR image. Marked thickening and fluid signal is seen along the ulnar attachments and ulnar aspect of the TFCC (*arrows*).

the subchondral marrow of the lunate, including marrow edema and subchondral cystic change, may develop as well (see Fig. 13). These may be difficult to distinguish from intraosseous ganglia; however, MR imaging can document the presence of the central tears of the TFC and the accompanying degeneration and degenerative tears of the lunate triquetral interosseous ligament.

Ulnocarpal abutment cannot be treated with simple partial debridement of the TFC. More extensive procedures, such as ulnar shortening or resection of the ulnar head, must be performed. After such procedures, improvement in some of the articular cartilage and bone marrow alterations may be identified [60]. In the study by Imaeda et al [60], there was focal abnormal signal intensity of the ulnar aspect of the lunate in 87% of wrists, of the radial aspects of the triquetrum in 43%, and of the radial aspects of the ulnar head in 10% before surgery. The signal intensity of the abnormalities was decreased on T1-weighted and decreased or increased on T2-weighted images. After surgery, the signal intensity of the lunate shifted from low through slightly low to normal on T1-weighted images and from low through high to normal on T2-weighted images.

Ulnar styloid impaction

This ulnar-sided wrist pain is caused by impaction between an excessively long ulnar styloid process and the triquetral bone [51,76]. One-time or repetitive impaction between the tip of the ulnar styloid process and the triquetral bone results in contusion, which leads to chondromalacia of the opposing articular surfaces, synovitis, and pain. If a single-event

trauma is forceful enough, fracture of the dorsal triquetral bone may occur. Impaction over a long period of time can lead to lunotriquetral instability. The diagnosis of this condition is made on the basis of radiographic evidence of an excessively long ulnar styloid process in combination with positive findings on a provocative clinical test. MR imaging may reveal the prominent ulnar styloid process, chondromalacia of the ulnar styloid process and proximal triquetral bone, associated marrow edema, and a lunate triquetral tear, if present (Fig. 15). Resection of all but the two most proximal millimeters of the styloid process (so as not to interfere with the TFC complex insertion) is the treatment of choice.

TFCC degenerative lesions

Signal within the TFC may be encountered commonly on T1-weighted and proton density-weighted MR images [44,71]. This signal can be mistaken for a tear. If such signal changes do not communicate with the inferior or superior surface of the TFC, and if it does not get bright on images with T2 contrast, it is not considered indicative of a tear. Such signal may diminish on images with T2 contrast, particularly if fat suppression is not applied. This signal pattern was studied in cadavers [44,71] and was believed to be attributable to degeneration, both mucinous and myxoid in character, and to the age of the person, increasing in frequency with age. Such alterations in signal intensity and their differentiation are similar to those problems that arise from degenerative-type signal that occurs in the glenoid labrum of the shoulder and in the meniscus of the knee.

Degenerative changes on the surface of the TFC may also be seen in asymptomatic individuals on MR imaging exam [44]. It is typically more evident on the proximal aspect of the TFC and in its more central portion. It occurs centrally as this is the thinner portion of the TFC and more proximally because of the greater stresses on this surface of the TFC biomechanically. These alterations on the ulnar surface of the TFC may be similar to those changes seen in patients with ulnocarpal abutment and may be accompanied by similar alterations in the distal portion of the ulna and of the inferior surface of the lunate [44].

Diagnostic performance

Tears of the TFC, when compared with arthrography and arthroscopy, have revealed a sensitivity of 0.92, specificity of 0.89, and accuracy of 0.91 [46]. Potter et al [77] assessed the diagnostic performance of MR imaging using thin-section 3D volume gradient-echo sequences. MR imaging was found to be sensitive and specific in the diagnosis

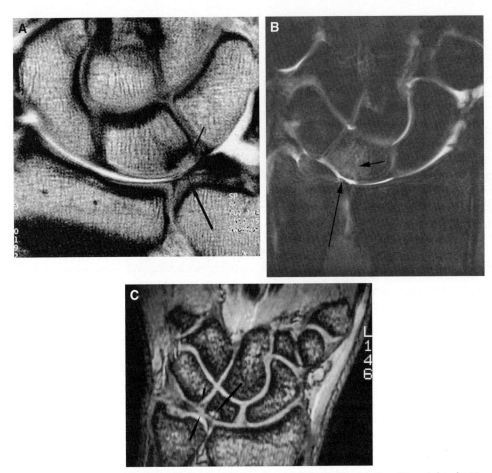

Fig. 13. Ulnar carpal impaction syndrome. (*A*) Early stage (stage 2B). High-resolution T1-weighted MR arthrogram reveals prominent thinning of the TFC undersurface (*long arrow*), with corresponding marrow alterations of the inferior medial aspect of the lunate (*short arrow*). (*B*) Late stage. Coronal T2 FSE image with fat saturation. A large central TFC defect is seen (*arrow*). There is marked chondromalacia of the infermedial lunate with associated marrow edema (*short arrow*). (*C*) Late stage (stage 2D). Note the wide central TFC defect (*short arrow*), cystic change in the inferomedial lunate (*long arrow*), and disrupted LT ligament (*arrowhead*).

and location of TFC tears when correlated with arthroscopy. The sensitivity of MR imaging for tears was 100% and the specificity was 90%. In a study by Oneson et al [73] of 56 patients who underwent arthroscopic evaluation of the TFC, using the Palmer classification for TFC pathology, the sensitivity for detecting central degenerative perforations was 91%. The sensitivity for detecting radial slitlike tears was 100% and 86% for observers 1 and 2. The sensitivity for detecting ulnar-sided avulsions was 25% and 50% for observers 1 and 2, indicating at least in this study that ulnar-sided avulsions can be more difficult to detect. In a British study by Johnstone and coworkers [78], however, results were less favorable when compared with arthroscopy. The sensitivity and specificity of MR imaging compared with arthroscopy were 0.8 and 0.7 for triangular fibrocartilage complex pathology. Another

study using cadavers [152] found that low field-strength extremity-only magnets may allow visualization of the triangular fibrocartilage and accurate assessment of a small number of complete tears. Observer experience may play a role in the accuracy of interpretation and predicting the location of the lesions.

In a recent study by Haims et al [72], MR imaging was not found to be sensitive in revealing injuries of the peripheral attachment of the triangular fibrocartilage complex. High signal intensity at the ulnar insertion of the triangular fibrocartilage complex as a marker for tear showed a sensitivity of 42%, a specificity of 63%, and an accuracy of 55%. The authors indicated, however, that all of the peripheral tears in this study were associated with synovitis at arthroscopy. It is possible that the finding of a focal synovitis at the ulnar attachment could be used as

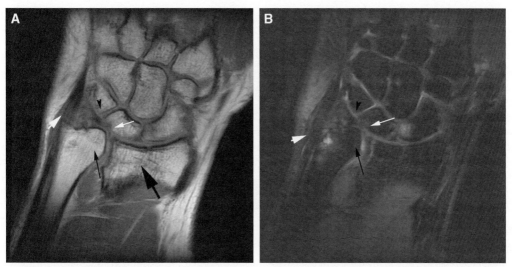

Fig. 14. Secondary ulnocarpal abutment. Coronal FSE PD (*A*) T2 with fat saturation (*B*). The ulna is positive (*black arrow*) owing to shortening from a previous distal radius fracture (*large arrow in A*). There is secondary ulnocarpal abutment. Note the TFC tear (*white arrow*), marrow change in the lunate, and LT tear (*arrowhead*). Note the tendinosis of the ECU (*short white arrow*).

a marker for peripheral tear. The authors believe that this focal synovitis could potentially be differentiated from fluid with the use of unenhanced and enhanced imaging [72].

MR arthrography may be of value in evaluating TFCC lesions, particularly in identifying defects on the ulnar aspect, where the anatomy is more complex and more ligamentous in nature. It may also help to outline partial tears of the undersurface. If MR imaging arthrography is performed, injection from the DRUJ may best outline such

partial-thickness defects. Schweitzer and colleagues [75] reported good initial results with indirect MR arthrography in evaluation of the TFCC, although a more recent study by this group revealed less promising results [74]. Herold and coworkers [79] evaluated indirect MR arthrography in detecting TFCC tears. The sensitivity and specificity in the detection of TFCC lesions were calculated as 100% and 77%. The accuracy was 93%. Small degenerative changes of the TFC fibers were most common (Palmer type IIA). In trauma patients, the tears

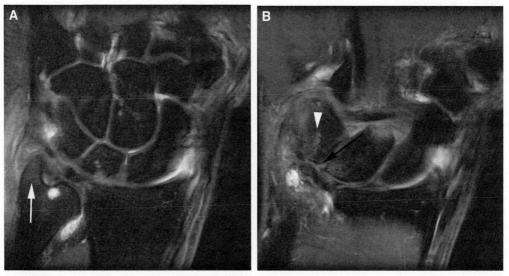

Fig. 15. Ulna styloid impingement coronal T2 FSE images with fat saturation. The ulna styloid is prominent in (*A*) (*arrow*). Note the edema in the triquetrum (*arrowhead*) and the LT tear (*long black arrow*). Abnormalities are also present in the TFCC undersurface and peripheral aspect.

occurred near the insertion of the TFCC at the ulna (Palmer type IB). No deficiency in the evaluation of ulnar-sided lesions was detected in this study.

Treatment

Treatment of TFC tears can often be performed arthroscopically. Unstable central fragments can be excised or debrided [80,81]. Peripheral separations may be treated with suture repair because of the more vascular nature of this region [82,83]. Tears associated with a positive ulnar variance can be treated with ulnar-shortening procedures described in the discussion of ulnocarpal impaction [84].

Other causes of ulnar-sided wrist pain

Other causes of ulnar-sided wrist pain that may mimic TFCC tears include pisiform-triquetral osteoarthritis, fractures of the hamate, DRUJ instability, radioulnar degenerative change, disorders of the extensor carpi ulnaris tendon (ECU) (see Fig. 14), and calcific tendonitis of the flexor carpi ulnaris tendon [85]. Recent assessment of MR imaging or MR arthrography for PTJ determined that it allows visualization of all anatomic structures of the PTJ [86]. Cartilaginous lesions and osteophytes were easily identified and were detected more often in the pisiform bone than in the triquetral bone. Communication of the PTJ with the radiocarpal joint was noted in 82% of wrists. MR arthrography improved the visualization of findings of osteoarthritis. Hamatolunate impingement is a less common cause of ulnar-sided wrist pain [87].

Instability of the distal radioulnar joint

Nathan and Schneider [88] emphasized the theory that instability of the DRUJ is caused by a deficiency or disruption of various components of the TFCC. Instability of the DRUJ may arise in relation to injury [89], may be part of a process associated with a fracture of the distal radius or of the styloid process of the ulna, or may accompany inflammatory processes, such as rheumatoid arthritis. The clinical manifestations of DRUJ instability include pain, weakness, loss of forearm rotation, and snapping. Dorsal instability predominates over volar instability. On physical exam a dorsal prominence of the ulnar head may be appreciated, especially in the position of forearm pronation.

The diagnosis, if not evident by clinical examination, can usually be made on the lateral radiograph with the wrist in neutral position [90]. However, if the distal radius is deformed by fracture, or proper positioning is precluded by intractable pain or a plaster cast, then axial imaging will provide a more accurate assessment of the congruity of the DRUJ [90]. Examinations that employ cross-sectional imaging, including CT and MR imaging, are advantageous over plain radiographic examination in the diagnosis of DRUJ instability.

Although CT [90–92] is generally considered the procedure of choice to make this diagnosis as it is more rapidly obtained and may be less expensive than MR imaging, the advantage of using MR imaging is that associated abnormalities, such as tears of the TFC, can be evaluated as well. Also, the dorsal and volar radioulnar ligaments can be directly visualized, especially on axial images [26,93]. Assessment of adjacent structures is also possible, such as the extensor carpi ulnaris tendon and other components of the TFCC that can be affected. Volar radioulnar ligament tears may be associated with dorsal instability.

Short TR/TE axial images through the DRUJ can be obtained rapidly and are satisfactory to demonstrate subluxation and dislocation (Fig. 16). In pronation, the distal ulna may rotate slightly dorsally and in supination slightly volarly. When imaging for DRUJ incongruity, scans are routinely obtained in pronation, supination, and neutral positions. Comparison views of the opposite side are helpful to diagnose minor degrees of instability.

Ligamentous injury

General features and pathophysiology

The ligaments of the wrist play a role in wrist stability. Intrinsic and extrinsic ligaments are important to wrist stability. Although the extrinsic volar radiocarpal ligaments are believed to be important factors in carpal stability, injuries to the intrinsic

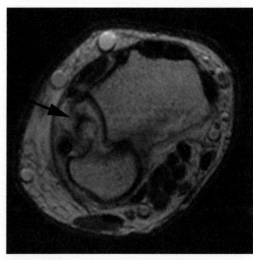

Fig. 16. Distal radioulnar joint (DRUJ) sublux. Axial MR image. Note volar subluxation of the DRUJ. The dorsal radioulnar ligament is stretched, irregular, and attenuated (*arrow*).

interossoeus ligaments of the wrist have been better documented with imaging techniques and may often be a cause of pain and dysfuntion in patients. Although MR imaging demonstrates the anatomy of the extrinsic ligaments [8,9,20], pathologic lesions of the intrinsic interosseous ligaments are more readily visualized (see references [7,26, 30,46,74,94–98]).

The wrist may be injured by a fall on the outstretched arm. In such a situation, it can undergo hyperextension, ulnar deviation, and internal supination. When there is ligamentous injury to the wrist, a spectrum of severity may result [2,99,100]. The first and most common ligamentous injuries occur on the radial side of the wrist. Mayfield [2,99,100] describes a pattern of progressively severe ligamentous injury as four stages of perilunar instability. According to Mayfield, stage 1 consists of tearing the volar extrinsic radioscaphoid ligament with elongation or partial tearing of the scapholunate interosseous ligament. With continued loading, total ligamentous failure occurs at the scapholunate joint, followed by failure of the radioscaphoidcapitate ligament or an avulsion fracture of the radial styloid (stage 2). If loading about the radial aspect of the wrist persists, then ligamentous disruption will occur at the lunate triquetral joint with radiolunate triquetral ligament and dorsal radiocarpal ligament disruption (stage 3). Finally, in stage 4, with a large load of prolonged duration, there occurs the ultimate failure of the dorsal radiocarpal ligament, which renders the lunate free to rotate volarly on its remaining volar ligamentous attachments.

Different schemas exist for classifying wrist instabilities. The carpus is considered unstable if it exhibits symptomatic malalignment [18]. Some authors have divided carpal instability into carpal instability dissociative (CID) and nondissociative forms (CIND) [101,102]. Nondissociative instability represents abnormalities of alignment or relationship of the carpal bones with intact interosseous ligaments, although there may be some attenuation of the palmar and dorsal radiocarpal and ulnocarpal ligaments. These are less common than dissociative instabilities, which include transcaphoid fractures and tears of the scapholunate and lunatotriquetral interosseous ligaments. These may occur in association with injuries to the palmar and dorsal extrinsic ligaments.

Instabilities may also be classified as static or dynamic [103–106]. Static instabilities are based on the presence of radiographically detectable carpal abnormalities. With dynamic instability the carpal alignment may be altered from normal to abnormal with certain movements of the wrist or with manipulation of the wrist during clinical exam. If these instabilities are classified anatomically there are three types of carpal instability [105,106]: lateral between the scaphoid and lunate, medial between the triquetrum and lunate and triquetrum and hamate (less common), and proximal when there is instability related to injury of the radius or massive radiocarpal disruption. Instabilities involving the scapholunate articulation may also produce a dorsal intercalated segmental instability pattern (DISI), and those between the lunate and triquetrum a volar segmental instability pattern (VISI). Static patterns of wrist instability, such as scapholunate dissociation and lunate triquetral dissociation with or without DISI or VISI, scapholunate advanced collapse (SLAC), and ulnar translocation, may often be identified on plain radiographic exam alone. Stress views and fluoroscopy may help identify some more subtle forms of static instability and some dynamic instability. MR imaging and MR arthrography can be helpful to identify some of the ligamentous and soft tissue injuries that occur the circumstances of wrist instability as well, more often in the static patterns. MR imaging has been found to be useful in the detection of injuries to the interosseous ligaments, particularly the scapholunate ligament and to a lesser degree the lunatotriquetral ligaments [10]. MR arthrography also has been of aid in diagnosing these abnormalities [14]. Dynamic or kinematic MR imaging [27,28] has been used over the years with variable success. Variable success has also been achieved with MR imaging and MR arthrography in evaluating injuries to the volar and dorsal radiocarpal ligaments [10,15,17].

Scapholunate instability

Scapholunate instability presents with pain, swelling, and tenderness over the dorsoradial aspect of the wrist. Tears of this ligament may be partial or complete. On MR imaging exam, complete tears (**Figs. 17 and 18**) appear as distinct areas of discontinuity within the ligament with increased signal intensity on images with T2-type contrast, or complete absence of the ligament [26,46,70]. Severe distortion of the morphology of ligament (fraying, thinning, or irregularity) may be reflective of ligamentous injury, and coursing of the central portion of the ligament in a direction other than horizontal may be considered abnormal. MR imaging arthrography may aid in revealing contrast extravasation through a complete defect (**Fig. 19**), or help to outline the aforementioned morphologic alterations. Fluid in the midcarpal joint is a sensitive but nonspecific finding of ligament tears [70]. In more advanced cases, widening of the scapholunate ligament articulation may be evident, particularly if at least two portions of the ligament are involved.

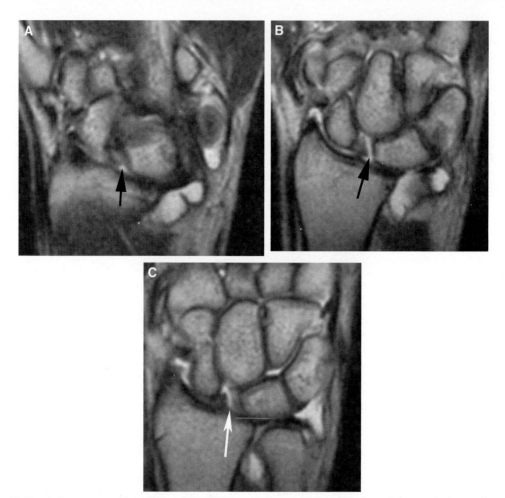

Fig. 17. Scapholunate tear. (*A–C*) Coronal T2- weighted images reveals widening of the scapholunate interval with an associated fluid-filled tear. The ligament is torn in the volar (*A*), central (*B*), and dorsal portions (*C*) (*arrows*).

Fluid pooling around a ligament and concomitant bone injury are other clues to injury. Ganglion cysts can also be a secondary finding of ligament derangement.

A partial tear may be diagnosed when there is focal thinning or irregularity or fluid signal in a portion of the ligament, more commonly in the volar portion (Fig. 20) where the weakest ligamentous attachments are located [107]. Considerable stretching (elongation) of the scapholunate ligament may also occur before or in the absence of a ligament tear [54,100], and this may also be observed as an abnormality on MR imaging exam. Partial tears and elongated but intact ligaments may be visualized with MR imaging in the presence of a normal conventional arthrogram (Fig. 21) [107]. Associated tears of the volar extrinsic radiocarpal ligaments may also be visualized with MR imaging (see Fig. 20), although less frequently than documented at arthroscopy and

surgery (see references [9,10,46,108]). Three-dimensional volumetric imaging [8] has been applied with some success in better defining these extrinsic ligament injuries with the aid of obliquely reformatted projections. MR arthrography may yield an increased sensitivity to scapholunate tears over MR imaging alone and conventional arthrography, especially more subtle injuries (see references [20,21,98,109–111]). This includes partial tears, which may show contrast leak or imbibition into a portion of an injured ligament (see Fig. 21) or better outline morphologic alterations or stretching. Installation of intraarticular contrast may also help outline dysfunctional ligaments that may have healed over with fibrosis and be scarred (Fig. 22). This latter process may be evident clinically but difficult to document with conventional MR imaging. MR arthrography may help outline the surfaces of the ligament and improve the detectability of this lesion.

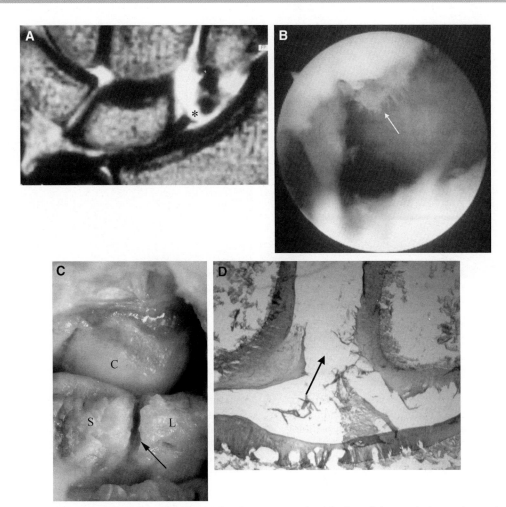

Fig. 18. Scapholunate tear. (*A*) Coronal T2- weighted image reveals widening of the scapholunate interval with an associated fluid-filled tear (*). (*B*) Arthroscopic view of an SL tear with frayed ligamentous edges (*arrow*). (*C*) Gross specimen of a scapholunate tear (*arrow*). C, capitate; L, lunate; S, scaphoid. (*D*) Corresponding histologic specimen (*arrow*).

There is controversy as to which portions of the ligament need to be injured for instability to occur. Mayfield has shown that the volar portion is injured first [2,99,100]. Most authors believe that the dorsal portion must be injured for instability to occur, or that both the volar and dorsal portion must be injured [112,113]. Complete scapholunate dissociation as seen on plain radiographic exam by way of a widened scapholunate interval requires a tear of the radioscaphoid as well as the volar and dorsal portions of the scapholunate ligament. MR imaging thus has the ability to show scapholunate injuries at an earlier stage than evident on plain radiographs. MR imaging also the ability to diagnose the site and the extent of involvement of these lesions (see Fig. 17) and thus differentiate those lesions that may involve only the central membranous portion and that may be of degenerative origin. These central lesions may be painful but not indicative of instability as would involvement of the other ligaments, particularly the dorsal portion. In this regard, MR imaging is of greater value than conventional arthrography, which cannot make this distinction. MR arthrography may, however, be of significant benefit in establishing the location and extent of such lesions (see Fig. 19) (see references [19,98,109,110,114]). Three-dimensional volumetric imaging may also aid in this diagnosis [7,13].

Disruption of the scapholunate articulation can be associated with dorsal intercalated segmental instability (DISI). The scaphoid and lunate are no longer linked. The lunate may collapse in a dorsiflexed posture, and the capitate will migrate proximally into the widened gap now present between the scaphoid and lunate. This is best demonstrated on a midplane sagittal MR imaging image (Fig. 23).

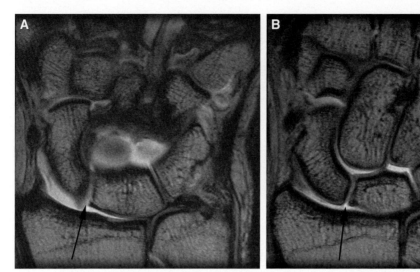

Fig. 19. Scapholunate tear. MR arthrography coronal T1-weighted MR arthrogram images. Note contrast outlining a tear in the volar (*A*) and midportion (*B*) of the scapholunate ligament (*arrows*).

The radius, lunate and capitate are no longer colinear but are shortened in a Z-like configuration [32]. The scaphoid will also rotate volarly. The advantage of MR imaging over plain radiographs is its tomographic nature; therefore, overlap from other carpal bones as would be present on plain radiographs is avoided and that associated ligament pathology is demonstrated. Measurement of scapholunate angles and capitolunate angles can be performed by evaluating successive sagittal sections. The scapholunate angle will increase greater than 70 degrees

(normal 30 to 60 degrees), and the capitolunate angle will be increased to greater than 30 degrees (normal 0 to 30 degrees) [115,116]. The lunate appears more dorsally tilted on MR images than on lateral radiographs, such that a DISI configuration may be simulated [116]. This occurred in patients with neutrally positioned and ulnarly deviated wrists. Subtle errors in the selection of the imaging plane did not substantially influence measurements. Thus caution must be taken in making this diagnosis based on MR images alone, and correlation with

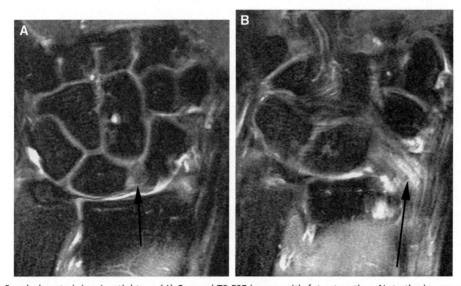

Fig. 20. Scapholunate injury/partial tear. (*A*) Coronal T2 FSE image with fat saturation. Note the increased signal and altered morphology of the volar portion of the scapholunate ligament (*arrow*). (*B*) Coronal T2 FSE image with fat saturation. Altered signal and morphology outlines an injury to the volar radiocarpal ligaments (*arrows*).

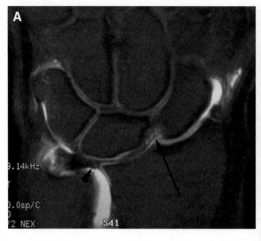 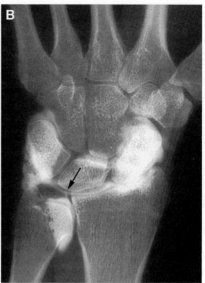

Fig. 21. (*A*) Coronal T1-weighted image after intraarticular contrast injection, with fat saturation. High signal contrast imbibes into the scapholunate ligament (*black arrow*). A small defect in the TFC was also noted (*small black arrow*). (*B*) Radiocarpal wrist arthrogram. The tear in the scapholunate ligament is not identified on the conventional arthrogram in this patient. The TFC tear is seen (*small black arrow*).

plain radiographs and the clinical status of the patients is necessary. Wrist positioning on MR imaging exam is also critical.

Scapholunate advance collapse (SLAC) represents the end-stage degenerative pattern in scapholunate insufficiency (**Fig. 24**) [117–120]. It also may be seen in similar fashion in nonunion of the scaphoid where it is known as scaphoid nonunion advanced collapse (SNAC) [121].

Lunate triquetral instability

There are different proposed etiologies for lunate triquetral instability [122]. Disruption of the lunate triquetral ligament may occur in the latter stages of

perilunar instability. It may present as an isolated injury in situations of perilunar instability, where the scapholunate component has healed, leaving only the lunatotriquetral tear. It may also present as a result of loading in maximal extension, radial deviation, and possibly pronation, indicating reverse perilunar instability. Finally, it may occur as part of the ulnocarpal abutment syndrome. Patients with

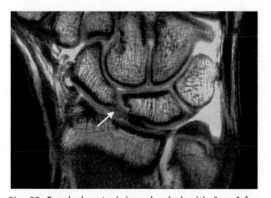

Fig. 22. Scapholunate injury, healed with "scar" formation. Intermediate signal is identified in the volar portion of a thickened scapholunate ligament (*arrow*). These findings can be likened to that seen in a healed partial ACL tear.

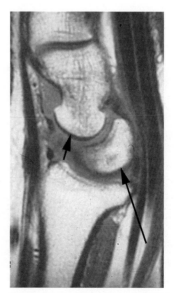

Fig. 23. Dorsal intercalated segmental instability (DISI). Sagittal T1-weighted image shows the dorsal tilt of the lunate (*long arrow*) and proximal migration of the capitate (*short arrow*).

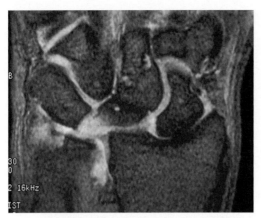

Fig. 24. Scapholunate advance collapse (SLAC): end stage of SL instability. The SL ligament is torn and there is widening of the interval. There is advanced radiocarpal arthritis, proximal migration of the capitate, and midcarpal arthritis.

lunate triquetral instability present with ulnar-sided pain.

Tears of the lunatotriquetral ligament are more difficult to detect than tears of the scapholunate ligament as it is a smaller ligament [26,46], but these lesions are less common. The most specific finding for a lunatotriquetral tears is discontinuity of the ligament with increased signal intensity on imaging sequences with T2-type contrast (Fig. 25). High signal contrast with MR arthrography may outline a defect in the lunate triquetral ligament as well (see Fig. 25). Absence of the ligament is a less useful

finding [70] as the lunate triqeutral ligament may be less reliably observed on MR imaging than the scapholunate ligament, although on thin-section 3D volumetric images this may be a more useful finding [7,31]. Changes in morphology are also less useful than they are in evaluating the scapholunate ligament. Fluid in the midcarpal joint is said to be a sensitive finding for lunatotriquetral tears as well [70]. A pitfall to be avoided is in the volar portion of the ligament. Here it attaches to the TFC and may appear discontinuous. Widening of the lunate triquetral articulation is not usually evident even in advanced cases [115].

Tears of the lunatotriquetral ligament may coexist with static and dynamic patterns of palmar midcarpal instability (VISI) (Fig. 26). In patients with volar intercalated segmental instability, the lunate is no longer linked to the triquetrum and follows the scaphoid. In this situation the lunate tends to be volarflexed with the wrist in a neutral position, and there is proximal and volar migration of the bones in the distal carpal row. Sagittal MR images will show the palmar tilting of the lunate and scaphoid (see Fig. 26). The scapholunate angle is less than 30 degrees, and the capitolunate angle may measure up to 30 degrees.

Patients with dynamic patterns of midcarpal instability may be normal at rest but present with a wrist clunk when moving from radial to ulnar deviation as a result of the proximal carpal row snapping suddenly from a palmar flexed position to a dorsal flexed position, instead of making a smooth

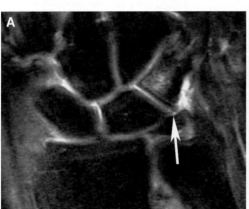

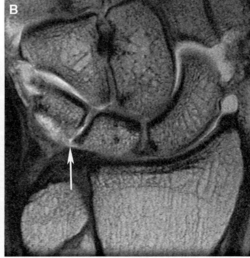

Fig. 25. Lunate triquetral ligament tear. (A) Coronal T2 FSE image with fat saturation Fluid signal delineates a tear in the lunate triquetral ligament (*arrow*). A contusion is noted in the triquetrum in this acute injury. (B) Coronal T1-weighted MR arthrogram in another patient also reveals a tear of the lunotriquetral ligament (*arrow*). Contrast injected by way of a radiocarpal injection extends through the LT tear into the midcarpal joint compartment.

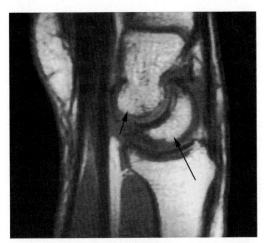

Fig. 26. Volar intercalated segmental instability (VISI). The lunate is volar flexed (*arrow*). There is proximal migration of the capitate (*small arrow*).

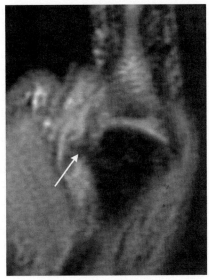

Fig. 28. Gamekeeper's thumb, Stener lesion. (*A*) Coronal fat-suppressed T2-weighted image shows a torn, retracted UCL lying superficial to the adductor aponeurosis (*arrow*). This gives the retracted ligament the appearance of a "yo-yo on a string."

synchronous transition [123,124]. Because of their complex motion, dynamic forms of carpal instability are still best documented with wrist fluoroscopy. Despite recent advances in the speed of exam and the use of different positioning devices [125], kinematic MR imaging is still unable to easily document such complex motion. This abnormality is thought to result from tear, laxity, or insufficiency of the ulnar limb of the arcuate ligament (V, deltoid). This ligament can be visualized with MR imaging [8,32,108] (see Fig. 2), although as yet there are no reports of the accuracy of MR imaging in depicting its disruption in patients with clinically evident

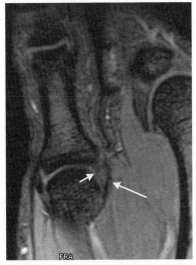

Fig. 27. Gamekeeper's thumb, nondisplaced ulnar collateral ligament tear. Coronal 3D GRE image of the first MCP joint reveals a focally disrupted distal UCL, outlined by high signal (*short arrow*), which remains beneath the adductor aponeurosis (*long arrow*).

midcarpal instability. MR imaging may also reveal degenerative changes on the proximal pole of the capitate in these patients [115].

Diagnostic performance

Zlatkin, Osterman, and coworkers [46,126] found a sensitivity, specificity, and accuracy of 0.80, 0.93, and 0.91 for SL tears compared with arthroscopy and surgery. For LT tears a sensitivity, specificity, and accuracy of 0.50, 0.81, and 0.70 was found when compared with arthroscopy and surgery. A later study of scapholunate tears alone, compared with arthroscopy, yielded a sensitivity of 0.76 and specificity of 0.60 [107]. In this study, arthrography (three phase) was also compared with arthroscopy. A sensitivity of 0.55 and specificity of 0.60 was found. MR imaging, in particular, was found to be more sensitive in the evaluation of partial tears and in determining the site, location, and extent of the ligament pathology. When patients had both studies performed there was an improvement in the specificity and positive predictive value. Schweitzer and coworkers [70] also compared MR imaging to arthrography and arthroscopy. Their results in evaluating scapholunate and lunte triquetral ligament injuries were less favorable.

A recent study by Manton and coworkers [95] assessed the accuracy of high-field MR imaging in the evaluation of partial ligament tears. They assessed primary signs and secondary signs potentially seen as mechanical sequelae of tears. This included osseous offset, arc disruption, or focal osteoarthritis The accuracy of the primary MR signs of partial tears was lower than that described in the literature for complete tears [sensitivity/specificity (kappa) = 0.56/0.56 (0.12) for scapholunate ligament tears and 0.31/0.76 (0.13) for lunate triquetral tears]. The secondary signs they studied showed a low sensitivity but high specificity, particularly for lunate triquetral ligament tears. Additionally, there was poor interobserver consistency for primary and secondary signs of partial ligament tears in this study.

Scheck et al [98] evaluated the benefit of MR arthrography in evaluation of the intercarpal ligaments. Using thin-section 3D volume images, there was better delineation of the wrist ligaments with MR arthrography. In addition, the sensitivity/ specificity and accuracy of noncontrast MR for the diagnosis of full-thickness ligamentous defects was 0.81/0.75/0.77. With MR arthrography there was improvement to 0.97/0.96/0.96.

Volar ligament injury

Tears of the volar ligaments are less commonly identified at MR exam. When seen, they may be characterized by increased signal intensity, irregularity and fraying, and corresponding high signal intensity on images with T2-type contrast (see Fig. 20). Most often such injuries may not be well seen at MR imaging, or areas of focal synovitis may be used as markers of such injury. The accuracy of MR imaging in determining tears in one study was 61% [126]. Recent improvements in resolution and MR arthrography [12,20] may improve the ability of MR imaging to evaluate these ligaments.

Treatment

Treatment of scapholunate instability is controversial. Advances continue to be made in direct scapholunate interosseous ligament reconstruction [127]. Early cases can be treated with pinning and ligamentous repair. Other forms of treatment include intercarpal fusions, such as fusion of the distal pole of the scaphoid to the trapezoid and trapezius (triscaphe fusion) [128,129] or capsulodesis [130]. These procedures can limit excessive scaphoid motion, promote wrist stability, and potentially prevent arthritis.

Lunatotriquetral instability can be treated with intercarpal fusion or with ulnar shortening and ligamentous repair if there is an ulna-positive variant. Arthroscopic techniques are developing as well [115,131]. If volar segmental instability pattern (VISI) is present, this may require repair of the dorsal radiocarpal ligaments as these may also be torn [132].

Thumb

Ulnar collateral ligament injury (gamekeeper's thumb)

Injury to the ulnar collateral ligament occurs from a radially directed force on the abducted thumb. Historically, the injury was described in Scottish gamekeepers. Ulnar collateral ligament injury involving the thumb is now most commonly associated with skiing and other sports-related activities [133–135]. Complete ulnar collateral ligament tear is detected clinically by the demonstration of MCP joint laxity with greater than 30 degrees of angulation at the joint. Stener first proposed that the torn ulnar collateral ligament may frequently become displaced so that it lies superficial to the adductor pollicis aponeurosis. This interposed aponeurosis, known as the Stener lesion, can inhibit proper healing of the ligament [136–138]. The incidence of Stener lesions is reported to be approximately 29%, but there is wide variation in the literature in this regard [136–141]. Nondisplaced ulnar collateral ligament tears are usually treated conservatively. Surgical intervention is usually reserved for Stener lesions. Avulsion fractures involving more than 20% of the articular surface may require pinning. Smaller fracture fragments are often excised (see references [139,140,142,143]).

The clinical diagnosis of Stener lesions may be difficult in the acute setting because of overlying soft tissue edema and hematoma. In the past, the lack of sufficient imaging required most hand surgeons to surgically explore suspected Stener lesions. Arthrography was used by some and demonstrated extravasation along the ulnar aspect of this joint when the ligament was torn. A filling defect indicated a Stener lesion [144–147].

MR imaging can detect the torn ligament and reveal displacement if present (see references [134,137,144,148–151]). One additional benefit of MR imaging in the assessment of these lesions is in the detection of associated clinically occult injuries involving bone or soft tissues. The normal ligament has a low signal, medial to the joint on coronal MR images. The adductor aponeurosis is visible as a paper-thin band of low signal superficial to the ligament from the distal half of the ligament over the base of the proximal phalanx. A nondisplaced tear appears as a discontinuity of the ligament without retraction (Fig. 27) and with the aponeurosis covering the distal end of the ligament.

In the presence of a Stener lesion the MR imaging findings include UCL disruption from the base of the proximal phalanx with retraction or folding of the ligament [137]. The retracted ligament lies superficial to the adductor aponeurosis, the proximal aspect of which abuts the folded ulnar collateral ligament, which appears as a round low signal structure on all pulse sequences. This characteristic MR appearance has been described as a "yo-yo on a string" (Fig. 28).

References

[1] Hobby JL, Dixon AK, Bearcroft PW, et al. MR imaging of the wrist: effect on clinical diagnosis and patient care. Radiology 2001;220(3): 589–93.

[2] Mayfield JK. Wrist ligamentous anatomy and pathogenesis of carpal instability. Orthop Clin North Am 1984;15(2):209–16.

[3] Taleisnik J. The ligaments of the wrist. J Hand Surg [Am] 1976;1(2):110–8.

[4] Berger RA, Linscheid RL, Berquist TH. Magnetic resonance imaging of the anterior radiocarpal ligaments. J Hand Surg [Am] 1994;19(2): 295–303.

[5] Berger RA. The ligaments of the wrist. A current overview of anatomy with considerations of their potential functions. Hand Clin 1997; 13(1):63–82.

[6] Berger RA, Landsmeer JM. The palmar radiocarpal ligaments: a study of adult and fetal human wrist joints. J Hand Surg [Am] 1990;15(6): 847–54.

[7] Smith DK. MR imaging of normal and injured wrist ligaments. Magn Reson Imaging Clin N Am 1995;3(2):229–48.

[8] Smith DK. Volar carpal ligaments of the wrist: normal appearance on multiplanar reconstructions of three-dimensional Fourier transform MR imaging. AJR Am J Roentgenol 1993; 161(2):353–7.

[9] Adler BD, Logan PM, Janzen DL, et al. Extrinsic radiocarpal ligaments: magnetic resonance imaging of normal wrists and scapholunate dissociation. Can Assoc Radiol J 1996;47(6):417–22.

[10] Timins ME, Jahnke JP, Krah SF, Erickson SJ, Carrera GF. MR imaging of the major carpal stabilizing ligaments: normal anatomy and clinical examples. Radiographics 1995;15(3):575–87.

[11] Johnston RB, Seiler JG, Miller EJ, Drvaric DM. The intrinsic and extrinsic ligaments of the wrist. A correlation of collagen typing and histologic appearance. J Hand Surg [Br] 1995; 20(6):750–4.

[12] Theumann NH, Pfirrmann CW, Antonio GE, et al. Extrinsic carpal ligaments: normal MR arthrographic appearance in cadavers. Radiology 2003;226(1):171–9.

[13] Totterman SM, Miller R, Wasserman B, Blebea JS, Rubens DJ, et al. Intrinsic and extrinsic carpal ligaments: evaluation by three-dimensional Fourier transform MR imaging. AJR Am J Roentgenol 1993;100(1):117–23.

[14] Berger RA. The anatomy of the scaphoid. Hand Clin 2001;17(4):525–32.

[15] Berger RA, Blair WF. The radioscapholunate ligament: a gross and histologic description. Anat Rec 1984;210(2):393–405.

[16] Berger RA, Kauer JM, Landsmeer JM. Radioscapholunate ligament: a gross anatomic and histologic study of fetal and adult wrists. J Hand Surg [Am] 1991;16(2):350–5.

[17] Mayfield JK, Johnson RP, Kilcoyne RF. The ligaments of the human wrist and their functional significance. Anat Rec 1976;186(3): 417–28.

[18] Gelberman RH, Cooney WP III, Szabo RM. Carpal instability. Instr Course Lect 2001; 50:123–34.

[19] Beaulieu CF, Ladd AL. MR arthrography of the wrist: scanning-room injection of the radiocarpal joint based on clinical landmarks. AJR Am J Roentgenol 1998;170(3):606–8.

[20] Brown RR, Fliszar E, Cotten A, Trudell D, Resnick D. Extrinsic and intrinsic ligaments of the wrist: normal and pathologic anatomy at MR arthrography with three-compartment enhancement. Radiographics 1998;18(3): 667–74.

[21] Zlatkin MB, Ouellette EA, Needell S. MR and MR arthrography of the intercarpal ligaments of the wrist. Histopathologic correlation. Paper presented at the annual meeting of the Society of Magnetic Resonance. New York, NY, 1996.

[22] Smith DK. Dorsal carpal ligaments of the wrist: normal appearance on multiplanar reconstructions of three-dimensional Fourier transform MR imaging. AJR Am J Roentgenol 1993; 161(1):119–25.

[23] Viegas SF. The dorsal ligaments of the wrist. Hand Clin 2001;17(1):65–75.

[24] Mizuseki T, Ikuta Y. The dorsal carpal ligaments: their anatomy and function. J Hand Surg [Br] 1989;14(1):91–8.

[25] DiMarcangelo MT, Smith PA. Use of magnetic resonance imaging to diagnose common wrist disorders. J Am Osteopath Assoc 2000;100(4): 228–31.

[26] Zlatkin MB, Greenan T. Magnetic resonance imaging of the wrist. Magn Reson Q 1992; 8(2):65–96.

[27] Berger RA. The anatomy of the ligaments of the wrist and distal radioulnar joints. Clin Orthop 2001;383:32–40.

[28] Berger RA. The gross and histologic anatomy of the scapholunate interosseous ligament. J Hand Surg [Am] 1996;21(2):170–8.

[29] Bogumill G. Anatomy of the wrist. In: Lichtman DM, Herbert A, editors. The wrist and its disorders. Philadelphia: W.B. Saunders; 1997. p. 34–48.

[30] Smith DK. Scapholunate interosseous ligament of the wrist: MR appearances in asymptomatic volunteers and arthrographically normal wrists. Radiology 1994;192(1):217–21.

[31] Smith DK, Snearly WN. Lunotriquetral interosseous ligament of the wrist: MR appearances in

asymptomatic volunteers and arthrographically normal wrists. Radiology 1994;191(1):199–202.

[32] Reicher MA, Kellerhouse LE. MRI of the wrist and hand. New York: Raven Press; 1990.

[33] Totterman SM, Miller RJ. Scapholunate ligament: normal MR appearance on three-dimensional gradient-recalled-echo images. Radiology 1996;200(1):237–41.

[34] Palmer AK, Werner FW. The triangular fibrocartilage complex of the wrist—anatomy and function. J Hand Surg [Am] 1981;6(2):153–62.

[35] Loftus JB, Palmer AK. Disorders of the distal radioulnar joint and TFCC. An overview. In: Lichtman DM, Alexander AH, editors. The wrist and its disorders. Philadelphia: W.B. Saunders; 1997.

[36] Benjamin M, Evans EJ, Pemberton DJ. Histological studies on the triangular fibrocartilage complex of the wrist. J Anat 1990;172:59–67.

[37] Prendergast N, Rauschning W. Normal anatomy of the hand and wrist. Magn Reson Imaging Clin N Am 1995;3(2):197–212.

[38] Totterman SM, Miller RJ. Triangular fibrocartilage complex: normal appearance on coronal three-dimensional gradient-recalled-echo MR images. Radiology 1995;195(2):521–7.

[39] Totterman SM, Miller RJ. MR imaging of the triangular fibrocartilage complex. Magn Reson Imaging Clin N Am 1995;3(2):213–28.

[40] Palmer AK, Werner FW. The triangular fibrocartilage complex of the wrist-anatomy and function. J Hand Surg [Am] 1981;6:153–62.

[41] Palmer AK, Glisson RR, Werner FW. Relationship between ulnar variance and triangular fibrocartilage complex thickness. J Hand Surg [Am] 1984;9(5):681–2.

[42] De Smet L. Ulnar variance: facts and fiction review article. Acta Orthop [Belg] 1994;60(1):1–9.

[43] Bednar MS, Arnoczky SP, Weiland AJ. The microvasculature of the triangular fibrocartilage complex: its clinical significance. J Hand Surg [Am] 1991;16(6):1101–5.

[44] Kang HS, Kindynis P, Brahme SK, et al. Triangular fibrocartilage and intercarpal ligaments of the wrist: MR imaging. Cadaveric study with gross pathologic and histologic correlation. Radiology 1991;181(2):401–4.

[45] Mikic Z. Age changes in the triangular fibrocartilage of the wrist joint. J Anat 1978;126:367–84.

[46] Zlatkin MB, Chao PC, Osterman AL, Schnall MD, Dalinka MK, Kressel HY. Chronic wrist pain: evaluation with high-resolution MR imaging. Radiology 1989;173(3):723–9.

[47] Totterman SM, Seo GS. MRI findings of scapholunate instabilities in coronal images: a short communication. Semin Musculoskelet Radiol 2001;5(3):251–6.

[48] Ekenstam F. Anatomy of the distal radioulnar joint. Clin Orthop 1992;275:14–8.

[49] Drobner WS, Hausman MR. The distal radioulnar joint. Hand Clin 1992;8(4):631–44.

[50] Chiang CC, Chang MC, Lin CF, Liu Y, Lo WH. Computerized tomography in the diagnosis of subluxation of the distal radioulnar joint. Zhonghua Yi Xue Za Zhi [Taipei] 1998;61(12):708–15.

[51] Cerezal L, del Pinal F, Abascal F, Garcia-Valtuille R, Pereda T, Canga A. Imaging findings in ulnar-sided wrist impaction syndromes. Radiographics 2002;22(1):105–21.

[52] De Smet L. Ulnar variance and its relationship to ligament injuries of the wrist. Acta Orthop [Belg] 1999;65(4):416–7.

[53] Escobedo EM, Bergman AG, Hunter JC. MR imaging of ulnar impaction. Skeletal Radiol 1995;24(2):85–90.

[54] Adolfsson L. Arthroscopic diagnosis of ligament lesions of the wrist. J Hand Surg [Br] 1994;19(4):505–12.

[55] Friedman SL, Palmer AK. The ulnar impaction syndrome. Hand Clin 1991;7(2):295–310.

[56] Oneson SR, Scales LM, Timins ME, Erickson SJ, Chamoy L. MR imaging interpretation of the Palmer classification of triangular fibrocartilage complex lesions. Radiographics 1996;16(1):97–106.

[57] Gilula LA, Palmer AK. Is it possible to diagnose a tear at arthrography or MR imaging? Radiology 1993;187(2):582.

[58] Steinborn M, Schurmann M, Staebler A, et al. MR imaging of ulnocarpal impaction after fracture of the distal radius. AJR Am J Roentgenol 2003;181(1):195–8.

[59] Tomaino MM. Ulnar impaction syndrome in the ulnar negative and neutral wrist. Diagnosis and pathoanatomy. J Hand Surg [Br] 1998;23(6):754–7.

[60] Imaeda T, Nakamura R, Shionoya K, Makino N. Ulnar impaction syndrome: MR imaging findings. Radiology 1996;201(2):495–500.

[61] Manaster BJ. The clinical efficacy of triple-injection wrist arthrography. Radiology 1991;178(1):267–70.

[62] Chidgey L. Histologic anatomy of the triangular fibrocartilage. Hand Clin 1991;14(4):624–7.

[63] Golimbu CN, Firooznia H, Melone CP Jr, Rafii M, Weinreb J, Leber C. Tears of the triangular fibrocartilage of the wrist: MR imaging. Radiology 1989;173(3):731–3.

[64] Melone CP Jr, Nathan R. Traumatic disruption of the triangular fibrocartilage complex. Pathoanatomy. Clin Orthop 1992;275:65–73.

[65] Millants P, De Smet L, Van Ransbeeck H. Outcome study of arthroscopic suturing of ulnar avulsions of the triangular fibrocartilage complex of the wrist. Chir Main 2002;21(5):298–300.

[66] Corso SJ, Savoie FH, Geissler WB, Whipple TL, Jiminez W, Jenkins N. Arthroscopic repair of peripheral avulsions of the triangular

fibrocartilage complex of the wrist: a multicenter study. Arthroscopy 1997;13(1):78–84.

[67] Hauck RM, Skahen J III, Palmer AK. Classification and treatment of ulnar styloid nonunion. J Hand Surg [Am] 1996;21(3):418–22.

[68] Mikic ZD. Treatment of acute injuries of the triangular fibrocartilage complex associated with distal radioulnar joint instability. J Hand Surg [Am] 1995;20(2):319–23.

[69] Fellinger M, Peicha G, Seibert FJ, Grechenig W. Radial avulsion of the triangular fibrocartilage complex in acute wrist trauma: a new technique for arthroscopic repair. Arthroscopy 1997; 13(3):370–4.

[70] Schweitzer ME, Brahme SK, Hodler J, et al. Chronic wrist pain: spin-echo and short tau inversion recovery MR imaging and conventional and MR arthrography. Radiology 1992; 182(1):205–11.

[71] Metz VM, Schratter M, Dock WI, et al. Age-associated changes of the triangular fibrocartilage of the wrist: evaluation of the diagnostic performance of MR imaging. Radiology 1992;184(1):217–20.

[72] Haims AH, Schweitzer ME, Morrison WB, et al. Limitations of MR imaging in the diagnosis of peripheral tears of the triangular fibrocartilage of the wrist. AJR Am J Roentgenol 2002; 178(2):419–22.

[73] Oneson SR, Timins ME, Scales LM, Erickson SJ, Chamoy L. MR imaging diagnosis of triangular fibrocartilage pathology with arthroscopic correlation. AJR Am J Roentgenol 1997; 168(6):1513–8.

[74] Haims AH, Schweitzer ME, Morrison WB, et al. Internal derangement of the wrist: indirect MR arthrography versus unenhanced MR imaging. Radiology 2003;227(3):701–7.

[75] Schweitzer ME, Natale P, Winalski CS, Culp R. Indirect wrist MR arthrography: the effects of passive motion versus active exercise. Skeletal Radiol 2000;29(1):10–4.

[76] Topper SM, Wood MB, Ruby LK. Ulnar styloid impaction syndrome. J Hand Surg [Am] 1997; 22(4):699–704.

[77] Potter HG, Asnis-Ernberg L, Weiland AJ, Hotchkiss RN, Peterson MG, McCormack RR Jr. The utility of high-resolution magnetic resonance imaging in the evaluation of the triangular fibrocartilage complex of the wrist. J Bone Joint Surg [Am] 1997;79(11):1675–84.

[78] Johnstone DJ, Thorogood S, Smith WH, Scott TD. A comparison of magnetic resonance imaging and arthroscopy in the investigation of chronic wrist pain. J Hand Surg [Br] 1997; 22(6):714–8.

[79] Herold T, Lenhart M, Held P, et al. Indirect MR arthrography of the wrist in the diagnosis of TFCC lesions [in German]. Rofo Fortschr Geb Rontgenstr Neuen Bildgeb Verfahr 2001; 173(11):1006–11.

[80] Osterman AL. Arthroscopic debridement of triangular fibrocartilage complex tears. Arthroscopy 1990;6(2):120–4.

[81] Baehser-Griffith P, Bednar JM, Osterman AL, Culp R. Arthroscopic repairs of triangular fibrocartilage complex tears. AORN J 1997;66(1): 101–2, 105–11; quiz 112, 115, 117–8.

[82] Zachee B, De Smet L, Fabry G. Arthroscopic suturing of TFCC lesions. Arthroscopy 1993; 9(2):242–3.

[83] Bednar JM, Osterman AL. The role of arthroscopy in the treatment of traumatic triangular fibrocartilage injuries. Hand Clin 1994;10(4): 605–14.

[84] Minami A, Kato H. Ulnar shortening for triangular fibrocartilage complex tears associated with ulnar positive variance. J Hand Surg [Am] 1998;23(5):904–8.

[85] Buterbaugh GA, Brown TR, Horn PC. Ulnar-sided wrist pain in athletes. Clin Sports Med 1998;17(3):567–83.

[86] Theumann NH, Pfirrmann CW, Chung CB, Antonio GE, Trudell DJ, Resnick D. Pisotriquetral joint: assessment with MR imaging and MR arthrography. Radiology 2002;222(3): 763–70.

[87] Thurston AJ, Stanley JK. Hamato-lunate impingement: an uncommon cause of ulnar-sided wrist pain. Arthroscopy 2000;16(5):540–4.

[88] Nathan R, Schneider LH. Classification of distal radioulnar joint disorders. Hand Clin 1991; 7(2):239–47.

[89] Nicolaidis SC, Hildreth DH, Lichtman DM. Acute injuries of the distal radioulnar joint. Hand Clin 2000;16(3):449–59.

[90] Mino DE, Palmer AK, Levinsohn EM. The role of radiography and computerized tomography in the diagnosis of subluxation and dislocation of the distal radioulnar joint. J Hand Surg [Am] 1983;8(1):23–31.

[91] King GJ, McMurtry RY, Rubenstein JD, Ogston NG. Computerized tomography of the distal radioulnar joint: correlation with ligamentous pathology in a cadaveric model. J Hand Surg [Am] 1986;11(5):711–7.

[92] Wechsler RJ, Wehbe MA, Rifkin MD, Edeiken J, Branch HM. Computed tomography diagnosis of distal radioulnar subluxation. Skeletal Radiol 1987;16(1):1–5.

[93] Steinbach LS, Smith DK. MRI of the wrist. Clin Imaging 2000;24(5):298–322.

[94] Daunt N. Magnetic resonance imaging of the wrist: anatomy and pathology of interosseous ligaments and the triangular fibrocartilage complex. Curr Probl Diagn Radiol 2002;31(4): 158–76.

[95] Manton GL, Schweitzer ME, Weishaupt D, et al. Partial interosseous ligament tears of the wrist: difficulty in utilizing either primary or secondary MRI signs. J Comput Assist Tomogr 2001; 25(5):671–6.

[96] Oneson SR, Scales LM, Erickson SJ, Timins ME. MR imaging of the painful wrist. Radiographics 1996;16(5):997–1008.

[97] Schadel-Hopfner M, Iwinska-Zelder J, Braus T, Bohringer G, Klose KJ, Gotzen L. MRI versus arthroscopy in the diagnosis of scapholunate ligament injury. J Hand Surg [Br] 2001;26(1): 17–21.

[98] Scheck RJ, Kubitzek C, Hierner R, et al. The scapholunate interosseous ligament in MR arthrography of the wrist: correlation with non-enhanced MRI and wrist arthroscopy. Skeletal Radiol 1997;26(5):263–71.

[99] Mayfield JK. Mechanism of carpal injuries. Clin Orthop 1980;149:45–54.

[100] Mayfield JK. Patterns of injury to carpal ligaments. A spectrum. Clin Orthop 1984;187: 36–42.

[101] Wright TW, Dobyns JH, Linzcheid RL, Macksoud W, Siegert J. Carpal instability nondissociative. J Hand Surg [Br] 1994;19(6): 763–73.

[102] Cooney WP, Dobyns JH, Linscheid RL. Arthroscopy of the wrist: anatomy and classification of carpal instability. Arthroscopy 1990;6(2): 133–40.

[103] Cassidy C, Ruby LK. Carpal instability. Instr Course Lect 2003;52:209–20.

[104] Miller RJ. Wrist MRI and carpal instability: what the surgeon needs to know, and the case for dynamic imaging. Semin Musculoskelet Radiol 2001;5(3):235–40.

[105] Taleisnik J. Classification of carpal instability. Bull Hosp Jt Dis Orthop Inst 1984;44(2): 511–31.

[106] Taleisnik J. Current concepts review. Carpal instability. J Bone Joint Surg [Am] 1988; 70(8):1262–8.

[107] Schofield BA, OE, Zlatkin MB, Murphy B. MRI correlation with scapholunate ligament tears. Paper presented at the annual meeting of the American Academy of Orthopedic Surgeons. Orlando, FL, 1995.

[108] Rominger MB, Bernreuter WK, Kenney PJ, Lee DH. MR imaging of anatomy and tears of wrist ligaments. Radiographics 1993;13(6): 1233–46; discussion 1247–8.

[109] Scheck RJ, Romagnolo A, Hierner R, Pfluger T, Whilhelm K, Hahn K. The carpal ligaments in MR arthrography of the wrist: correlation with standard MRI and wrist arthroscopy. J Magn Reson Imaging 1999;9(3):468–74.

[110] Steinbach LS, Palmer WE, Schweitzer ME. Special focus session. MR arthrography. Radiographics 2002;22(5):1223–46.

[111] Zanetti M, Bram J, Hodler J. Triangular fibrocartilage and intercarpal ligaments of the wrist: does MR arthrography improve standard MRI? J Magn Reson Imaging 1997;7(3):590–4.

[112] Linscheid RL, Dobyns JH, Beabout JW, Bryan RS. Traumatic instability of the wrist:

diagnosis, classification, and pathomechanics. J Bone Joint Surg [Am] 2002;84(1):142.

[113] Ruby LK, An KN, Linscheid RL, Cooney WP 3rd, Chao EY. The effect of scapholunate ligament section on scapholunate motion. J Hand Surg [Am] 1987;12(5 Pt 1):767–71.

[114] Kovanlikaya I, Camli D, Cakmakci H, et al. Diagnostic value of MR arthrography in detection of intrinsic carpal ligament lesions: use of cine-MR arthrography as a new approach. Eur Radiol 1997;7(9):1441–5.

[115] Brody GSD. The wrist and hand. In: Stoller D, editor. Magnetic resonance imaging in orthopedics and sports medecine. Philadelphia: J.P. Lippincott; 1993. p. 683–807.

[116] Zanetti M, Hodler J, Gilula LA. Assessment of dorsal or ventral intercalated segmental instability configurations of the wrist: reliability of sagittal MR images. Radiology 1998;206(2): 339–45.

[117] Stabler A, Heuck A, Reiser M. Imaging of the hand: degeneration, impingement and overuse. Eur J Radiol 1997;25(2):118–28.

[118] Resnick D. SLAC wrist. J Hand Surg [Am] 1985; 10(1):154–5.

[119] Watson HK, Ballet FL. The SLAC wrist: scapholunate advanced collapse pattern of degenerative arthritis. J Hand Surg [Am] 1984;9(3): 358–65.

[120] O'Meeghan CJ, Stuart W, Mamo V, Stanley JK, Trail IA. The natural history of an untreated isolated scapholunate interosseus ligament injury. J Hand Surg [Br] 2003;28(4):307–10.

[121] Osterman AL, Mikulics M. Scaphoid nonunion. Hand Clin 1988;4(3):437–55.

[122] Weiss LE, Taras JS, Sweet S, Osterman AL. Lunotriquetral injuries in the athlete. Hand Clin 2000;16(3):433–8.

[123] Brown DE, Lichtman DM. Midcarpal instability. Hand Clin 1987;3(1):135–40.

[124] Lichtman DM, Bruckner JD, Culp RW, Alexander CE. Palmar midcarpal instability: results of surgical reconstruction. J Hand Surg [Am] 1993;18(2):307–15.

[125] Ton ER, Pattynama PM, Bloem JL, Obermann WR. Interosseous ligaments: device for applying stress in wrist MR imaging. Radiology 1995;196(3):863–4.

[126] Osterman AL, Zlatkin MB. Magnetic resonance imaging in patients with chronic wrist pain. Presented at the forty-fifth annual meeting of the American Society for Surgery of the Hand. Toronto, Canada, 1990.

[127] Walsh JJ, Berger RA, Cooney WP. Current status of scapholunate interosseous ligament injuries. J Am Acad Orthop Surg 2002;10(1): 32–42.

[128] Watson HK, Ryu J, Akelman E. Limited triscaphoid intercarpal arthrodesis for rotatory subluxation of the scaphoid. J Bone Joint Surg [Am] 1986;68(3):345–9.

[129] Watson HK, Weinzweig J, Zeppieri J. The natural progression of scaphoid instability. Hand Clin 1997;13(1):39–49.

[130] Lavernia CJ, Cohen MS, Taleisnik J. Treatment of scapholunate dissociation by ligamentous repair and capsulodesis. J Hand Surg [Am] 1992;17(2):354–9.

[131] Moskal MJ, Savoie FH III, Field LD. Arthroscopic capsulodesis of the lunotriquetral joint. Clin Sports Med 2001;20(1):141–53 [ix–x.].

[132] Viegas SF. Ulnar-sided wrist pain and instability. Instr Course Lect 1998;47:215–8.

[133] Heim D. The skier's thumb. Acta Orthop [Belg] 1999;65(4):440–6.

[134] Plancher KD, et al. Role of MR imaging in the management of "skier's thumb" injuries. Magn Reson Imaging Clin N Am 1999;7(1):73–84 [viii.].

[135] Engkvist O, Balkfors B, Lindsjo U. Thumb injuries in downhill skiing. Int J Sports Med 1982;3(1):50–5.

[136] Kaplan SJ. The Stener lesion revisited: a case report. J Hand Surg [Am] 1998;23(5):833–6.

[137] Haramati N, et al. MRI of the Stener lesion. Skeletal Radiol 1995;24(7):515–8.

[138] Stener B. Skeletal injuries associated with rupture of the ulnar collateral ligament of the metacarpophalangeal joint of the thumb. A clinical and anatomical study. Acta Chir Scand 1963;125:583–6.

[139] Fairhurst M, Hansen L. Treatment of "gamekeeper's thumb" by reconstruction of the ulnar collateral ligament. J Hand Surg [Br] 2002; 27(6):542–5.

[140] Melone CP Jr, Beldner S, Basuk RS. Thumb collateral ligament injuries. An anatomic basis for treatment. Hand Clin 2000;16(3): 345–57.

[141] Salvi V. Rupture of the ulnar collateral ligament of the metacarpophalangeal joint of the thumb (Stener's lesion). Panminerva Med 1968;10(4): 159–63.

[142] Kozin SH, Bishop AT. Gamekeeper's thumb. Early diagnosis and treatment. Orthop Rev 1994;23(10):797–804.

[143] Hintermann B, et al. Skier's thumb—the significance of bony injuries. Am J Sports Med 1993; 21(6):800–4.

[144] Vasenius J, Nieminen O, Lohman M. Late reconstruction of the ulnar collateral ligament of the thumb MP joint with free tendon graft—a new technique. J Hand Surg [Am] 2003;28(Suppl 1):44.

[145] Engel J, et al. Arthrography as a method of diagnosing tear of the ulnar collateral ligament of the metacarpophalangeal joint of the thumb ("gamekeeper's thumb"). J Trauma 1979;19(2): 106–9.

[146] Bowers WH, Hurst LC. Gamekeeper's thumb. Evaluation by arthrography and stress roentgenography. J Bone Joint Surg [Am] 1977; 59(4):519–24.

[147] Resnick D, Danzig LA. Arthrographic evaluation of injuries of the first metacarpophalangeal joint: gamekeeper's thumb. Am J Roentgenol 1976;126(5):1046–52.

[148] Romano WM, et al. The spectrum of ulnar collateral ligament injuries as viewed on magnetic resonance imaging of the metacarpophalangeal joint of the thumb. Can Assoc Radiol J 2003; 54(4):243–8.

[149] Lohman M, et al. MR imaging in chronic rupture of the ulnar collateral ligament of the thumb. Acta Radiol 2001;42(1):10–4.

[150] Ahn JM, et al. Gamekeeper thumb: comparison of MR arthrography with conventional arthrography and MR imaging in cadavers. Radiology 1998;206(3):737–44.

[151] Hinke DH, et al. Ulnar collateral ligament of the thumb: MR findings in cadavers, volunteers, and patients with ligamentous injury (gamekeeper's thumb). AJR Am J Roentgenol 1994;163(6):1431–4.

[152] Ahn JM, Broun RR, Kwak SM, Kang HS, Mutrle C, Botte MJ, et al. Evaluation of the triangular fibric cortilage and the scaphalunate and lunctriquetal ligaments in cadavers with low-field-strength extremity-only magnet. Comparison of available imaging sequences and macroscopic findings. Invest Radiol 1998; 33:401–6.

RADIOLOGIC CLINICS OF NORTH AMERICA

Radiol Clin N Am 44 (2006) 625–642

MR Imaging: Arthropathies and Infectious Conditions of the Elbow, Wrist, and Hand

Marlena Jbara, MD*, Madhavi Patnana, MD, Faaiza Kazmi, MD, Javier Beltran, MD

- Rheumatoid arthritis
- Seronegative spondyloarthropathy
- Gout
- Synovial osteochondromatosis
- Pigmented villonodular synovitis
- Tenosynovitis
- de Quervain's tenosynovitis
- Infectious tenosynovitis
- Osteoarthritis
- Neuropathic arthropathy

- Sarcoidosis
- Amyloid arthropathy
- Hemophilic arthropathy
- Osteomyelitis
- Septic arthritis
- Septic olecranon bursitis
- Pyomyositis
- Mycobacteria
- Cat scratch disease
- References

The superior soft tissue contrast and multiplanar capability of MR imaging has contributed to earlier diagnosis and implementation of effective treatment for a variety of arthropathies and infectious conditions of the elbow, wrist, and hand. Because of overlapping clinical signs and symptoms, MR imaging plays an important role in delineating the features and staging of each of these conditions. This article discusses the seropositive and seronegative inflammatory arthropathies, with emphasis on early detection and surveillance, as well as gout, synovial osteochondromatosis, pigmented villonodular synovitis, tenosynovitis, and de Quervain's tenosynovitis. Certain noninflammatory arthritides that can affect the upper extremity, such as osteoarthritis, neuropathic arthropathy, sarcoidosis, amyloid and hemophilic arthropathies, are also briefly discussed. Infectious conditions including osteomyelitis, pyomyositis, septic olecranon bursitis, tuberculosis, and cat scratch disease, with emphasis on MR imaging characteristics, are reviewed.

Rheumatoid arthritis

Rheumatoid arthritis is a very common disease that affects up to 1% of the world population. The disease predominates in the elderly population but can occur at any age. Synovitis, which progresses to joint space destruction and long-term disability, is known to begin as early as 2 years after disease onset [1–3]. MR imaging has emerged as the most sensitive means of identifying rheumatoid arthritis (RA) in its earliest stages [4–9]. The use of disease-modifying antirheumatic drugs early in the

This article was previously published in *Magnetic Resonance Imaging Clinics of North America* 2004; 12:361–379.

Department of Radiology, Maimonides Medical Center, 4802 10th Avenue, Brooklyn, NY 11219, USA

* Corresponding author.

E-mail address: jamalito1027@aol.com (M. Jbara).

doi:10.1016/j.rcl.2006.04.009

course of the disease has led to a need to accurately identify the acute synovitis associated with early RA [10]. The ability to detect joint effusions, capsular distension, bony erosion, and bone marrow edema, and dynamic imaging to differentiate active from inactive RA, firmly establish the role of MR imaging in the evaluation of disease activity.

Numerous studies support interrogation of the wrist, metacarpophalangeal (MCP), and proximal interphalangeal (PIP) joints of the hand because these are the presenting sites in most patients with RA [11]. Synovial lined joints, bursae, and tendon sheaths are the principal sites of inflammation in early RA. Hyperemia resulting from an increase in the number and permeability of local capillary beds can be exploited to aid in the early detection of synovitis [12]. Periarticular contrast enhancement is an additional tool that may be used in the diagnosis of early inflammatory arthropathy [3,4]. Dynamic imaging is being investigated as a quantitative tool for evaluating the degree of inflammation based on synovial volume and dynamic perfusion [3].

Synovitis represents an inflammatory process that facilitates the ingress of antigens, antibodies, and cytokines resulting in structural joint damage. Gadolinium-diethylenetriamine pentaacetic acid (Gd-DTPA), a paramagnetic contrast agent, diffuses freely into the interstitium, allowing differentiation between synovial proliferation and joint effusion [13–15]. The conspicuity of lesions can be augmented using fat suppression imaging techniques [16,17]. The presence of periarticular joint enhancement, bone marrow edema, and erosions may predict joint damage and assess treatment outcome [18–20].

MR imaging reveals manifestations of synovitis that include increased signal on fluid-sensitive sequences conforming to areas that are invested by synovium. In the more advanced stages of RA, the synovium becomes hypertrophied, with villous transformation, and invades the joint, beginning at the marginal or bare areas of the joint (Fig. 1). *Bare area* refers to the intra-articular cortical bone within the joint capsule, lined by synovium but devoid of hyaline articular cartilage. An inflammatory pannus may also manifest as increased signal on fluid-sensitive sequences and may be difficult to delineate from an articular effusion (Fig. 2). Similarly, on T1-weighted sequences the low-signal pannus may blend imperceptibly with the effusion. The use of Gd-DTPA may help to differentiate the hypervascular synovium because the inflamed synovium and pannus can be easily differentiated from effusion. Enhancement of the synovium occurs rapidly between 60 and 120 seconds [21]. After this period, equilibrium occurs between the synovium and the effusion in which the Gd-DTPA diffuses from the synovium into the articular space, thus equalizing the intensity of the pannus with the effusion [21,22]. Therefore, imaging within the first minutes after injection yields the highest level of conspicuity of inflamed synovium versus effusion (Fig. 3).

Manually identifying and quantifying the synovial volumes has been proposed as a method to determine the extent of disease. Increased synovial volume may predict the location and development of bony erosions. Additionally, volumes of synovial membrane are significantly higher in MCP, PIP, and distal interphalangeal (DIP) joints in patients with inflammatory arthritis (Fig. 4) [23]. However, this technique is limited [24,25] by an over- or underestimation of the synovial volume based on a manual outlining of the synovium;

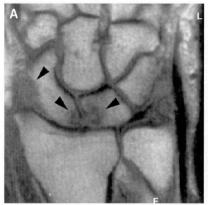
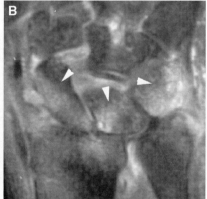

Fig. 1. (*A*) Coronal T1-weighted image through the wrist and hand demonstrates marginal bone erosion of the scaphoid, base of lunate, and triquetral bones (*black arrowheads*). (*B*) Gd-DTPA-enhanced fat-suppressed T1-weighted coronal image demonstrates bone marrow edema adjacent to the erosions with pannus contrast enhancement in a patient with RA (*white arrowheads*). Note the contrast enhancement of the ulna styloid, extensor carpi ulnaris tendon sheath, and adjacent pannus.

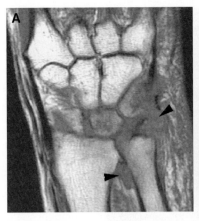
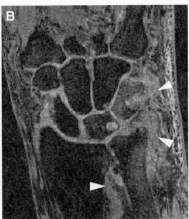

Fig. 2. (*A*) Coronal T1-weighted image through the wrist with heterogeneous low-signal intensity within the lunate and triquetrum. Note the heterogeneous low signal in the distal radioulnar joint and ulna styloid recess in a patient with RA. (*black arrowheads*). (*B*) Coronal fat-suppressed T1-weighted Gd-DTPA-enhanced image through the wrist demonstrating pannus enhancement in the ulna styloid recess and distal radioulnar joint in a patient with RA (*white arrowheads*). Note the erosions of the waist of the triquetral bone. A subchondral cyst is noted at the base of the lunate.

the process, therefore, is time-consuming and has limited clinical value.

Patterns of periarticular enhancement have also been studied as a tool to prospectively grade and classify patients with inflammatory arthropathy. The generation of Gd-DTPA enhancement curves parallels clinical indicators of inflammation. In addition, the technique is reproducible and may be an effective way to follow patients with a known diagnosis of RA [21]. However, enhancement patterns of the radiocarpal joint have been studied in normal subjects, and there is a considerable overlap because periarticular enhancement can be seen frequently in healthy volunteers [26]. Partik et al [26] found that 44% of the healthy subjects that were investigated demonstrated at least mild enhancement in the region of the prestyloid recess of the radiocarpal joint. Also, contrast enhancement is nonspecific and overlapping findings exist among non-rheumatoid arthritides, viral arthritis, and normal [4,27,28].

Bone marrow edema has been found to be predictive of a future site of erosion [8,29]. McQueen et al [18] identified the presence of edema to be a pre-erosive state, with a sixfold increased risk of erosion within 1 year. It has been suggested that the erosive process may be reversible, and early intervention may be warranted to prevent joint damage [6,29]. The presence of edema may be more specific for inflammatory arthropathy [8,29,30].

Qualitatively, the presence of erosions and bone marrow edema can be used to predict and evaluate treatment response. Erosive bony changes are more specific of early RA than synovitis and can be diagnosed using MR imaging as early as 4 months after

symptom onset [8,18,29,31]. Numerous investigators have demonstrated early sites of erosions in the common locations, which include the triquetrum, capitate, scaphoid waist, and the radial aspect of the second and third MCP joints [8,32,33].

Many findings and complications from RA have been extensively studied using MR imaging. Tenosynovitis from inflammation of the extensor carpi ulnaris tendon sheath as it passes the ulnar styloid is a well-recognized cause of ulnar styloid erosion. In addition, synovial cyst formation is easily identified using MR imaging, with heterogeneous internal signal representing the synovial fronds. A variety of pathology directly related to inflammation of the tendons, tendon sheaths, bursae, and soft tissues also can be evaluated with MR imaging (Figs. 5, 6).

Seronegative spondyloarthropathy

Ankylosing spondylitis (AS), the prototype of the spondyloarthropathies, includes the following group of disorders: psoriatic arthritis, Reiter's disease, enteropathic arthritis, and undifferentiated types of spondyloarthropathy. These diseases have a variety of systemic manifestations but share involvement of the axial skeleton. Skeletal involvement primarily manifests through sacroiliitis and spondylodiscitis. The main imaging findings that discriminate these conditions from RA are the distribution of disease with an axial predilection and the enthesitis, which characterizes this group of diseases.

Rheumatoid arthritis shares many of the previously discussed features with the seronegative group, including soft tissue swelling, periarticular

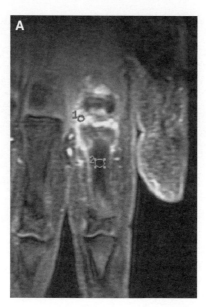

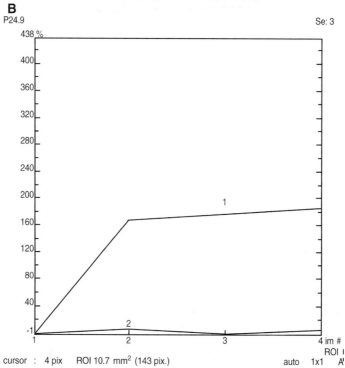

Fig. 3. (*A*) Coronal fat-suppressed T1-weighted Gd-DTPA-enhanced image through the second MCP with range of intensity (ROI) cursor (*1*) placed over the inflamed synovium and ROI cursor (*2*) over bone marrow in a patient with RA. (*B*) Linear graph depicting ROI measurements versus time. The rapid contrast enhancement in the first minute compared with the bone marrow provides assessment of inflammatory activity within the syrovium.

effusion, joint effusion, synovial pannus, increased synovial volumes, bone marrow edema, periarticular contrast enhancement, and marginal erosions [30]. Extrapolation of data from studies of sacroiliitis with identification of findings consistent with active inflammatory enthesitis, however, may allow the radiologist to offer a more specific differential diagnosis [34]. Moreover, subclinical joint involvement of patients with psoriasis has been studied, and data suggest that early MR imaging examinations, before symptomatic joint involvement occurs, may be able to identify lesions at an earlier

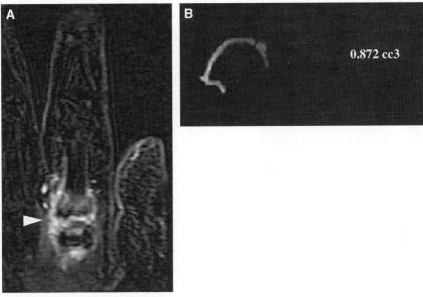

Fig. 4. (A) Coronal fat-suppressed T1-weighted Gd-DTPA-enhanced image through the second MCP joint demonstrating pannus enhancement (*white arrowhead*) in a patient with RA. (B) After manual outlining of the pannus, a volume-rendered analysis can be quantified. 0.872 cc³.

point in disease progression. Offidani et al [35] found that 68% of patients with skin manifestations of psoriasis and no clinical evidence of hand involvement had at least one imaging finding consistent with arthritis.

However, the overlap in imaging findings between RA and seronegative arthropathies has led some authors to conclude that RA and seronegative disorders cannot be differentiated (Fig. 7). Savnik et al [30] found synovial volumes in the MCP, PIP, and DIP joints and the number of joints with effusion to be higher in both groups, as well as bone marrow edema and erosion; and they concluded that there were no MR imaging differences between the rheumatoid and seronegative groups. Patients with arthralgia were also studied, and interestingly, no bone marrow edema was detected in this group. Jevtic et al [34] described distinctive radiologic features in patients with RA as opposed to those with seronegative spondyloarthritis and concluded that the latter group shows a distinctive extra-articular pattern of disease with dactylitis, enthesopathy, and extracapsular inflammatory change.

The visualization of enthesopathy on MR imaging may be subtle, and inspection of the insertions of ligaments, tendons, and muscles on short tau inversion recovery (STIR) or fat-suppressed T2-weighted images may suggest the diagnosis. Enthesitis involving the elbow with the olecranon and bicipital insertion of the proximal radius being affected is reportedly rare [36,37].

Gout

Gout is a metabolic disease that occurs in adults between 50 and 70 years of age. The first metatarsophalangeal joint is invariably affected and other common sites include the hands, wrists, elbows, and knees. There is an increase in serum urate, leading to deposition of monosodium urate crystals, known as *tophi*, within and around joints. Acute, subacute, and chronic phases of the disease exist

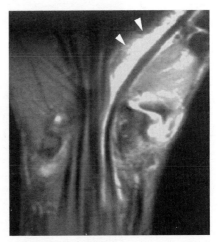

Fig. 5. Coronal T2-weighted fat-suppressed image through the wrist with tenosynovitis of the flexor pollicis longus. Note the shaggy, hypertrophied synovium (*white arrowheads*).

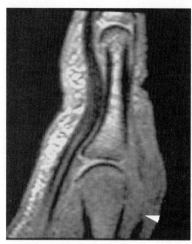

Fig. 6. Sagittal gradient recalled echo image through the second ray demonstrates a full thickness tear through the extensor digitorum tendon (*white arrowhead*).

in which many patients remain asymptomatic after acute episodes for varying periods of time. Usually acute gouty arthritis can be diagnosed clinically with laboratory correlation; however, chronic gout may require further evaluation by imaging. Tophi occur as soft tissue masses around the joint and may have adjacent intra- or juxta-articular bone erosions that may be eccentrically located. In the elbow particularly, gout has extra-articular manifestations, most commonly with olecranon bursitis [38]. As a rule of thumb, osteoporosis and joint space narrowing are not present until late in the course of the disease.

Gouty tophi are made up of a combination of crystals, hemosiderin, protein, and fibrous tissue, which result in varying signal intensity characteristics on MR imaging [39]. Tophi may induce a granulomatous response and are usually isointense to muscle on T1-weighted images and low- to intermediate heterogeneous-signal on T2-weighted images (Fig. 8) [40,41]. After injection of Gd-DTPA, T1-weighted fat-suppressed images demonstrate homogeneous intense enhancement of the soft tissue tophus.

Synovial osteochondromatosis

Primary synovial osteochondromatosis manifests by synovial proliferation and metaplasia, with production of numerous cartilaginous or osteocartilaginous nodules within the joints, bursae, or tendon sheaths. The most common sites of occurrence are the knee, followed by the elbow, hip, and shoulder [42]. This condition usually presents with progressively limited range of motion, pain, and swelling that may eventually lead to early osteoarthritis. Synovial osteochondromatosis occurs between the fourth and fifth decades of life, more often in men than women. Treatment usually includes surgical removal of the intra-articular bodies, but these bodies may recur. In contrast, secondary osteochondromatosis, which occurs following trauma, tends to have fewer intra-articular bodies that vary more in size.

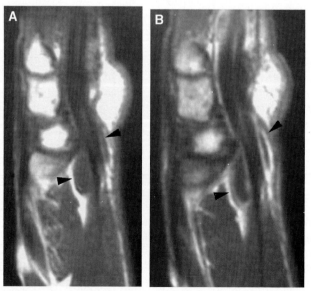

Fig. 7. (*A*) Sagittal T2-weighted image demonstrates tenosynovitis of the common flexor tendons with hypertrophied synovium (*black arrowheads*) in a patient with psoriasis. (*B*) Sagittal T1-weighted Gd-DTPA-enhanced image demonstrates the synovitis (*black arrowheads*) in a patient with psoriasis.

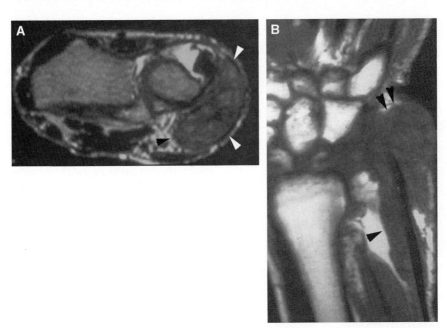

Fig. 8. (*A*) Axial T2-weighted image through the wrist demonstrates a large tophus displacing the extensor carpi ulnaris tendon dorsally (*arrowheads*). (*B*) Coronal T1-weighted image demonstrates the gouty tophus (*double arrowheads*) and thick inflamed synovium along the extensor carpi ulnaris tendon sheath (*arrowhead*).

MR imaging findings in primary synovial osteo-chondromatosis demonstrate the nonosseous synovial lesions as isointense or slightly hyperintense periarticular masses relative to skeletal muscle on T1-weighted images and hyperintense to muscle on T2-weighted images. On post-gadolinium images, there may be septations and peripheral or septal enhancement of chondral lesions. If calcification is present within chondroid masses, small signal voids are seen on all pulse sequences. Joint effusions are an infrequent finding. Mature bone and fatty marrow within intra-articular bodies demonstrate central areas of high-signal intensity on T1-weighted images [43]. MR imaging of the elbow exhibits these bodies in one of three locations including the coronoid and olecranon fossae and within the annular recess. Intra-articular bodies usually adhere to synovium and are rarely seen free within the joint space. Synovial proliferation may manifest as low signal on T2-weighted sequences and typically blooms on gradient-echo imaging [38].

Pigmented villonodular synovitis

Pigmented villonodular synovitis (PVNS) and giant cell tumors are a part of a spectrum of benign proliferative disorders of the synovium that affect tendon sheaths, joints, and bursae [44]. PVNS occurs more frequently in the knee and hip and less commonly in the ankle, shoulder, and elbow [43]. Shoulder involvement tends to occur in older patients without evidence of joint effusion [45]. PVNS occurs between the third and fourth decades of life and equally affect both males and females. Clinical symptoms in PVNS include progressive pain, stiffness, and swelling of the joint involved. Malignant transformation is extremely rare, although it has been reported [46]. Histologically, there is synovial thickening with accumulation of hemosiderin. Chronic lesions demonstrate fibrosis, chronic inflammation, and hyalinization [47]. There is a subtype of PVNS called *nodular synovitis*, which is believed to be part of the spectrum of giant cell tumors of the tendon sheath. Nodular synovitis is a condition that usually occurs focally within a joint and less frequently demonstrates hemosiderin deposition [38].

MR imaging findings in PVNS classically demonstrate diffuse or nodular thickening of the synovium. Synovial lesions manifest as low- to intermediate-signal intensity relative to muscle on T1-weighted images [48]. These lesions are low in signal on T2-weighted images because of hemosiderin, which "blooms" on gradient-echo images, particularly in chronic lesions and at high field strengths. There may be patchy high signal within the lesions on T1- and T2-weighted pulse sequences, which are secondary to fat, effusion, edema, or inflammation. Joint effusions may occur most commonly in the knee joint. On post-gadolinium T1-weighted sequences obtained during the active or early phase of PVNS there is homogeneous

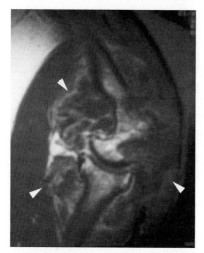

Fig. 9. Sagittal T2-weighted spin-echo image through the elbow demonstrates nodular low-signal masses. Note the well-defined pressure erosions on the volar and dorsal aspects of the capitellum in this patient with PVNS (*white arrowheads*).

or peripheral synovial enhancement. Abnormal synovial tissue may extend into the articular space, periarticular tissues, adjacent joints, or adjacent bursae. Lytic subchondral lesions may show varying signal intensity depending on the presence of hemosiderin, fluid, or soft tissue [43]. As described previously with synovial osteochondromatosis, synovial proliferation also may manifest as low signal on T2-weighted sequences and typically blooming on gradient-echo imaging. Similar MR imaging findings are seen in the subtype, nodular synovitis, although the signal varies within these focal lesions (Fig. 9) [38].

Tenosynovitis

Tenosynovitis refers to the inflammation that occurs in one or more tendons as part of either an overuse syndrome from repetitive activity or secondary to adjacent osseous pathology such as fractures, ganglia, osteoarthritis, or systemic inflammatory disorders. Generally, tenosynovitis is diagnosed clinically, but MR imaging aids in distinguishing tenosynovitis from simple tendinosis, which is important in regard to patient treatment. For instance, the initial approach to both simple tendinosis and tenosynovitis is to prescribe rest and anti-inflammatory medications. However, if tenosynovitis does not improve despite these measures, systemic steroids or even surgical debridement may be warranted [49]. The most commonly affected tendons in tenosynovitis of the wrist include the flexor carpi radialis and the flexor carpi ulnaris [50]. Tenosynovitis manifests on MR imaging as fluid within the tendon sheath, with or without tendon sheath thickening. Low-signal intensity within the sheath indicates fibrosis, which has a poorer clinical prognosis and is usually seen in chronic tenosynovitis [50].

de Quervain's tenosynovitis

de Quervain's tenosynovitis occurs more often in women and may occur bilaterally in up to 30% of cases [51]. de Quervain's disease affects the extensor pollicis longus and the abductor pollicis brevis tendons simultaneously, located on the radial aspect (Fig. 10). Patients usually present with pain and swelling above the radial styloid, which worsens with activity and improves with rest. A more complicated course can develop with the presence of

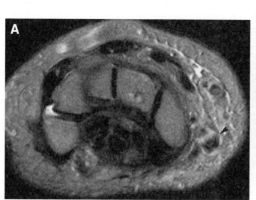
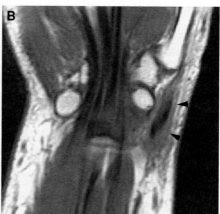

Fig. 10. (*A*) Axial T2-weighted fat-suppressed image demonstrates tendinosis and surrounding tenosynovitis of the extensor pollicis brevis and abductor pollicis longus in a patient with de Quervain's tenosynovitis (*arrowhead*). (*B*) Coronal T1-weighted image demonstrates tendinosis extensor pollicis brevis and abductor pollicis longus with tenosynovitis (*black arrowheads*) in a patient with de Quervain's tenosynovitis.

soft tissue ganglia or stenosis of the fibro-osseous tunnel [51].

Infectious tenosynovitis

Infectious tenosynovitis consists of gonococcal tenosynovitis and nongonococcal infectious tenosynovitis caused by such organisms as *Staphylococcus aureus*, *Pasteurella multocida*, *Eikenella corrodens*, and *Mycobacterium* sp, resulting from wounds and injuries, bites, or as a result of intravenous drug abuse. Gonococcal tenosynovitis usually occurs in teenagers and young adults, more frequently in females especially during pregnancy or after menstruation, and affects the dorsum of the wrist, hand, and ankle [52,53]. The diagnosis of tenosynovitis secondary to infection from *Mycobacterium* is often delayed because of the lack of clinical suspicion and the extended time required for culture and sensitivity [54]. This delay in diagnosis has been recently discussed in patients who have been exposed to *Mycobacterium marinum* through abrasions of the hand and fingers. Documenting a patient's history of exposure to contaminated water can facilitate the diagnosis [54].

Osteoarthritis

Osteoarthritis is a degenerative joint disease that equally affects males and females and increases in incidence with advancing age. The most common locations are the hip, medial compartment of the knee, spine, and hand. Multifocal asymmetric cartilage loss is the diagnostic hallmark of osteoarthritis, which is best observed on MR arthrography [55]. However, if there is joint effusion, indirect MR arthrography with intravenous Gd-DTPA injection and passive exercise (the unaffected arm moves the arm to be imaged) can be useful [38,55]. Active elbow movement of the arm to be imaged is less desirable because of an increase in intra-articular pressure that will result in decreased diffusion of contrast into the joint space to be imaged. Gradient-echo imaging is the most commonly used sequence in the evaluation of cartilage loss. Ancillary sequences include fast spin-echo T2-weighted imaging with long echo times (TE) and approximately 160 milliseconds short inversion time inversion recovery sequences, fast spin-echo imaging with a TE of 85 milliseconds and fat suppression, spectroscopy, and magnetization transfer imaging [38,56].

Osteophytes in the elbow are seen typically in the region of the coronoid process on axial imaging and along the dorsal aspect of the olecranon on sagittal imaging. Geodes and subchondral cysts may produce imaging characteristics that vary, ranging from cysts that appear benign to irregular masses. The irregular appearance may result from bone bruising or edema surrounding the cyst [38]. Synovial proliferation occurs in osteoarthritis and, therefore, does not always signify an inflammatory arthropathy [57]. The normal synovium shows as a barely noticeable line less than 1 mm in size [58]. In the elbow joint, synovial proliferation on MR imaging may exhibit subtle nodular filling defects or septae, usually on the radial aspect. Post-gadolinium imaging is an alternative method to evaluate for synovial proliferation [59,60].

Neuropathic arthropathy

Neuropathic arthropathy, or *Charcot joint*, is attributed to various distributions of articular lesions related to central or peripheral neurologic disorders that consist of tabes dorsalis, syringomyelia, meningomyelocele, multiple sclerosis, trauma, diabetes mellitus, and alcoholism. Recurrent injury resulting from loss of sensation contributes to the pathogenesis of this disease [61]. Central disorders such as syringomyelia tend to affect the upper extremity joints, particularly the shoulder. On the other hand, in diabetic or alcoholic patients, neuropathic arthropathy tends to involve the tarsal or metatarsal joints. MR imaging demonstrates early changes that simulate those of osteoarthritis. In more advanced stages, there is subchondral bone depression, absorption, or fragmentation, sclerosis, osteophyte formation, intra-articular bony fragments, joint debris, subluxation, joint effusion, and bony fractures [43].

Sarcoidosis

Sarcoidosis is characterized by the occurrence of noncaseating granulomas affecting tissues in different organ systems including the lungs, skin, lymph nodes, eyes, and the musculoskeletal system. Involvement of the latter is seen in approximately 1% to 13% of patients with sarcoidosis [62], although the cause for this inflammatory disorder is not clear. Sarcoidosis manifests in the musculoskeletal system in a variety of forms including osseous lesions in small and large bones and in the calvarium, as well as sarcoidal myopathy and arthropathy. Sarcoidal abnormalities that can be appreciated on MR imaging are infiltration of the bone marrow and soft tissue, focal and diffuse lesions in the muscle, intramuscular masses in addition to tendinopathy, and tenosynovitis.

Small bone sarcoidosis is demonstrated on MR imaging by granulomatous marrow lesions, which can appear aggressive, with permeation of the cortex and extension into the adjacent soft tissues

(Fig. 11). Fine perpendicular lines resembling periostitis extending from the cortex may be seen on MR imaging [63]. MR imaging also can help to differentiate gouty tophi from sarcoidal nodules in evaluating dactylitis in a patient with both gout and sarcoidosis. Typically, gouty tophi are hypointense whereas sarcoidal nodules are hyperintense on intermediate-density–weighted MR imaging [64,65].

MR imaging of large bone sarcoidosis produces a variety of appearances, and characterization of the signal intensity and morphology at various stages of the disease requires further investigation. In one study [63] large bone sarcoidal lesions can look like "cannonball-like" intramedullary lesions, confluent irregular marrow infiltration, ill-defined discrete lesions with a "starry sky" appearance, or diffuse, patchy intramedullary lesions. These lesions demonstrate varying signal intensities, with decreased signal intensity on T1-weighted images. Mostly there is increased signal intensity, although sometimes a low signal can also be seen on inversion-recovery, T2-weighted, and fat-saturated proton density-weighted MR images, and these lesions may enhance on post-gadolinium images [63]. Focal areas of fat-type signal intensity within the intramedullary bone lesions may be identified and can be useful in distinguishing sarcoidal lesions from osseous metastases. The principal differential considerations include osseous metastases, lymphoma, and myeloma, rarely infection such as tuberculosis or serous atrophy of AIDS, anorexia nervosa, or cancer. In some patients these sarcoidal lesions resolve on follow-up MR imaging, showing a signal intensity similar to that of fat or fibrosis [63].

One type of sarcoidal arthropathy is manifested in Lofgren syndrome in which patients exhibit bilateral hilar lymphadenopathy, erythema nodosum, and arthralgias. Symptoms within the first six months demonstrate polyarticular involvement affecting the knees, ankles, proximal interphalangeal joints of the hands, wrists, and elbows, and patients complain of pain and stiffness. Joint effusions and monoarthritis are not common in this diagnosis, rather, it is believed arthralgia is the result of circulating cytokines as opposed to granulomatous disease [66,67].

There is a second form of sarcoidal arthropathy seen generally in 10%–35% of sarcoidosis patients, more frequently in females, and separately from patients with Lofgren syndrome [68]. This condition is referred to as *granulomatous arthritis* and manifests with chronic, transient, or relapsing sarcoidal arthropathy. This second form of sarcoidal arthropathy occurs 6 months after the diagnosis of sarcoidosis and is usually associated with cutaneous sarcoidosis but not with erythema nodosum [66]. Granulomatous arthritis consists of symptoms including pain involving two or three joints such as the ankles, knees, proximal interphalangeal joints, and less frequently the wrists or shoulders. The fingers appear "sausage-like." MR images of sarcoidal arthropathy are nonspecific and may exhibit findings consistent with tenosynovitis, tendonitis, bursitis, and synovitis; therefore, a synovial or soft tissue biopsy may be necessary to confirm a granulomatous cause [66,69].

Sarcoidal myopathy may manifest as multiple, bilateral, focal nodular intramuscular masses at the musculotendinous junction, usually in the lower extremities [70,71]. MR findings demonstrate soft tissue masses described as having a "dark star" appearance with peripheral high-signal and central low-signal intensity on T2-weighted and post-gadolinium images [71]. Certain MR findings in sarcoidal myopathy are more nonspecific such as proximal muscle atrophy with fatty replacement. Other soft tissue lesions, including subcutaneous granulomatous infiltration, skin nodules, and sarcoidal soft tissue masses with lymphadenopathy, exhibit high-signal intensity on water-sensitive images, low-signal intensity on T1-weighted images, and enhancement on post-gadolinium images. The differential diagnosis would consist of tophus, pannus, and xanthoma, as well as other benign or malignant soft tissue masses [63].

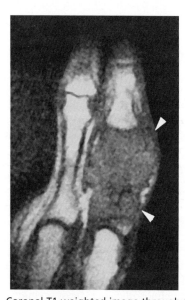

Fig. 11. Coronal T1-weighted image through the second ray demonstrates an expansile low-signal lesion within the second proximal phalanx, which destroys the cortex (*arrowheads*) in this patient with sarcoidosis.

Amyloid arthropathy

Amyloidosis can be divided into various subtypes. Primary amyloidosis develops without a coexisting disease, usually involves specific mesenchymal tissue, and is associated with multiple myeloma. Secondary amyloidosis occurs with other chronic diseases such as rheumatoid arthritis, inflammatory processes including Crohn's disease, neoplastic entities, sepsis, cystic fibrosis, and familial Mediterranean fever [72]. Other classifications of amyloidosis include heredofamilial amyloid syndromes, senile amyloidosis, localized amyloid tumors, and amyloidosis of chronic hemodialysis. A few cases of patients with coexisting plasma cell myeloma and amyloidosis have demonstrated tumor-like lesions in the bone containing amyloid associated with plasma cell infiltration and, at times, calcification within the lesion [72].

Amyloid arthropathy occurs as a result of accumulation of fibrous serum protein amyloid within the musculoskeletal system resulting from the inability to be filtered through glomerular membranes. β2-microglobulin is another form of amyloid, which can lead to bilateral shoulder pain and carpal tunnel syndrome and can cause lytic bony lesions, referred to as *amyloidomas*[73,74]. Amyloid arthropathy has similar characteristics such as inflammatory arthritides in the shoulder and other large joints. MR imaging demonstrates joint effusion and abnormal soft tissue material, which lines the synovial membrane or can fill subchondral lesions and involve soft tissue surrounding the joint with a low to intermediate signal on T1- and T2-weighted images [75,76].

Hemophilic arthropathy

Hemophilic arthropathy caused by hemophilia A and B (Christmas disease) involves recurrent bleeding into synovial joints, usually occurring in the knee, ankle, elbow, and shoulder bilaterally. Repetitive bleeding within the same joint causes arthritic changes such as chronic inflammation and synovial fibrosis, siderosis, and hyperplasia. Chronic bleeding into adjacent muscles can lead to contractures and soft tissue pseudotumors [43]. MR evaluation of hemophilic arthropathy demonstrates low-signal intensity on all MR sequences, particularly on gradient-echo imaging because of the presence of hemosiderin [77]. Synovial hyperplasia can also be visualized on MR images.

Osteomyelitis

Osteomyelitis represents the inflammatory response of the bone secondary to infection with pyogenic organisms. Osteomyelitis can be further divided based on the mechanism of acquisition, such as hematogenous spread versus direct seeding of the bone [78]. In hematogenous osteomyelitis, the most common site of acquisition is the highly vascular metaphysis of growing bones, primarily affecting children (Fig. 12). *S aureus* is the most common causative agent. Other organisms include *Enterobacteriaceae* organisms, group A and B *Streptococcus* sp, and *Haemophilus influenzae*. There is a bimodal distribution of acute hematogenous osteomyelitis that occurs in children younger than 3 years of age and older than 7 years of age [38]. In the older group, infection is facilitated by the acute angle of the vessel, with the distal metaphysis predisposing the vessels to thrombosis. As a result, the bone is subject to localized necrosis and subsequent bacterial seeding [78].

Direct osteomyelitis occurs secondary to the inoculation of organisms from direct trauma (puncture wounds), foreign bodies, open fractures, and surgery, although this mechanism is seen more

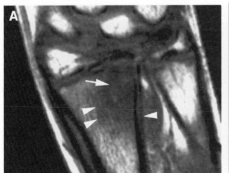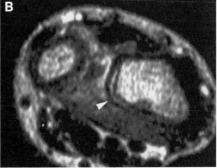

Fig. 12. (A) Coronal T1-weighted image through the wrist demonstrates focal low-signal intensity in the metaphysis of the radius (*arrow*) surrounded by reactive edema (*double arrowheads*) in this patient with hematogenous osteomyelitis. Periosteal reaction parallels the cortex (*arrowhead*). (B) Axial T2-weighted image (same patient as in A) demonstrates the periostitis along the distal radius as linear high signal within the surrounding low-signal periosteal reaction (*arrowhead*).

often in adolescents and adults [79]. Symptoms of direct inoculation osteomyelitis are more localized than those of hematogenous osteomyelitis and tend to involve multiple organisms. In direct osteomyelitis, the causative agents generally include *S aureus*, *Enterobacter* sp, and *Pseudomonas* sp. In patients with sickle cell anemia, *S aureus* and *Salmonella* sp are the common agents. Human bites (*S aureus*, *Bacillus funformis*) and animal bites (*P multocida*, *S aureus*, and *S epidermidis*) also are common causes of osteomyelitis from direct implantation [79]. The infection may begin in the soft tissues, the periosteum, or cortical or medullary bone.

Contiguous spread is defined as infection of osseous structures from the spread of infection from adjacent soft tissues. This is most often seen in debilitated patients, diabetics, and in patients on corticosteroids [79]. The disease process starts as a cellulitis followed by tissue involvement, osteitis, and progresses into the bone marrow producing an osteomyelitis.

MR imaging of osteomyelitis is useful not only for evaluating bone involvement but also to identify abscess formation, adjacent soft tissue involvement, and areas of necrosis. A radiograph with normal findings is typical in the first week of acute hematogenous osteomyelitis; however, in the next 7 to 14 days, osteopenia, fine linear periosteal reaction, and permeative or "moth-eaten" bone destruction can be seen on radiographs [79]. MR imaging demonstrates replacement of the fat by bone marrow edema, which is exhibited by high-signal intensity on T1-weighted images. Elevation of the periosteum can occur, and this is shown as a linear low-signal intensity paralleling the cortex on all pulse sequences. The potential space between the periosteum and cortical bone normally has intermediate signal intensity on T1-weighted images and high-signal intensity on STIR images. Cortical destruction is shown as a focal interruption of the cortical line and is demonstrated by low-signal intensity on all pulse sequences.

A cloaca, which is an opening through the periosteum that allows pus from the infected bone to decompress into surrounding soft tissues, can also be seen. On STIR images, the cloaca is seen as a high-signal intensity defect crossing the low-signal periosteal line [79]. The cloaca may then develop into an abscess or sinus tract identified as a channel between the infected bone and the skin surface. An abscess is low-signal intensity on T1-weighted and high-signal intensity on T2-weighted images. Using intravenous gadolinium, enhancement of the wall of the cavity can be seen, with low signal centrally representing pus and debris. Cellulitis will show diffuse contrast enhancement limited to the subcutaneous soft tissues. Osteomyelitis from contiguous spread will demonstrate enhancement extending from soft tissue ulceration through the cortical bone.

Septic arthritis

There are approximately 20,000 cases of septic arthritis per year in the United States [80]. Bacterial pathogens include gonococcal and nongonococcal species. In patients with septic arthritis, *Neisseria gonorrhoeae* is the microbe found most frequently (75% of cases) in the younger, sexually active population, and *S aureus* is most common in adults and children older than 2 years of age. *S viridans*, *S pneumoniae*, and group B streptococci are responsible for 20% of cases, and aerobic gram-negative rods account for 20% to 25% of cases [80]. Lyme disease (*Borrelia burgdorferi*), viruses (eg, HIV, lymphocytic choriomeningitis virus, hepatitis B virus, rubella virus), mycobacteria, fungi (eg, *Histoplasma* sp, *Sporothrix schenckii*, *Coccidioides immitis*, *Blastomyces* sp) may produce a nonsuppurative joint infection [80], and there can be polymicrobial joint infections.

Septic arthritis of the upper extremity, particularly the elbow, accounts for approximately 3% to 13% of all cases [38]. This entity is more commonly seen in the pediatric population and in patients who are immunocompromised or have an underlying chronic synovitis such as rheumatoid arthritis. Other predisposing factors include diabetes, corticosteroid treatment, debilitating diseases, and intravenous drug abuse [79]. Symptoms include pain, swelling, and decreased range of motion. MR imaging findings include the presence of a joint effusion with synovial hyperemia, and swelling with shaggy rim enhancement on post-gadolinium T1-weighted images. The joint effusion and synovitis are low-signal intensity on T1-weighted images and high-signal intensity on T2-weighted images. Many other noninfectious conditions have similar nonspecific manifestations; therefore, aspiration with culture is a necessary adjunct to the clinical, laboratory, and imaging findings. Other findings include cartilage destruction, bony erosions, and subchondral edema [38]. MR imaging also can be useful in evaluating for complications of septic arthritis such as osteomyelitis.

Septic olecranon bursitis

The majority of olecranon bursitis cases result from inflammatory arthropathies, with 25% of cases being infectious in origin. Septic olecranon bursitis is most commonly seen in adults, with men being more affected than women in a ratio of approximately 9:1 [81]. Patients can present with pain, swelling, erythema, localized tenderness in the region of the olecranon process, and loss of function. Some patients experience fever, an elevated white blood cell count, or an elevated sedimentation rate. The most common causative agent is *S aureus.* Less common agents include streptococcus, gram-negative species, mycobacteria, and *Sporothorix* sp. Patients who are immunocompromised do not appear to be at greater risk of developing septic bursitis.

Olecranon bursitis usually is a straightforward clinical diagnosis, with MR imaging reserved for more complex cases to exclude osteomyelitis in patients refractory to antibiotic therapy. Fluid within the olecranon bursa signifies a bursitis (Fig. 13). T1-weighted post-gadolinium images can sometimes demonstrate fluid in the olecranon bursa, with a thick, enhancing irregular rim signifying synovial proliferation, a common finding in the inflammatory arthropathies [38]. Associated cellulitis is often demonstrated on MR imaging with edema identified as high-signal on T2-weighted images and ill-defined enhancement on T1-weighted post-gadolinium images in the soft tissues adjacent to the fluid-filled olecranon bursa [38]. Findings of osteomyelitis involving the adjacent olecranon process include cortical irregularity and destruction, low-signal intensity on T1-weighted imaging, increased signal intensity on T2-weighted imaging, and enhancement on fat-suppressed T1-weighted post-gadolinium imaging. [79] Septic arthritis is a rare complication of olecranon bursitis secondary to the lack of direct communication with the elbow joint.

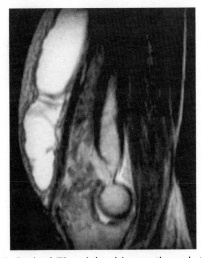

Fig. 13. Sagittal T2-weighted image through the elbow demonstrates an enlarged olecranon bursa, which compresses the triceps tendon in this patient with olecranon bursitis.

Pyomyositis

Pyomyositis, or infection of the muscle, may be caused by penetrating injury or hematogenous spread, but the exact pathogenesis of pyomyositis is uncertain. Tropical pyomyositis is described in association with previous blunt muscle trauma, nutritional deficiencies, and parasitic infections. Nontropical pyomyositis typically affects those patients who are immunocompromised by HIV infection, cancer, diabetes, dermatomyositis, or other debilitating illnesses. *S aureus* is the most common causative agent, with streptococcal species being less common [38].

Pyomyositis typically presents as a localized infection of muscle, and pain, swelling, fever, leukocytosis and elevated erythrocyte sedimentation rate may be present. The involved muscles may eventually develop a firm, wooden texture on palpation. In a study of three cases [82], muscle biopsy specimens revealed a myopathy with multiple areas of muscle fiber necrosis surrounded by neutrophils, mononuclear inflammatory cells, and gram-positive cocci.

On MR imaging, there is diffuse muscle involvement with the triceps muscle most commonly involved in the upper extremity [83]. On T2-weighted images, there is increased signal intensity throughout the affected muscle, and the muscle is often enlarged, with high-signal intensity fluid in the fascial planes [79]. Often, intramuscular abscesses can be seen as high-signal fluid-filled cavities with a thick low-signal rind on T2-weighted images. On a T1-weighted sequence, there is low-signal intensity centrally with an enhancing rim on post-gadolinium imaging.

Mycobacteria

Tuberculosis (TB) remains a global problem predominantly in immigrant, indigent, and inner city populations, and in immunocompromised (eg, AIDS) patients caused by *Mycobacterium tuberculosis.* The disease manifests by the formation of tubercles and caseous necrosis. *M tuberculosis* bacilli are aerosolized, infecting the pulmonary alveoli, and producing an exudative response within the alveoli, with extension to lymph nodes. Extrapulmonary disease (pleura, lymph nodes, bones, gastrointestinal tract, or urinary tract) is present in 15% of non-HIV patients and up to 70% of HIV-positive patients with tuberculosis. Bone and joint involvement of TB accounts for 10% of all cases of extrapulmonary TB.

Musculoskeletal involvement of TB can mimic other rheumatic disorders, therefore it is important to suggest the diagnosis when pertinent. In the musculoskeletal system, tuberculosis can cause spondylitis (Pott's disease), peripheral arthritis, osteomyelitis, tenosynovitis, bursitis, and Poncet's disease (aseptic inflammatory polyarthritis in the presence of active TB, usually involving the lungs). In any bursal location, dystrophic calcification may appear. Tuberculous spondylitis is the most common manifestation of musculoskeletal involvement, although that is beyond the scope of this article. Changes in extraspinal sites, such as the hip, knee, wrist, and elbow, also may occur.

Since the advent of antituberculosis medications approximately 40 years ago, tuberculosis infections of the wrist are rare and account for approximately 2% of skeletal TB manifestations [84]. *M marinum* is the most common type of mycobacterium that can infect the hand and results in tenosynovitis [54]. *M kansasii*, as well, has the potential to develop deep infections of the hand. Another causative agent includes sporotrichosis, which can only be differentiated from *Mycobacterium* sp based on biopsy [85]. Infections of the hand can present in various ways, most commonly as the compound palmar ganglion, which is a tenosynovial infection involving the flexor tendon sheaths. Tuberculous dactylitis involving the short tubular bones of the hands and feet occurs especially frequently in children. In addition to soft tissue swelling, periostitis of phalanges, metacarpals, or metatarsals may be seen. Wrist joint infection involving both capsule and carpal bones is another manifestation [84].

TB infections of the carpal bones and wrist are usually chronic, with loss of function and decreased range of motion occurring as indolent processes. Soft tissue swelling may occur before joint space narrowing and osteoporosis. This chronicity often distinguishes tuberculous infections from other pyogenic infections [84]. Most cases of tuberculous infection of the wrist exhibit tenosynovitis with or without arthritis and osteomyelitis. The flexor tendon sheath and the radioulnar bursae are the most common sites of tenosynovitis [57]. Although there are no pathognomonic signs of tuberculous infection of the wrist, suggestive findings include soft tissue swelling, periosteal reaction, osteoporosis, subchondral cysts, abscess formation, joint-space narrowing, and bony destruction [86].

MR imaging findings may show synovitis, synovial effusion, early erosions, intra- and extra-articular abscess, pannus formation, and bursitis. Radiologic evaluation may support a diagnosis of TB infection, demonstrating destructive osseous changes and associated soft-tissue masses with rim enhancement, but radiologic evaluation by itself is of limited value [87]. Tuberculous bursal infection usually results from hematogenous spread of infection. The presence of enlarged bursae with wall

thickening suggests the diagnosis of TB, with bursae surrounding the hip, which is the most common site of affliction (Fig. 14) [57], and these enlarged bursae may contain rice bodies. Laboratory tests that can be helpful in making a clinical diagnosis of tuberculous infection include a leukocyte count, erythrocyte sedimentation rate, purified protein derivative skin test, biopsy, histologic staining, and cultures. An adequate biopsy sample from the wrist requires synovium and tissues from nearby cystic lesions [88].

Tuberculous infection of the elbow joint is less frequently involved compared with other joints. These infections are chronic and slowly progressive and may be mistaken for monoarticular rheumatoid arthritis if there is no history of pulmonary tuberculosis. Approximately two thirds of patients with tuberculous infection of the upper extremity have no history of lung involvement [84]. TB tenosynovitis is difficult to diagnose, and the most sensitive method is open biopsy, which demonstrates caseating granulomas. It is important to note, however, that other diseases such as sarcoidosis or atypical mycobacterium arthritis can also produce granulomatous lesions. Accurate diagnosis with administration of the appropriate medication regimen is important in preventing deleterious sequelae of tuberculous infection. Complications include fibrous ankylosis, advanced joint

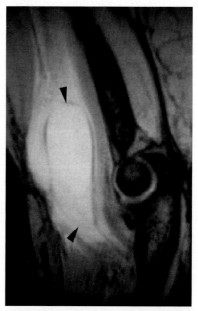

Fig. 14. Sagittal gradient recalled echo image through the elbow demonstrates an enlarged pear-shaped bicipitoradialis septic bursitis (*arrowheads*) with surrounding inflammatory changes in this patient with tuberculosis.

destruction with ruptured tendons, and spontaneous radiocarpal and intercarpal fusions [88].

Cat scratch disease

Cat scratch disease is a disease caused by *Bartonella henselae* and *Afipia felis*. Symptoms can be mild to severe and may include malaise, or anorexia, or both. It is a self-limiting benign disorder, except in immunosuppressive patients. In healthy individuals, it usually resolves spontaneously over 2 to 5 months. Most patients have a history of exposure to a cat, although there have been reports of occurrence after exposure to squirrels, dogs, goats, crab claws, and barbed wire. Within 3 to 10 days after exposure, a small skin lesion such as a macule, papule, or vesicle may appear. In 1 to 2 weeks, edema and tenderness manifest in regional lymph nodes that drain the area of exposure. Some patients have a mildly elevated leukocytosis.

The necrotic nodes are often mistaken clinically for soft tissue sarcomas or other neoplasms. The diagnosis of cat scratch disease should be considered in relatively young patients who manifest with lymphadenopathy in the upper extremity and head and neck region, with a history of cat exposure [89]. On MR images, an ill-defined mass with surrounding edema in the epitrochlear region along the nodal chain indicates epitrochlear lymphadenopathy (Fig. 15). On T2-weighted images, the lymph nodes are high signal but have a nonspecific appearance. Definitive diagnosis can be made by excisional node biopsy or fine needle aspiration. Patients can be treated with cephalexin or

doxycycline. Even without antibiotic treatment, however, the adenopathy will resolve spontaneously in 3 weeks to several months [89].

In conclusion, there are a wide variety of arthropathic conditions, including those of infectious and noninfectious origins, that affect the elbow, hand, and wrist. MR imaging allows for accurate, early diagnosis and evaluation because it is capable of superior soft tissue contrast and multiplanar imaging. In addition, the role of MR imaging in the evaluation of treatment outcome is invaluable, which fortifies it as a diagnostic and therapeutic tool available to the clinician. MR imaging is a tremendously growing field. With further investigation and continuing research, new MR imaging sequences and techniques will aid in more sensitive and specific diagnoses in the near future.

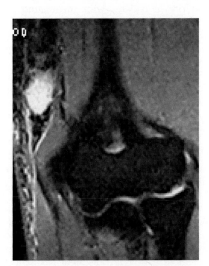

Fig. 15. Coronal STIR image through the elbow demonstrates an enlarged epitrochlear lymph node with inflammatory changes within the adjacent subcutaneous soft tissues in this patient with cat scratch disease.

References

[1] Fuchs HA, Kaye JJ, Callahan LF, Nance EP, Pincus T. Evidence of significant radiographic damage in rheumatoid arthritis within the first 2 years of disease. J Rheumatol 1989;16:585–91.
[2] Brook A, Corbett M. Radiographic changes in early rheumatoid arthritis. Ann Rheum Dis 1977;36:71–3.
[3] Sugimoto H, Hyodoh TA. Early stage rheumatoid arthritis: prospective study of the effectiveness of MR imaging for diagnosis. Radiology 2000; 216:569–75.
[4] Sugimoto H, Takeda A, Masuyama J, Furuse M. Early-stage rheumatoid arthritis: diagnostic accuracy of MR imaging. Radiology 1996;198:185–92.
[5] McQueen FM. Magnetic resonance imaging in early inflammatory arthritis: what is its role? J Rheumatol 2000;39:700–6.
[6] Peterfly CG. Magnetic resonance imaging in rheumatoid arthritis: current status and future directions. J Rheumatol 2001;28:1134–42.
[7] Goupille P, Roulot B, Akoka S, Avimadje AM, Garaud P, Naccache L, et al. Magnetic resonance imaging: a valuable method for the detection of synovial inflammation in rheumatoid arthritis. J Rheumatol 2001;28:35–40.
[8] McQueen FM, Stewart N, Crabbe J, Robinson E, Yeoman S, Tan PL, et al. Magnetic resonance imaging of the wrist in early rheumatoid arthritis reveals a high prevalence of erosions at four months after symptom onset. Ann Rheum Dis 1998;57:350–6.
[9] Boutry N, Larde A, Lapegue F, Solau-Gervais E, Flipo R, Cotton A. Magnetic resonance imaging appearance of the hands and feet in patients with early rheumatoid arthritis. J Rheumatol 2003; 30:671–9.
[10] Herburn B. What is a disease modifying antirheumatic drug? J Rheumatol 1988;15(Suppl 16): S40–2.

[11] Jacoby RK, Jayson MI, Cosh JA. Onset, early stages, and prognosis of rheumatoid arthritis. BMJ 1973;2:96–100.

[12] Firestein GS. Starving the synovium: angiogenesis and inflammation in rheumatoid arthritis. J Clin Invest 1999;103:3–4.

[13] Kursunoglu-Bramhe S, Riccio T, Weisman MH, Resnick D, Zvaifler N, Sanders ME, et al. Rheumatoid knee: role of gadopentetate-enhanced MR imaging. Radiology 1990;176:831–5.

[14] Konig H, Sieper J, Wolf KJ. Rheumatoid arthritis: evaluation of hypervascular and fibrous pannus with dynamic MR imaging enhanced with Gd-DTPA. Radiology 1990;176:473–7.

[15] Bjorkengren AG, Geborek P, Rydholm U, Holtas S, Petterson H. MR imaging of the knee in acute rheumatoid arthritis: synovial uptake of gadolinium-DOTA. AJR 1990;155:329–32.

[16] Nakahara N, Uetani M, Hayashi K, Kawahara Y, Matsumoto T, Oda J. Gadolinium-enhanced MR imaging of the wrist in rheumatoid arthritis: value of fat suppression sequences. Skeletal Radiol 1996;25:639–47.

[17] Huh YM, Suh JS, Jeong EK, Lee SK, Lee JS, Choi BW, et al. Role of the inflamed volume of the wrist in defining remission of rheumatoid arthritis with gadolinium-enhanced 3D-SPGR MR imaging. J Magn Reson Imaging 1999;10:202–8.

[18] McQueen FM, Stewart N, Crabbe J, Robinson E, Yeoman S, Tan PL, et al. Magnetic resonance imaging of the wrist in early rheumatoid arthritis reveals progression of erosions despite clinical improvement. Ann Rheum Dis 1999;58:156–63.

[19] Ostergaard M, Hansen M, Stoltenberg M, Gideon P, Klarlund M, Jensen KE, et al. Magnetic resonance imaging-determined synovial membrane volume as a marker of disease activity and a predictor of progressive joint destruction in the wrists of patients with rheumatoid arthritis. Arthritis Rheum 1999;42:918–29.

[20] McGonagle D, Gibbon W, O'Connor P, Green M, Pease C, Ridgway J, et al. An anatomical explanation for good-prognosis rheumatoid arthritis. Lancet 1999;353:123–4.

[21] Cimmino MA, Innocenti S, Livrone F, Magnaguagno F, Silvestri E, Garlaschi G. Dynamic gadolinium-enhanced MRI of the wrist in patients with rheumatoid arthritis can discriminate active from inactive disease. Arthritis Rheum 2003;48:1207–13.

[22] Yamato M, Tamai K, Yamaguchi T, Ohno W. MRI of the knee in rheumatoid arthritis: Gd-DTPA perfusion dynamics. J Comput Assist Tomogr 1993;17:781–5.

[23] Savnik A, Malmskov H, Thomsen HS, Graff LB, Nielsen H, Danneskiold-Samsoe B, et al. Magnetic resonance imaging of the wrist and finger joints in patients with inflammatory joint disease. J Rheumatol 2001;28:2193–200.

[24] Ostergaard M, Gideon P, Hendriksen O, Lorenzen I. Synovial volume-marker of disease severity in rheumatoid arthritis? Quantification by MRI. Scand J Rheumatol 1994;23:197–202.

[25] Polisson RP, Schoenberg OI, Fischman A, Rubin R, Simon LS, Rosenthal D, et al. Use of magnetic resonance imaging and positron emission tomography in the assessment of synovial volume and glucose metabolism in patients with rheumatoid arthritis. Arthritis Rheum 1995; 38:819–25.

[26] Partik B, Rand T, Pretterklieber ML, Voracek M, Hoermann M, Helbich TH. Patterns of gadopentetate-enhanced MR imaging of radiocarpal joints of healthy subjects. AJR Am J Roentgenol 2002;179:193–7.

[27] Tonolli-Serabian I, Poet JL, Dufour M, Carasset S, Mattei JP, Roux H. Magnetic resonance imaging of the wrist in rheumatoid arthritis: comparison with other inflammatory joint disease and control subjects. Clin Rheumatol 1996;15:137–42.

[28] Reiser MF, Bongartz GP, Erlemann R, Schneider M, Pauly T, Sittek H, et al. Gadolinium-DTPA in rheumatoid arthritis and related diseases: first results with dynamic magnetic resonance imaging. Skeletal Radiol 1989;18:591–7.

[29] McGonagle D, Conaghan PG, O'Connor P, Gibbon W, Green M, Wakefield R, et al. The relationship between synovitis and bone changes in early untreated rheumatoid arthritis. Arthritis Rheum 1999;42:1706–11.

[30] Savnik A, Malmskov H, Thomsen HS, Graff LB, Nielsen H, Danneskiold-Samsoe B, et al. MRI of the wrist and finger joints in inflammatory joint diseases at 1-year interval: MRI features to predict bone erosions. Eur Radiol 2002; 12:1203–10.

[31] McGonagle D, Green MJ, Proudman S, Richardson C, Veale D, O'Connor P, et al. The majority of patients with rheumatoid arthritis have erosive disease at presentation when magnetic imaging resonance of the dominant hand is employed. Br J Rheumatol 1997;36(Suppl 1): S121.

[32] Pierre-Jerome C, Bekkelund SI, Mellgren SI, Torbergsen T, Husby G, Nordstrom R. The rheumatoid wrist: bilateral MR analysis of rheumatoid lesions in axial plane in a female population. Clin Rheumatol 1997;16:80–6.

[33] Conaghan P, Edmonds J, Emery P, Genant H, Gibbon W, Klarlund M, et al. Magnetic resonance imaging in rheumatoid arthritis: summary of OMERACT activities, current status, and plans. J Rheumatol 2001;28:1158–62.

[34] Jevtic V, Watt I, Rozman B, Kos-Golja M, Demsar F, Jarb O. Distinctive radiological features of small hand joints in rheumatoid arthritis and seronegative spondyloarthritis demonstrated by contrast enhanced (Gd-DTPA) magnetic resonance imaging. Skeletal Radiol 1995;24(5):351–5.

[35] Offidani A, Cellini A, Valeri G, Giovagnoni A. Subclinical joint involvement in psoriasis:

magnetic resonance imaging and X-ray findings. Acta Derm Venereol 1998;78(6):463–5.

[36] Scarpa R, Ames PRJ, Valle G, Lubrano E, Oriente P. A rare enthesopathy in psoriasis oligoarthritis. Acta Derm Venereol 1994;186:74–5.

[37] Smith DL, Campbell SM, Wernick R. Tumoral enthesopathy: a juxtacortical osteosarcoma simulation. J Rheumatol 1991;18:1631–4.

[38] Schweitzer M, Morrison WB. Arthropathies and inflammatory conditions of the elbow. Magn Reson Imaging Clin N Am 1997;5(3):603–17.

[39] Mille LJ, Pruett SW, Losada R, Fruauff A, Sagerman P. Tophaceous gout of the lumbar spine: MR findings. J Comput Assist Tomogr 1996;20:1004–5.

[40] Chen CKH, Yeh LR, Pan HB, Yang CF, Lu YC, Wang JS, et al. Intra-articular gouty tophi of the knee: CT and MR imaging in 12 patients. Skeletal Radiol 1999;28:75–80.

[41] Yu JS, Chung C, Recht M, Dailiana T, Jurdi R. MR imaging of tophaceous gout. AJR Am J Roentgenol 1997;168:523–7.

[42] Burrafato V, Campanacci DA, Franchi A, Capanna R. Synovial chondromatosis in a lumbar apophyseal joint. Skeletal Radiol 1999; 27:385–7.

[43] Llauger J, Palmer J, Roson N, Bague S, Camins A, Cremades R. Nonseptic monoarthritis: imaging features with clinical and histopathologic correlation. Radiographics 2000;20:S263–78.

[44] Llauger J, Palmer J, Roson N, Cremades R, Bague S. Pigmented villonodular synovitis and giant cell tumors of the tendon sheath. AJR Am J Roentgenol 1999;172:1087–91.

[45] Dowart RH, Genant HK, Johnston WH, Morris JM. Pigmented villonodular synovitis of the shoulder: radiologic-pathologic assessment. AJR Am J Roentgenol 1984;143:886–8.

[46] Khalil RK, Unni KK. Malignancy in pigmented villonodular synovitis. Skeletal Radiol 1998; 27:392–5.

[47] Dowart RH, Genant HK, Johnston WH, Morris JM. Pigmented villonodular synovitis of synovial joints: clinical, pathologic, and radiologic features. AJR Am J Roentgenol 1984; 143:877–85.

[48] Jelinek JS, Kransdorf MJ, Utz JA, Bency BH Jr, Thomson JD, Heekin RD, et al. Imaging of pigmented villonodular synovitis with emphasis on MR imaging. AJR Am J Roentgenol 1989; 152:337–42.

[49] Pretorius ES, Epstein RE, Dalinka MK. MR imaging of the wrist. Radiol Clin North Am 1997; 35(1):145–62.

[50] Klug JD. MR diagnosis of tenosynovitis about the wrist. MRI Clin North Am 1995;3:305–12.

[51] Stern PJ. Tendinitis, overuse syndromes, and tendon injuries. Hand Clin 1990;6:467–76.

[52] Krieger LE, Schnall SB, Holtom PD, Costigan W. Acute gonococcal flexor tenosynovitis. Orthopedics 1997;20(7):649–50.

[53] Schaefer RA, Enzenauer RJ, Pruitt A, Corpe RS. Acute gonococcal flexor tenosynovitis in an adolescent male with pharyngitis: a case report and literature review. Clin Orthop 1992;281:212–5.

[54] Amrami K, Sundaram M, Shin A, Bishop A. *Mycobacterium marinum* infections of the distal upper extremities: clinical course and imaging findings in two cases with delayed diagnosis. Skeletal Radiol 2003;32:546–9.

[55] Beltran J, Noto AM, McGhee RB, Freedy RM, McCalla MS. Infections of the musculoskeletal system: high field strength MR imaging. Radiology 1987;164:449–54.

[56] Hughes TH, Sartoris DJ, Schweitzer ME, Resnick DL. Pigmented villonodular synovitis: MRI characteristics. Skeletal Radiol 1995; 24:7–12.

[57] Jaovisidha S, Chen C, Ryu KN, Siriwongpairat P, Pekanan P, Sartoris DJ, et al. Tuberculous tenosynovitis and bursitis: imaging findings in 21 cases. Radiology 1996;201:507–13.

[58] Broderick LS, Turner DA, Renfrew DL, Schnitzer TJ, Huff JP, Harris C. Severity of articular cartilage abnormality in patients with osteoarthritis: evaluation with fast spin-echo MR vs arthroscopy. AJR Am J Roentgenol 1994; 162:99–103.

[59] Gupta NC, Prezio JA. Radionuclide imaging in osteomyelitis. Semin Nucl Med 1988;18:287–99.

[60] Ho G, Su EY. Antibiotic therapy of septic bursitis. Arthritis Rheum 1981;24:905–11.

[61] Resnick D. Neuro-arthropathy. In: Resnick D, Niwayama G, editors. Diagnosis of bone and joint disorders. Philadelphia: WB Saunders; 1981. p. 2422–49.

[62] James DG, Neville E, Carstairs LS. Bone and joint sarcoidosis. Semin Arthritis Rheum 1976; 6:53–81.

[63] Moore SL, Teirstein AE. Musculoskeletal sarcoidosis: spectrum of appearances at MR imaging. Radiographics 2003;23:1389–99.

[64] Popp JD, Bidgood WD, Edwards NL. Magnetic resonance imaging of tophaceous gout in the hands and wrists. Semin Arthritis Rheum 1996; 25:282–9.

[65] Resnick D, Niwayama G. Gouty arthritis. In: Resnick D, Niwayama G, editors. Diagnosis of bone and joint disorders. 3rd edition. Philadelphia: WB Saunders; 1995. p. 1511–55.

[66] Murphy EP, McEvoy A, Conneely OM, Bresnihan B, FitzGerald O. Involvement of the nuclear orphan receptor NURR1 in the regulation of corticotropin-releasing hormone expression and actions in human inflammatory arthritis. Arthritis Rheum 2001;44:782–93.

[67] Visser H, Vos K, Zanelli E, Verduyn W, Schreuder GM, Speyer I, et al. Sarcoid arthritis: clinical characteristics, diagnostic aspects, and risk factors. Ann Rheum Dis 2002;61:499–504.

[68] Resnick D, Niwayama G. Sarcoidosis. In: Resnick D, Niwayama G, editors. Diagnosis of

bone and joint disorders. 3rd edition. Philadelphia: WB Saunders; 1995. p. 4333–52.

[69] Fuss M, Pepersack T, Gillet C, Karmali R, Corvilain J. Calcium and vitamin D metabolism in granulomatous disease. Clin Rheumatol 1992;11:28–36.

[70] Otake S, Ishigaki T. Muscular sarcoidosis. Semin Musculoskelet Radiol 2001;5:167–70.

[71] Otake S. Sarcoidosis involving skeletal muscle: imaging findings and relative value of imaging procedures. AJR Am J Roentgenol 1994;162:369–75.

[72] Resnick D. Plasma cell dyscrasias and dysgammaglobulinemias. In: Resnick D, Niwayama G, editors. Diagnosis of bone and joint disorders. 3rd edition. Philadelphia: WB Saunders; 1996. p. 602–5.

[73] Gejyo F, Odani S, Yamada T, Honma N, Saito H, Suzuki Y, et al. Beta 2-microglobulin: a new form of amyloid protein associated with chronic hemodialysis. Kidney Int 1986;30:385–90.

[74] Ross LV, Ross GJ, Mesgarzadeh M, Edmond PR, Bonakdarpour A. Hemodialysis-related amyloidomas of bone. Radiology 1991;178:263–5.

[75] Cobby MJ, Adler RS, Swartz R, Martel W. Dialysis-related amyloid arthropathy: MR findings in four patients. AJR Am J Roentgenol 1991; 157:1023–7.

[76] Weissman BN. Imaging of arthritis. In: Weissman BN, editor. Syllabus: a categorical course in musculoskeletal radiology. Oak Brook, IL: Radiological Society of North America; 1993. p. 37–50.

[77] Yulish BS, Lieberman JM, Strandjord SE, Bryan PJ, Mulopulos GP, Modic MT. Hemophilic arthropathy: assessment with MR imaging. Radiology 1987;164:759–62.

[78] Butters KP, Morrey BF. Septic arthritis. In: Morrey BF, editor. The elbow and its disorders. 2nd edition. Philadelphia: WB Saunders; 1994. p. 784–91.

[79] Schweitzer M, Morrison WB. Arthropathies and inflammatory conditions of the elbow. Magn Reson Imaging Clin N Am 1997;5:603–17.

[80] Kaplan PA, Helms CA, Anderson MW, Major NM. Musculoskeletal MRI. Philadelphia: WB Saunders; 2001. p. 101–16.

[81] Brusch JL. Septic arthritis. Available at: http://www.emedicine.com. Accessed October 21, 2002.

[82] Hoffmeyer P, Chalmers A, Price GE. Septic olecranon bursitis in a general hospital population. CMAJ Canadian Medical Association Journal 1980;122:874–6.

[83] Meena AK, Rajashekar S, et al. Pyomyositis: clinical and MRI characteristics report of three cases. Neurol India 1999;47:4.

[84] Gordon BA, Martinez S, Collins AJ. Pyomyositis: characterisitics at CT and MR imaging. Radiology 1995;197:279–86.

[85] Jeong GK, Lester B. *Mycobacterium tuberculosis* infection of the wrist. Am J Orthop 2001;30: 411–4.

[86] Gunther SF, Levy CS. Mycobacterial infections. Hand Clin 1989;5:591–8.

[87] Vesfeld GA, Solomon A. A diagnostic approach to tuberculosis of bones and joints. J Bone Joint Surg Br 1982;64:446–9.

[88] Asaka T, Takizawa Y, Kariya T, Nitta E, Yasuda T, Fujita M, et al. Tuberculosis tenosynovitis in the elbow joint. Intern Med 1996; 35:162–5.

[89] Robins RHC. Tuberculosis of wrist and hand. Br J Surg 1967;54:211–8.

RADIOLOGIC
CLINICS
OF NORTH AMERICA

Radiol Clin N Am 44 (2006) 643–648

Index

Note: Page numbers of article titles are in **boldface** type.

Moving?

Make sure your subscription moves with you!

To notify us of your new address, find your **Clinics Account Number** (located on your mailing label above your name), and contact customer service at:

E-mail: elspcs@elsevier.com

800-654-2452 (subscribers in the U.S. & Canada)
407-345-4000 (subscribers outside of the U.S. & Canada)

Fax number: 407-363-9661

Elsevier Periodicals Customer Service
6277 Sea Harbor Drive
Orlando, FL 32887-4800

*To ensure uninterrupted delivery of your subscription, please notify us at least 4 weeks in advance of move.